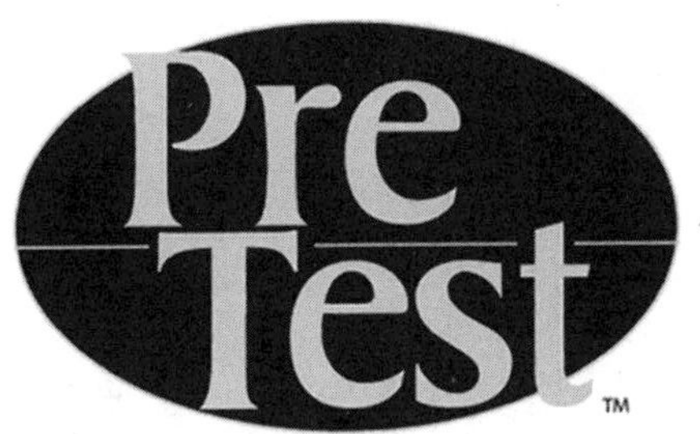

Biochemistry and Genetics

PreTest™ Self-Assessment and Review

Notice

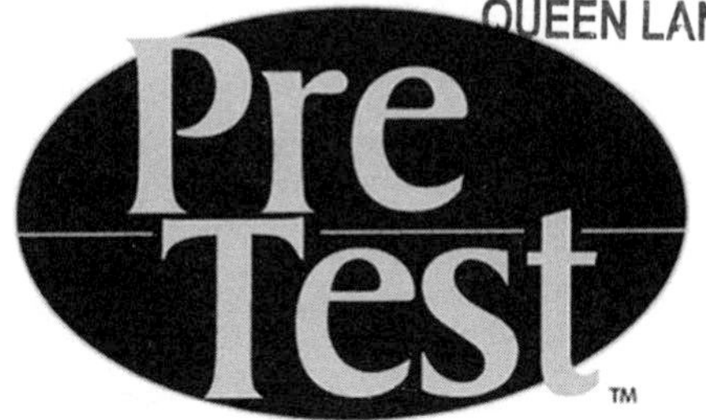

Biochemistry and Genetics

PreTest™ Self-Assessment and Review

Third Edition

Golder N. Wilson MD, PhD
Clinical Professor, Texas Tech University
KinderGenome Pediatric Genetics, Dallas, Texas

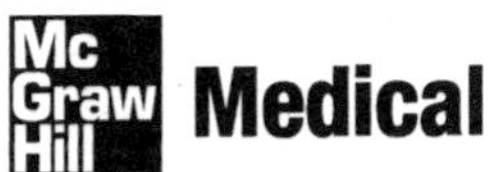

New York Chicago San Francisco Lisbon London Madrid Mexico City
Milan New Delhi San Juan Seoul Singapore Sydney Toronto

The McGraw-Hill Companies

Biochemistry and Genetics: PreTest™ Self-Assessment and Review, Third Edition

1 2 3 4 5 6 7 8 9 0 DOC/DOC 0 9 8 7

ISBN-13: 978-0-07-147183-1
ISBN-10: 0-07-147183-9

This book was set in Berkeley by International Typesetting and Composition.
The editors were Catherine A. Johnson and Regina Y. Brown.
The production supervisor was Sherri Souffrance.
Project management was provided by International Typesetting and Composition.
The cover designer was Maria Scharf.
Cover photo: DNA helices.
Cover photo credit: Lawrence Lawry/Photo Researchers, Inc.
RR Donnelley was printer and binder.

This book is printed on acid-free paper.

Library of Congress Cataloging-in-Publication Data

Wilson, Golder.
Biochemistry and genetics : PreTest self-assessment and review / Golder N. Wilson.—3rd ed.
p. ; cm.
Includes bibliographical references and index.
ISBN-13: 978-0-07-147183-1 (pbk. : alk. paper)
ISBN-10: 0-07-147183-9 (pbk. : alk. paper)
1. Biochemistry—Examinations, questions, etc. 2. Genetics—Examinations, questions, etc. I. Title.
[DNLM: 1. Biochemistry—Examination Questions. 2. Genetics, Medical—Examination Questions. QU 18.2 W748b 2007]
QP518.5.P74 2007
612′.015076—dc22 2007000524

Student Reviewers

Daniel Krochmal
University of Michigan Medical School
Class of 2006

Sunitha J. Moonthungal
St. George's University
Class of 2006

David Scoville
University of Kansas School of Medicine
Class of 2008

Contents

Preface ix
Introduction x
Note Concerning Disease Examples xi
Abbreviations xii

High-Yield Facts

High-Yield Facts in Biochemistry and Genetics 1

STORAGE AND EXPRESSION OF GENETIC INFORMATION

DNA Structure, Replication, and Repair

Questions 59
Answers 75

Gene Expression and Regulation

Questions 93
Answers 119

ACID-BASE EQUILIBRIA, AMINO ACIDS, AND PROTEIN STRUCTURE/FUNCTION

Acid-Base Equilibria, Amino Acids, and Protein Structure

Questions 147
Answers 163

Protein Structure/Function

Questions 183
Answers 196

Intermediary Metabolism

Carbohydrate Metabolism

Questions 209
Answers 223

Bioenergetics and Energy Metabolism

Questions 239
Answers 251

Lipid, Amino Acid, and Nucleotide Metabolism

Questions 263
Answers 284

Nutrition

Vitamins and Minerals

Questions 309
Answers 320

Hormones and Integrated Metabolism

Questions 337
Answers 351

Inheritance Mechanisms and Biochemical Genetics

Inheritance Mechanisms/Risk Calculations

Questions 373
Answers 395

Genetic and Biochemical Diagnosis

Questions 419
Answers 442

Bibliography 469
Appendix 471
Index 485

Preface

The new edition of *Biochemistry and Genetics PreTest: Self-Assessment and Review* is based in part on earlier editions prepared by Golder N. Wilson, MD, PhD, Department of Pediatrics, Texas Tech University Health Sciences Center, Cheryl Ingram-Smith, PhD, and Kerry S. Smith, PhD, Department of Genetics, Biochemistry, and Life Science Studies Clemson University Clemson, South Carolina, and by Francis J. Chlapowski, PhD, Department of Biochemistry and Molecular Biology, University of Massachusetts Medical School. All questions are in single-best-answer format and a large number are analogous to those of the United States Medical Licensing Examination (USMLE), Step 1. Questions are updated to the most current editions of leading textbooks in medical biochemistry and medical genetics.

Introduction

Each PreTest Self-Assessment and Review allows medical students to comprehensively and conveniently assess and review their knowledge of a particular basic science, in this instance biochemistry and genetics. The 500 questions parallel the format and degree of difficulty of the questions found in the United States Medical Licensing Examination (USMLE) Step 1. The Appendix lists subjects from the USMLE guidelines and shows the relevant question numbers from this PreTest book that relate to these subjects.

Each question is accompanied by an answer, a paragraph explanation, and a specific page reference to an appropriate textbook. A bibliography listing sources can be found at the end of this text, and a list of abbreviations used in the text follows this introduction. Over 200 clinical disorders or processes are discussed and related to biochemical and/or genetic mechanisms (see the appendix for a list of disease examples). For genetic disorders, a McKusick number is included that allows the reader to immediately access information about the disorder using the Online Mendelian Inheritance in Man Internet site *(http://www.ncbi.nlm.nih.gov/omim/)*.

An effective way to use this PreTest is to allow yourself 1 minute to answer each question in a given chapter. As you proceed, indicate your answer beside each question. By following this suggestion, you approximate the time limits imposed by the USMLE Step 1 examination. After you finish going through the questions in the section, spend as much time as you need verifying your answers and carefully reading the explanations provided. Pay special attention to the explanations for the questions you answered incorrectly—but read every explanation. The authors of this material have designed the explanations to reinforce and supplement the information tested by the questions. If you feel you need further information about the material covered, consult and study the text or online references indicated.

The high-yield facts in this book are provided to facilitate rapid review of biochemistry and genetics. Key concepts and diagrams are arranged before each section, and it is anticipated that the reader will use the key concepts as a "memory jog" before proceeding through the questions.

Note Concerning Disease Examples

This book provides over 130 disease examples (see Appendix) to illustrate the broad application of biochemistry and genetics to medicine. These include more common chromosomal or multifactorial disorders (Down syndrome, cleft palate, diabetes mellitus) that have incidences ranging from 1 in 200 to 1 in 2000–3000 to less common single gene disorders (cystic fibrosis, glycogen storage diseases) with incidences of 1 in 1600 to 1 per million individuals). Students can ignore clinical information about these rarer diseases since such knowledge is not tested in first/second-year biochemistry/genetic courses or USLME I examinations. The examples are provided to place basic science knowledge in clinical context and to demonstrate the broad range of organ systems and medical specialties that are impacted by genetic/biochemical disease. More relevant to examination are much-used disease prototypes like diabetes, cleft palate, Down/Turner syndromes, sickle cell anemia, phenylketonuria (PKU): students may need to match them with underlying biochemical/genetic mechanisms.

Abbreviations

ACAT	acyl CoA–cholesterol acyl transferase
ACTH	adrenocorticotropic hormone
ADP	adenosine diphosphate
AMP	adenosine monophosphate
ATP	adenosine triphosphate
ATPase	adenosine triphosphatase
CAP	catabolite activator protein
CDP	cytidine diphosphate
CMP	cytidine monophosphate (cytidylic acid)
CoA	coenzyme A
cyclic AMP	adenosine 3′,5′-cyclic monophosphate (3′,5′-cyclic adenylic acid)
DHAP	dihydroxyacetone phosphate
DNA	deoxyribonucleic acid
DNP	2,4-dinitrophenol
DPG	diphosphoglycerate
dTMP	deoxythymidine monophosphate
dUMP	deoxyuridine monophosphate
EF	elongation factor
FAD (FADH)	flavin adenine dinucleotide (reduced form)
FMN	flavin mononucleotide
FSH	follicle-stimulating hormone
GDP	guanosine diphosphate
GMP	guanosine 5′-monophosphate (guanylic acid)
GTP	guanosine triphosphate
hCG	human chorionic gonadotropin
HDL	high-density lipoprotein
HGPRT	hypoxanthine-guanine phosphoribosyl-transferase
HMG CoA	3-hydroxy-3-methylglutaryl coenzyme A
hnRNA	heterogeneous RNA of the nucleus
IDL	intermediate-density lipoprotein
IMP	inosine 5′-monophosphate (inosinic acid)
IP_3	inositol 1,4,5-triphosphate
LDH	lactate dehydrogenase
LDL	low-density lipoprotein

LH	luteinizing hormone
mRNA	messenger RNA
MSH	melanocyte-stimulating hormone
NAD (NADH)	nicotinamide adenine dinucleotide (reduced form)
NADP (NADPH)	nicotinamide adenine dinucleotide phosphate (reduced form)
PGH	pituitary growth hormone
P_i	inorganic orthophosphate
PP_i	inorganic pyrophosphate
PRPP	5-phosphoribosylpyrophosphate
RNA	ribonucleic acid
RQ	respiratory quotient
rRNA	ribosomal RNA
TMP	thymidine monophosphate
TPP	thymidine pyrophosphate
tRNA	transfer RNA
TSH	thyroid-stimulating hormone
TTP	thymidine triphosphate
UDP	uridine diphosphate
UMP	uridine monophosphate
UTP	uridine triphosphate
VLDL	very-low-density lipoprotein

High-Yield Facts in Biochemistry and Genetics

DNA STRUCTURE, REPLICATION, AND REPAIR

Key concepts: DNA structure (Murray, pp 314–340. Scriver, pp 3–45. Lewis, pp 171–184.)

- DeoxyriboNucleic Acid (DNA) is the chemical basis of genes and chromosomes, its structure providing information for cell division, embryogenesis, and heredity. Changes in DNA structure cause human variation and genetic disease, providing the basis for DNA diagnosis.
- Each DNA strand is a sequence of the GATC deoxyribonucleotide units shown in Fig. 1A, remembered from the sci-fi film *Gattaca*.
- DNA strands are directional and are diagrammed with the free triphosphate of the 5'-sugar-carbon (5'-end) at the left and the 3'-end to the right (Fig. 1B). The 2-deoxyribose in DNA contrasts with the 2' and 3' hydroxyls of ribose (in ribonucleic acid [RNA]) that are susceptible to base hydrolysis.
- DNA in eukaryotic cells is a double helix with the strands oriented in opposite directions (antiparallel—Fig. 2A), with sugar-phosphate links on the outside and complementary base-pairing on the inside (Fig. 2B); uncompacted DNA duplex has a length of 3.4 nm per 10 base pairs (bp).
- DNA duplexes can be denatured or "melted" into component single strands at a temperature (T_m) that is proportionate to the fidelity of A-T or G-C base-pairing and the percentage of 3-bond G-C pairs (Fig. 2B); the reverse process of renaturation underlies DNA replication, transcription, or repair in that one DNA strand serves as guide or template for its complementary strand.
- The human haploid genome contains 3×10^9 bp, 70% as unique or low-copy DNA (transcribed euchromatin with an estimated 30,000 genes) and 30% as repetitive DNA (including nontranscribed heterochromatin at chromosome centromeres, telomeres, and satellites).
- DNA is compacted some 8000-fold in eukaryotic cells, associating with histone octamers (two H2A-H2B dimers plus two H3/H4 dimers) and

Base Formula	Base X = H	Nucleoside X = ribose or deoxyribose	Nucleotide, where X = ribose phosphate
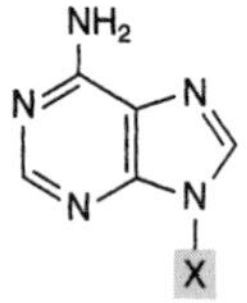 NH_2, N, N, N, N, X	Adenine A	Adenosine A	Adenosine monophosphate AMP
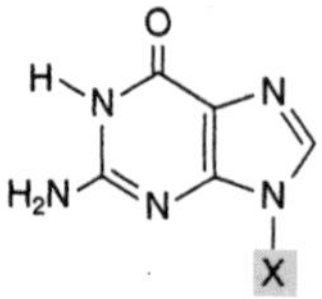 O, H, N, N, H_2N, N, N, X	Guanine G	Guanosine G	Guanosine monophosphate GMP
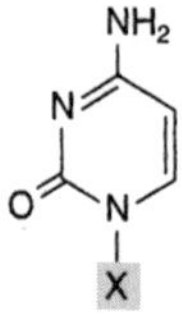 NH_2, N, O, N, X	Cytosine C	Cytidine C	Cytidine monophosphate CMP
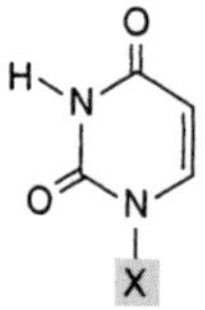 O, H, N, O, N, X	Uracil U	Uridine U	Uridine monophosphate UMP
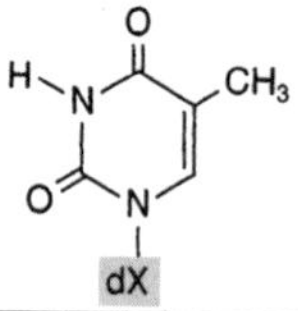 O, H, N, CH_3, O, N, dX	Thymine T	Thymidine T	Thymidine monophosphate TMP

Figure 1 (A)

Bases, nucleotides, and nucleosides.

(A: Reproduced, with permission, from Murray RK, Granner DK, Mayes PA, Rodwell VW: Harper's Biochemistry. 26/e. New York, McGraw-Hill, 2003: 288.)

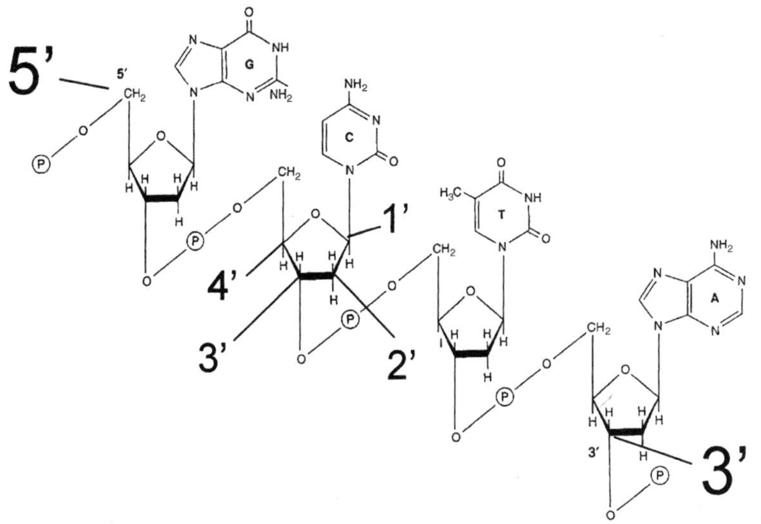

Figure 1 (B)

DNA strand showing 5' to 3' direction of phosphodiester linkages. The pictured strand could also be diagramed as pGpCpTpA.

(B: Adapted, with permission, from Murray RK, Granner DK, Mayes PA, Rodwell VW: Harper's Biochemistry. 26/e. New York, McGraw-Hill, 2003: 304.)

histone H1 to form nucleosomes (10 nm), chromatin fibrils (30 nm), chromosome loops (300 nm), and chromosomes; the average human chromosome (haploid number 23) contains a DNA duplex of 1.3×10^8 bp (4 cm compacted to 1.4 mm) and 1300 genes.

- DNA is modified by methylation and its associated histones by acetylation, methylation, and other processes; these alterations constitute a second code for genetic regulation, a process known as epigenesis.

Key concepts: DNA replication and repair (Murray, pp 314–340. Scriver, pp 3–45. Lewis, pp 171–184.)

- Copying of DNA is synchronous during cell division (DNA replication) and continuous when needed to replace altered bases or broken strands (DNA repair).
- DNA replication is effected by DNA polymerase I, a complex of helicases and topoisomerases for duplex DNA unwinding, primase for initiating DNA copying with RNA primer, DNA binding proteins for single-strand

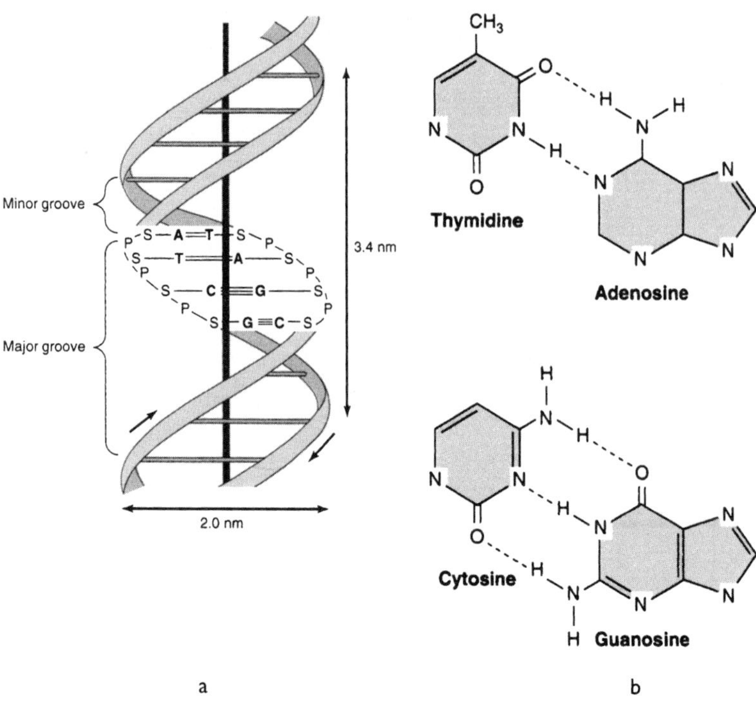

Figure 2
(A) Structure of DNA (B form) showing the double helix with antiparallel strands (arrows). One complete turn (3.4 nm) includes 10 base pairs (bp). A, adenine; C, cytidine; G, guanine; T, thymine; P, phosphate; S, deoxyribose sugar; (B) Base pairing showing two hydrogen bonds (broken lines) between A and T and three bonds between C and G. *(Reproduced with permission, from Murray RK, Granner DK, Mayes PA, Rodwell VW: Harper's Biochemistry. 26/e. New York, McGraw-Hill, 2003: 305.)*

maintenance or proofreading, and ligase for sealing nicks between nascent strands and Okazaki fragments (Fig. 3).

- DNA synthesis occurs during the synthetic or S phase of the cell cycle, after the growth or gap 1 (G1) phase and before the gap 2 (G2) and mitosis (M) phases. The cycle is coordinated by a protein cascade of cyclin-dependent protein kinases (CDKs), cyclins (cyclin D1 is a product of the

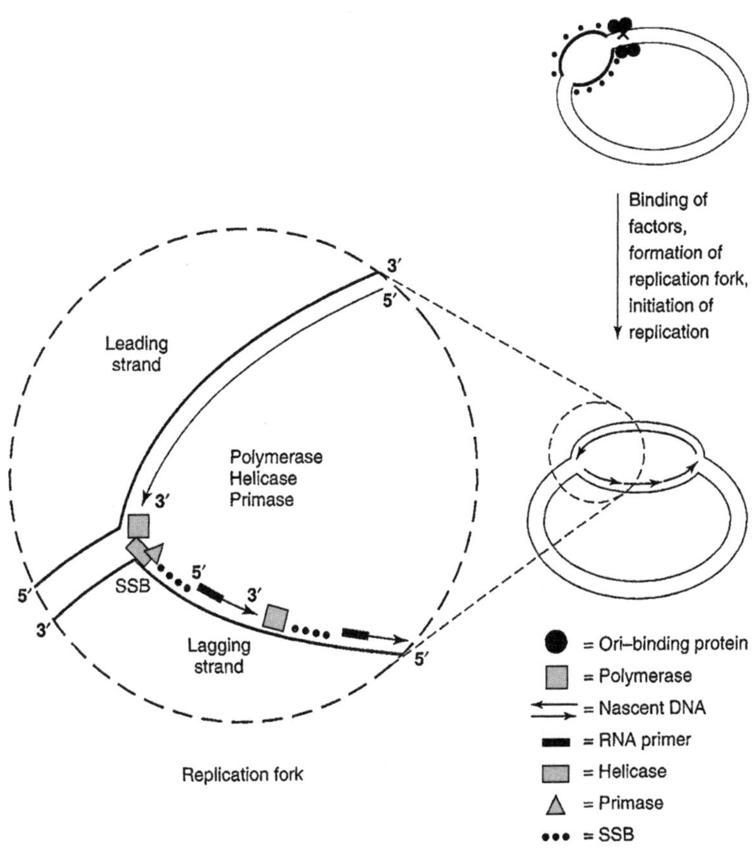

Figure 3

DNA replication fork demonstrating asymmetry with continuous DNA polymerization (long arrow) on the leading strand and discontinuous DNA polymerization/ligation of Okazaki fragments on the lagging strand (short arrows). The asymmetry is necessary for unidirectional replication along antiparallel DNA strands because nature provides only 5' to 3' DNA polymerases. The diagram shows circular bacterial or mitochondrial DNA, but can be extrapolated to linear chromosomes by imagining the same steps of origin recognition, denaturation of AT-rich regions, and asymmetric DNA synthesis at multiple chromosomal origins.

(Reproduced with permission, from Murray RK, Granner DK, Mayes PA, Rodwell VW: Harper's Biochemistry. 26/e. New York, McGraw-Hill, 2003: 327.)

bcl or B-cell lymphoma oncogene), and transcription factors including E2F and Rb (retinoblastoma protein).

- Maintenance of the primary DNA code responsible for accurate protein synthesis and function requires proofreading at the time of DNA replication and DNA repair (about 10^{16} cell divisions per lifetime and 6×10^9 bp per cell means 6×10^{25} bp replicated per lifetime-error or damage rates of even 1 per 10^{20} bp would yield almost a million mutations per individual).
- Specific DNA repair processes (Table 1) exist for each of the four types of DNA damage: (1) depurination or other modification of DNA bases (radiation, chemical agents), (2) two-base alterations (thymine-thymine dimers with ultraviolet light), (3) strand breaks (radiation, free radicals), and (4) cross-linkage of DNA with its associated proteins (chemical agents).
- Four checkpoint controls monitor DNA and chromosome integrity during the cell cycle—checks for damaged DNA at G1 and G2, incomplete replication in S, and improper spindle alignment at M. Irreparable damage halts cell cycle progression and initiates cell death (apoptosis). The tumor suppressor gene p53, mutated in Li-Fraumeni tumor syndrome and several human cancers, has a key role in G1/G2 checkpoint controls.
- Enzymes for DNA synthesis and repair are used *in vitro* for DNA engineering, allowing isolation or "cloning" of mammalian DNA segments by placing them in simpler, rapidly replicating bacterial or viral genomes.

GENE EXPRESSION AND REGULATION

Key concepts: Gene expression (Murray, pp 374–395. Scriver, pp 3–45. Lewis, pp 205–216.)

- RNA is polymerized (transcribed) using one strand of DNA as template, RNA polymerase enzyme, DNA sequence signals (promoters, enhancers), and DNA-binding or polymerase-associated proteins (transcription factors). Alterations in DNA sequence or its expression produce genetic disease.
- Three major RNA polymerases in eukaryotic cells include RNA polymerase I that transcribes ribosomal RNA (rRNA), RNA polymerase II that transcribes messenger RNA (mRNA), and RNA polymerase III that transcribes transfer (tRNA) and small nuclear RNAs (snRNAs).
- Primary transcription of heterogenous (Hn) RNA is followed by RNA processing, involving RNA splicing to remove introns, 7-methyl-guanine

TABLE 1. TYPES OF DNA REPAIR

Type of Repair	Type of DNA Damage	Mechanism (*Associated Processes*)
Mismatch repair	Copying errors—single base or 2 to 5-base unpaired loops*	Exonuclease digestion of damaged strand relative to methylated A within GATC site; strand replaced by DNA polymerase and ligase (*defective in hereditary nonpolyposis colon cancer-HNPCC*)
Base excision-repair	Chemical or radiation change/removal of a base as in depurination or cytosine to uracil*	*N*-Glycosidases remove abnormal bases, apurinic or apyrimidinic endonuclease recognizes damaged sites and removes the sugar, and a new nucleotide is inserted using DNA polymerase and ligase.
Nucleotide excision-repair	Chemical or radiation damage to DNA segment*	A special exonuclease excises 27–29 nucleotides from the damaged strand followed by special DNA polymerases and ligase (*damage by UV light, cigarette smoking; defective in xeroderma pigmentosum*)
Double-strand break repair	Ionizing radiation, chemotherapy, oxidative free radicals	Proteins bind to and unwind the duplex DNA ends. These are joined by uneven base pairing, trimmed by exonuclease, and sealed by ligase (*part of the physiologic process of immunoglobulin gene rearrangement*)

*These processes can occur spontaneously or in response to agents, exposures, and specific genetic conditions.

(Modified, with permission, from Murray RK, Granner DK, Mayes PA, Rodwell VW: Harper's Biochemistry. 26/e. New York, McGraw-Hill, 2003: 336.)

capping on the 5'-end, polyadenylation to add ~200 adenosines at the 3'-end, and transport to the cytoplasm, yielding a contiguous mRNA template for protein translation (Fig. 4A).

- Small nuclear RNAs (snRNAs) are a diverse family of 21-30 nucleotides RNAs that includes small nucleolar RNAs (snoRNAs), small interfering RNAs (siRNAs), and microRNAs (miRNAs), numbering over 1000 in humans.
- SnRNAs are often processed from double-stranded or hairpin (stem-loop) structures and in turn may regulate splicing of mRNA, setting up complex cascades of snRNA processing regulating splicing of particular mRNAs that are thought to regulate one-third of human genes.
- RNA polymerase II acts as a transcription complex of 50 different proteins that include transcription factors and activators/coactivators that chemically modify the polymerase or associated factors (phosphorylation or dephosphorylation is common). Small molecules may change RNA

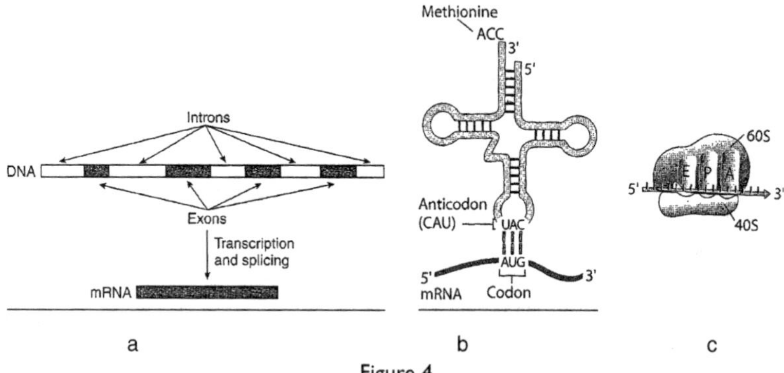

Figure 4

(A) RNA splicing removes introns from the HnRNA primary transcript to produce mRNA for export to the cytoplasm; (B) Specific tRNAs are "charged" with their specific amino acid using aminoacyl-tRNA synthetase and ATP, mediating code-specific insertion of amino acids through binding of their specific anticodon to mRNA codons on the ribosome; (C) Ribosomes composed of 60/40s ribosomal RNAs and multiple proteins provide exit (E), peptidyl (P) and aminoacyl (A) sites that accomplish protein synthesis using energy from GTP hydrolysis.

(Reproduced, with permission, from Bhushan V, Le T. First Aid for the USMLE Step 1: 2006. New York, McGraw-Hill, 2006: 80–81.)

polymerase specificity through cell membrane-nucleus-transcription factor activation/deactivation that is called signal transduction.

- Transfer RNAs are 75–90 bp single strands with clover-leaf shapes that include specific 3-bp anticodon sites and 3'-CCA ends that are charged with specific amino acids using aminoacyl-tRNA synthetase and ATP (Fig. 4B).
- Translation involves conversion of processed mRNA into protein using transfer RNA intermediaries (Fig. 4A&B), catalytic sites on ribosomes (Fig. 4C), and the genetic code (see Table 2).
- The genetic code (Table 2) is unambiguous, degenerate, nonoverlapping, and universal (with exceptions of mitochondria, mycoplasma, and archaeobacteria that have unusual tRNAs).
- Initiation of protein synthesis involves binding of ribosomes, mRNA, and over 10 initiation factors such as eIF-1, eIF-2, eIF-3. The initiator codon

TABLE 2. THE GENETIC CODE (CODON ASSIGNMENTS IN MESSENGER RNA)

First Nucleotide	Second Nucleotide				Third Nucleotide
	U	C	A	G	
	Phe	Ser	Tyr	Cys	U
	Phe	Ser	Tyr	Cys	C
U	Leu	Ser	Term	Term	A
	Leu	Ser	Term	Trp	G
	Leu	Pro	His	Arg	U
	Leu	Pro	His	Arg	C
C	Leu	Pro	Gln	Arg	A
	Leu	Pro	Gln	Arg	G
	lle	Thr	Asn	Ser	U
	lle	Thr	Asn	Ser	C
A	lle	Thr	Lys	Arg	A
	Met	Thr	Lys	Arg	G
	Val	Ala	Asp	Gly	U
	Val	Ala	Asp	Gly	C
G	Val	Ala	Glu	Gly	A
	Val	Ala	Glu	Gly	G

(Reproduced, with permission, from Murray RK, Granner DK, Mayes PA, Rodwell VW: Harper's Biochemistry. 26/e. New York, McGraw-Hill, 2003: 359.)

AUG (specifying methionine) and poly (A) tail of the mRNA are important for protein synthesis initiation.

- Elongation of protein (peptide bond) synthesis involves successive binding and shifting of aminoacyltRNAs from A (aminoacyl), to P (peptidyl) to E (exit) sites on the ribosome; these translocation steps are powered by GTP hydrolysis (Fig. 4C).

Key concepts: Gene regulation (Murray, pp 374–395. Scriver, pp 3–45. Lewis, pp 205–216.)

- DNA sequence elements that regulate transcription efficiency include promoters (e.g., the TATA box), enhancers, repressors or silencers, and RNA termination signals (e.g., the AAUAAA DNA sequence).
- Alternative processing can produce different mRNAs and different proteins by using different combinations of splice donor, splice acceptor, and polyadenylation sites (see Fig. 5).
- Changes in the primary genetic code (mutations) can occur as single bp substitutions (silent, missense, nonsense mutations) or as 1–3 bp insertions/deletions that can change the frame of codon reading (frameshift mutations—see Fig. 6).
- Single bp substitutions at the third positions of codons cause silent mutations with no amino acid change due to tRNA "wobble," while those at first or second codon positions may change the coded amino acid (missense mutations—see Fig. 6)
- Human disease can result from (1) mutations that alter the primary genetic code with resulting changes in gene and protein sequence or (2) mutations that alter the complex "second code"—epigenetic changes in chromatin (DNA/histone) structure/conformation, small RNAs, or the numerous protein factors that regulate RNA transcription, RNA processing, and protein synthesis.

ACID-BASE EQUILIBRIA, AMINO ACIDS, AND PROTEIN STRUCTURE/FUNCTION

Key concepts: Acid-base equilibria and protein structure (Murray, pp 5–13. Scriver, pp 3–45. Lewis, pp 185–204.)

- Water has a dipolar structure that solvates organic molecules through formation of hydrogen bonds.
- The polar environment of aqueous solutions stabilizes organic molecules by hydrogen bonding (e.g., CHO–H–OH), electrostatic interaction

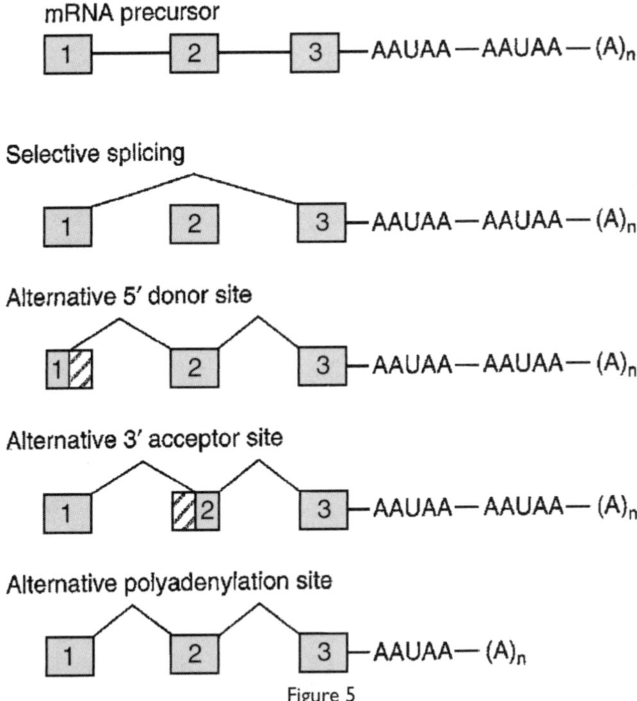

Figure 5

Alternative processing of messenger RNA precursors through use of selective 5-'donor, 3'-acceptor, or polyadenylation sites.

(Reproduced, with permission, from Murray RK, Granner DK, Mayes PA, Rodwell VW: Harper's Biochemistry. 26/e. New York, McGraw-Hill, 2003: 354.)

(e.g., R–NH3$^+$ ——$^-$OOC–CHR), hydrophobic interactions (e.g., bases inside DNA helix), and van der Waal forces (transient dipolarity over short atomic distances).

- Solvated organic molecules (e.g., amino acids of proteins, nucleotide bases of DNA, RNA; lipids and complex carbohydrates) interact with water as acids (proton or H^+ donors) or bases (proton acceptors like hydroxyl ion OH^-).
- The tendency of acids to dissociate into anion (A^-) and proton (H^+) is measured by the dissociation constant (Ka); this equilibrium can be

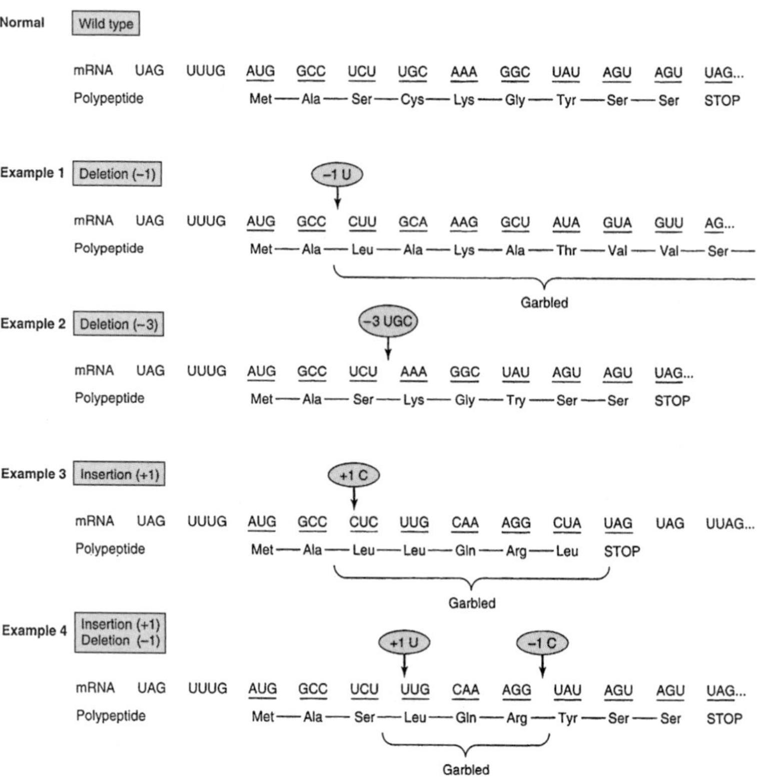

Figure 6
Effects of gene mutation on mRNA and protein products.
(Reproduced, with permission, from Murray RK, Granner DK, Mayes PA, Rodwell VW: Harper's Biochemistry. 26/e. New York, McGraw-Hill, 2003.)

arranged as the Henderson-Hasselbach equation (brackets [ ] indicate concentrations):

$$HA \leftrightarrows H^+ + A^- \quad \text{and} \quad K_a = \frac{[H^+][A^-]}{[HA]}$$

$$\text{Rearranging:} \quad [H^+] = \frac{K_a[HA]}{[A^-]}$$

Taking the –log of both sides of the equation yields:

$$-\log[H^+] = -\log K_a - \frac{\log[HA]}{[A^-]}$$

Using the symbol pN for $-\log_{10}$ [N]:

$$pH = pK_a + \log\frac{[A^-]}{HA}$$

(note that the unprotonated form is up)

- Weak acids with low dissociation constants (e.g. $H_2CO_2 \rightarrow HCO_3^-$) with pK of 6.4 act to buffer changes in pH in biological fluids like that outside of cells (pH range 7.35–7.45).
- Amino acids are Zwitterions with dual charges from carboxyl (COO^-) and amino (NH_3^+) groups that react to form peptide bonds (RCO–NHR); peptides (short amino acid chains) and longer polypeptide proteins are also important buffers through their amino acid side groups (Table 3).
- Interaction of side groups and other factors convert linear amino acid sequences (primary structures) into helical or β-sheet segments (secondary structures) to three-dimensional conformations (tertiary structures) with functional regions (domains—see Fig. 7).
- Tertiary protein structures comprising one peptide chain can associate with other peptide chains (subunits) to form quaternary structures.
- Tertiary and quaternary structures are stabilized by the aqueous forces described in concept number 2 above and by covalent links like disulfide (-S-S-) bonds.

PROTEIN STRUCTURE/FUNCTION

Key concepts: Protein structure/function (Murray, pp 21–39. Scriver, pp 3–45. Lewis, pp 185–204.)

- The folding of proteins into tertiary and quaternary structures is stepwise, thermodynamically favored, and assisted by auxiliary proteins like chaperones, disulfidases, and proline cis-trans isomerases.
- Protein conformation provides a diversity of protein function illustrated by the fibrils of collagen or fibrillin, ligand binding like heme/bisphosphoroglycerate with hemoglobin, and assembly of catalytic sites for enzymes.

TABLE 3. L-α-AMINO ACIDS PRESENT IN PROTEINS

Name	Symbol	Structural formula
With apliphatic side chains		
Glycine	Gly [G]	H–CH(–NH_3^+)–COO^-
Alanine	Ala [A]	CH_3–CH(–NH_3^+)–COO^-
Valine	Val [V]	$(H_3C)_2$CH–CH(–NH_3^+)–COO^-
Leucine	Leu [L]	$(H_3C)_2$CH–CH_2–CH(–NH_3^+)–COO^-
Isoleucine	Ile [I]	CH_3–CH_2–CH(CH_3)–CH(–NH_3^+)–COO^-
With side chains containing hydroxylic (OH) groups		
Serine	Ser [S]	CH_2(OH)–CH(–NH_3^+)–COO^-
Threonine	Thr [T]	CH_3–CH(OH)–CH(–NH_3^+)–COO^-
Tyrosine	Tyr [Y]	See below.
With side chains containing sulfur atoms		
Cysteine	Cys [C]	CH_2(SH)–CH(–NH_3^+)–COO^-
Methionine	Met [M]	CH_2(S–CH_3)–CH_2–CH(–NH_3^+)–COO^-
With side chains containing Acidic groups or their amides		
Aspartic acid	Asp [D]	$^-$OOC–CH_2–CH(–NH_3^+)–COO^-
Asparagine	Asn [N]	H_2N–C(=O)–CH_2–CH(–NH_3^+)–COO^-
Glutamic acid	Glu [E]	$^-$OOC–CH_2–CH_2–CH(–NH_3^+)–COO^-
Glutamine	Gln [Q]	H_2N–C(=O)–CH_2–CH_2–CH(–NH_3^+)–COO^-

Name	Symbol	Structural formula
With side chains containing basic groups		
Arginine	Arg [R]	H–N(–C(=NH_2^+)–NH_2)–CH_2–CH_2–CH_2–CH(–NH_3^+)–COO^-
Lysine	Lys [K]	CH_2(NH_3^+)–CH_2–CH_2–CH_2–CH(–NH_3^+)–COO^-
Histidine	His [H]	(imidazole ring, HN, N)–CH_2–CH(–NH_3^+)–COO^-
Containing aromatic rings		
Histidine	His [H]	See above.
Phenylalanine	Phe [F]	(benzene ring)–CH_2–CH(–NH_3^+)–COO^-
Tyrosine	Tyr [Y]	HO–(benzene ring)–CH_2–CH(–NH_3^+)–COO^-
Tryptophan	Trp [W]	(indole ring, N–H)–CH_2–CH(–NH_3^+)–COO^-
Imino acid		
Proline	Pro [P]	(pyrrolidine ring, $\overset{+}{N}H_2$)–COO^-

(Modified, with permission, from Murray RK, Granner DK, Mayes PA, Rodwell VW: Harper's Biochemistry. 26/e. New York, McGraw-Hill, 2003: 15.)

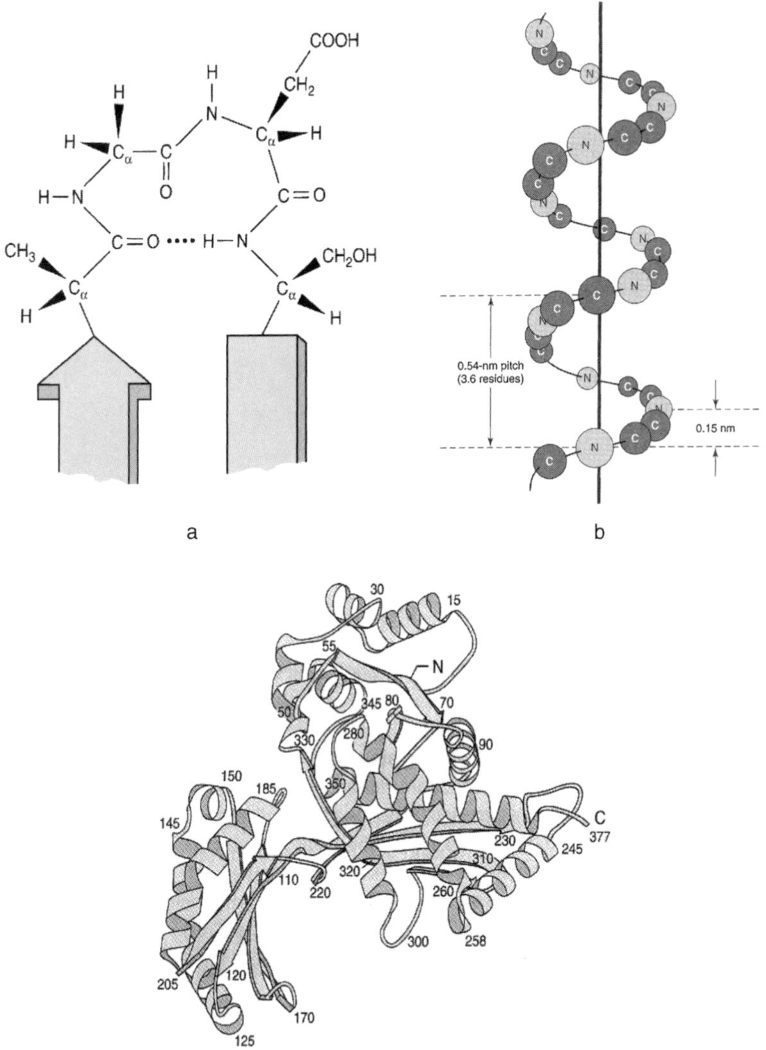

Figure 7

X Levels of protein structure: (A) Primary structure of OC-NC peptide bonds shown as a turn within a secondary structure of antiparallel β-sheets. The four residue segment Ala-Gly-Asp-Ser is stabilized by a hydrogen bond (dotted line); (B) Orientation of the core C and N atoms within a peptide segment with α-helical secondary structure; (C) Tertiary structure of a bacterial enzyme illustrating the folding of sequential amino acid molecules (numbers) to form a three-dimensional protein scaffold with helical and β-sheet domains.

(Reproduced, with permission, from Murray RK, Granner DK, Mayes PA, Rodwell VW: Harper's Biochemistry. 26/e. New York, McGraw-Hill, 2003.)

- Influence of small molecules on protein conformation/function is exemplified by the Bohr effect on the hemoglobin saturation curve (Fig. 8) or initiation of signal transduction cascades by molecules like cyclic adenosine monophosphate (AMP).
- Amounts of proteins may be measured by reaction with specific antibodies (e.g., Western blotting or enzyme-linked immunosorbent assays [ELISA]) or, for enzyme proteins, by their rates of conversion of substrates to products (enzyme catalysis).
- Enzymes lower the activation energy for reactions of substrates (precursors) to products; the amino acid side groups within enzyme catalytic sites lower energy by forming substrate-enzyme intermediates (transition states).

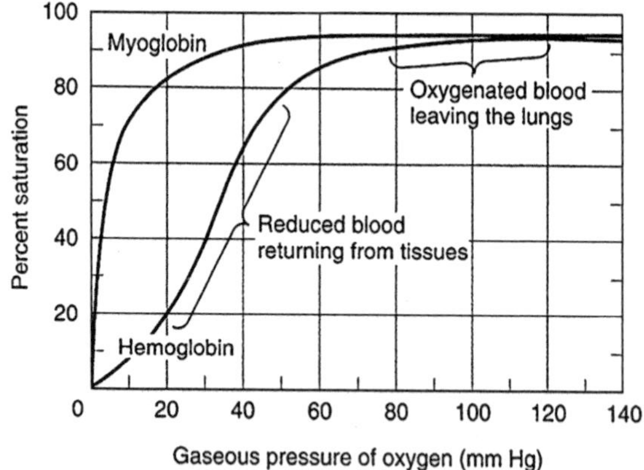

Figure 8

Oxygen binding curves of both hemoglobin and myoglobin. The arterial oxygen tension of blood leaving the lungs is about 100 mm Hg compared to 40 mm for veins returning blood from tissues or 20 mm within capillary beds of actively metabolizing tissues like muscle. The contrast in percent oxygen saturation between hemoglobin (~30%) and myoglobin (~90%) percent oxygen saturation in the 20–40 mm Hg oxygen tension region of the curve (the oxygen tension of peripheral tissues) illustrates that greater release of oxygen at low tensions made possible by the subunit structure of hemoglobin.

(Reproduced with permission, from Murray RK, Granner DK, Mayes PA, Rodwell VW: Harper's Biochemistry. 26/e. New York, McGraw-Hill, 2003: 42.)

- Enzyme assays use initial rate conditions with excess substrate such that the initial velocity (v_i) of substrate reaction is proportionate to enzyme concentration.
- For a given amount of enzyme, the relation between reaction velocity *V* and substrate concentration *S* is given by the Michaelis-Menton equation and its reciprocal (plotted in Fig. 9):

$$V_i = \frac{V_{max}[S]}{K_m + [S]} \text{ and } \frac{1}{V_i} = \frac{K_m + [S]}{V_{max}[S]} \text{ or } \frac{1}{V_i} = \frac{K_m}{V_{max}} \times \frac{1}{[S]} + \frac{1}{V_{max}}$$

The Michaelis constant K_m is defined as the substrate concentration giving one-half the maximal reaction velocity, and can be viewed as a binding constant—substrates with high affinity for the enzyme catalytic site have low K_m values and vice versa.

As *S* increases and becomes much greater than the K_m, *V* approaches its maximal velocity V_{max}:

$$V = \frac{V_{max}[S]}{[S]} = V_{max}$$

Substrates with higher affinity (lower K_m) will thus saturate enzyme catalytic sites and achieve V_{max} at lower concentrations

- Because the Michaelis-Menton equation shows that attainment of V_{max} is a hyperbolic curve (Fig. 9A), use of the reciprocal Lineweaver-Burk equation shown above provides an easy graphical determination of V_{max} and K_m as shown in Fig. 9B. The reciprocal of velocity 1/V is plotted on the *y* axis against the reciprocal of substrate concentration 1/S on the *x* axis. Direct graphic determination of V_{max} is made by measuring the *y* intercept ($= 1/V_{max}$ when $1/S = 0$). Direct graphic measurement of the K_m is made by measuring the *x* intercept ($= -1/K_m$ when $1/V = 0$). The slope is K_m/V_{max}.
- The reciprocal Lineweaver-Burk plot constructed by measuring enzyme velocities with and without inhibitor distinguishes competitive inhibition from noncompetitive inhibition (Fig. 10). A competitive inhibitor will have similar structure to the substrate and compete for enzyme catalytic sites, changing the effective K_m but not the V_{max} (Fig. 10A). A simple noncompetitive inhibitor does not resemble substrate in structure and will not compete for its binding at the enzyme catalytic site—thus changing V_{max} but not K_m (Fig. 10B).

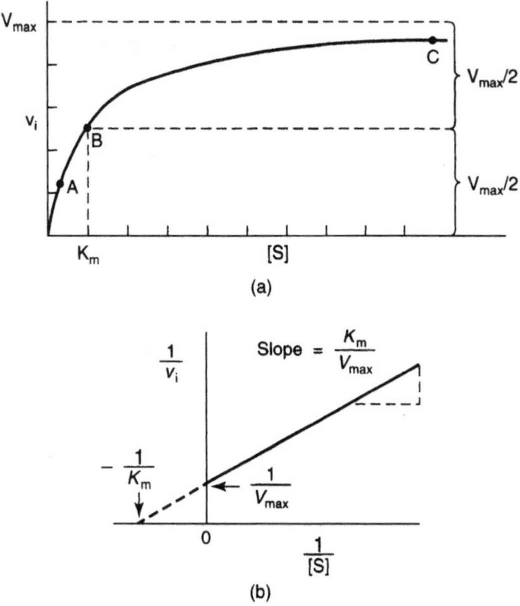

Figure 9

(A) Effect of substrate concentration on the initial velocity of an enzyme-catalyzed reaction. (B) Double reciprocal or Lineweaver-Burk plot of $1/v_i$ versus $1/[S]$ that can be used to evaluate K_m and V_{max}.

(Reproduced, with permission, from Murray RK, Granner DK, Mayes PA, Rodwell VW: Harper's Biochemistry. 26/e. New York, McGraw-Hill, 2003: 64, 66.)

INTERMEDIARY METABOLISM

Key concepts: Intermediary metabolism (Murray, pp 122–129. Scriver, pp 3–45.)

- Metabolism involves breakdown (catabolism) of dietary carbohydrates, fat, and protein to glucose, fatty acids glycerol, and amino acids, respectively, providing energy for biosynthesis (anabolism) and organ function.
- Common metabolic diseases involve nutrient, vitamin, or hormone deficiencies that reflect interaction of genes and environment (multifactorial determination), exemplified by marasmus, rickets, or diabetes mellitus.
- Rarer metabolic diseases (inborn errors of metabolism) result from specific enzyme deficiencies and exhibit autosomal or X-linked recessive

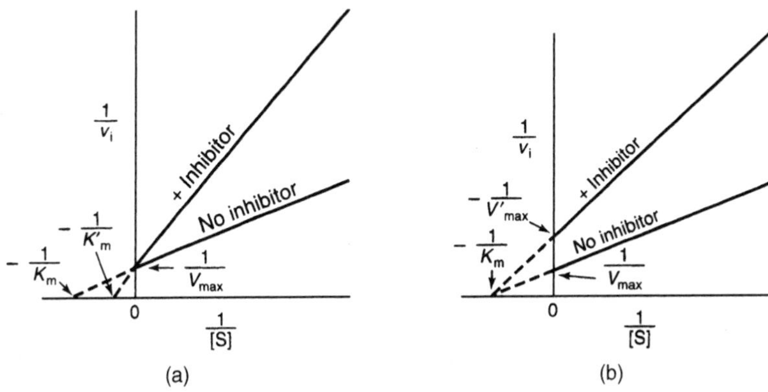

Figure 10
(a) Lineweaver-Burk plot of competitive inhibition. Note the complete relief of inhibition at high [S] (i.e., low 1/[S] concentrations; (b) Lineweaver-Burk plot for simple noncompetitive inhibition. Note the change in V_{max} with identical K_m
(Reproduced, with permission, from Murray RK, Granner DK, Mayes PA, Rodwell VW: Harper's Biochemistry. 26/e. New York, McGraw-Hill, 2003: 68, 69.)

inheritance; accumulation or deficiency of small molecules often produces acute catastrophic disease (acidosis, seizures, coma) while accumulation of larger molecules often produces chronic disease (storage disease).

- The enzyme and cofactor deficiencies of inborn errors of metabolism can be defined in terms of substrate excess and product deficit, guiding diagnostic tests (blood amino acids, urine organic acids) and therapies (substrate avoidance and product or vitamin supplementation through the diet).
- Metabolic pathways are highly compartmentalized as enzyme complexes (e.g., the pyruvate dehydrogenase with >30 peptides) or organelles (e.g., citric acid cycle enzymes in the mitochondrial matrix); even the cytoplasm is a liquid crystal of heterogenous enzyme associations rather than a homogenous protein solution.
- The entry and flow (flux) of metabolites in pathways is controlled through compartmentalization, irreversibility of certain enzyme steps, binding of substrates by low K_m, first-step pathway enzymes, and regulatory/rate-limiting enzymes that are activated or inhibited by small molecules (allosteric modifiers) or hormones.

CARBOHYDRATES, CARBOHYDRATE, AND GLYCOGEN METABOLISM

Key concepts: Carbohydrate structures and glycoproteins (Murray, Chaps. 16–20; Scriver, Chaps. 67–73)

- Carbohydrates (sugars), and particularly glucose, are important metabolic fuels for mammals, particularly during fetal development.
- Glucose is the common currency of carbohydrate metabolism, synthesized in plant photosynthesis, ingested and absorbed into animal bloodstreams, and converted from other sugars in the liver (Fig. 11).
- Monosaccharides include 3-carbon trioses (glyceraldehyde), 5-carbon pentoses (ribose, arabinose, xylose), and 6-carbon hexoses (glucose, galactose, mannose); each group has many isomers (same structural formulae but different arrangement of CHO groups).
- The 4 optically active carbons of hexoses with CH = O (aldehyde group) at carbon 1 (C1) produce 16 isomers including glucose; these include dexto (D) or levo (L) conformations at C4 (optical isomers), formation of 4 carbon (furan) or 5 carbon (pyran) rings through C1-O-C4 or C1-O-C5 bonds, and upward (β) or downward (α) conformations of the C1-hydroxyl group after ring formation (anomers).
- Important monosaccharides with a C = O group at C2 (ketoses) include fructose (6 carbons), xylulose or ribulose (5 carbons), and dihydroxyacetone (3 carbons).
- Disaccharides can be formed between various sugar isomers, including lactose (β-D-galactose-C1-O-C4-β-D-glucose = β-D-galactose-[1 → 4]-β-D-glucose), maltose (α-D-glucose-[1 → 4]-α-D-glucose), or sucrose (α-D-glucose-[1 → 2]-β-D-fructose).
- Longer sugar chains (polysaccharides) are composed of single sugars (e.g., starch, amylopectin, and glycogen with α-D-glucose 1 → 4 links and 1 → 6 branches) or multiple sugars (e.g., mucopolysaccharides or heparin with glucuronic acid, acetylglucosamine, iduronic acid groups, etc.).
- Sugars may be added to amino acid side chains on proteins to form glycoproteins, illustrated by influenza virus hemagglutinins, coagulation proteins (like thrombin), surface antigens (like the ABO blood groups), or glycosylated hemoglobin A_{1c} formed during hyperglycemia from uncontrolled diabetes mellitus.

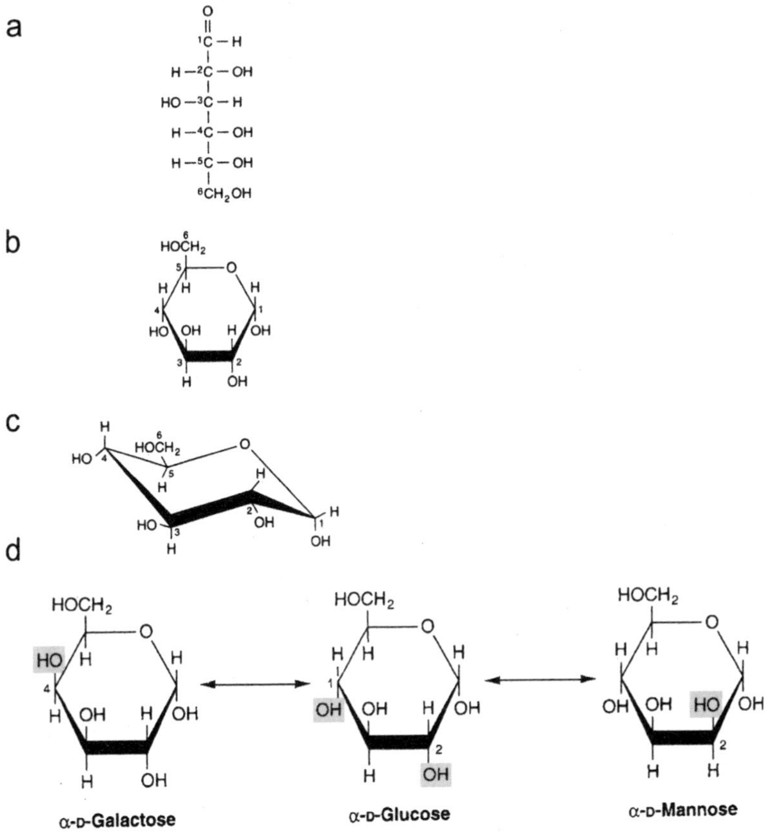

a

b

c

d

α-D-Galactose

α-D-Glucose

α-D-Mannose

Figure 11

D-Glucose in (A) straight chain form; (B) With C1-O-C5 ring formation to yield C1 hydroxyl orientation (arrow) as α anomer; (C) Actual structural conformation of α-D-glucose as Haworth projection showing –OH (and $-CH_2OH$) groups in most stable position (in plane with ring) except for C1 α-hydroxyl (arrow–note that C1 β-hydroxyl would be in plane, accounting for 62% β, 38% α anomers of D-glucose in water solution); (D) Biologically important epimers of D-glucose shown as α-anomers (galactose and mannose will include hydroxyls out of ring plane in Haworth projection, accounting for decreased stability and potential energy release when converted to glucose as "ground state" of animal metabolism.

(Reproduced, with permission, from Murray RK, Granner DK, Mayes PA, Rodwell VW: Harper's Biochemistry. 26/e. New York, McGraw-Hill, 2003: 104.)

Key concepts: Carbohydrate metabolism (Murray, pp 102–110, 130–172. Scriver, pp 1407–1666.)

- Major themes of human carbohydrate metabolism include the distribution of glucose to tissues, metabolism to lactate in anaerobic tissues, metabolism to pyruvate and acetyl coenzyme A (acetyl CoA) in aerobic tissues, and generation of energy (ATP) through the citric acid cycle and oxidative phosphorylation (ox-phos).
- Glucose, fructose, and galactose are the main carbohydrates absorbed from dietary starch, sucrose, and lactose, respectively; fructose and galactose are converted to glucose in liver (mainly) and deficiencies in their conversion cause essential fructosemia and galactosemia.
- Glycolysis (Fig. 12) is the main path of glucose metabolism (and of dietary fructose or galactose), producing lactate in anaerobic tissues (brain, muscle, gastrointestinal tract, retina, skin, and erythrocytes with no mitochondria).
- Aerobic tissues like heart, liver, or kidney glycolyze glucose to pyruvate, convert pyruvate to acetyl CoA via pyruvate dehydrogenase (PDH), and effect complete oxidation to carbon dioxide and water using the citric acid cycle (CAC) and ox-phos.
- Aerobic tissues oxidize lactate when oxygen is plentiful and ox-phos is effective, but produce lactic acidosis under circumstances of hypoxia, cardiopulmonary failure, exercise fatigue, or ox-phos interruption (PDH or thiamine cofactor deficiencies, PDH inhibitors (arsenate, mercurate ions), mitochondrial diseases, alcoholism with thiamine deficiency.
- Deficiencies of glycolytic enzymes have predominant effects in anaerobic tissues including hemolytic anemias or myopathies.
- The pentose phosphate pathway is an alternative route for glucose metabolism that generates reducing equivalents of NADPH for steroid/fatty acid synthesis and ribose for nucleotide formation.
- The citric acid cycle (CAC) is a final common pathway for carbohydrate, lipid, and amino acid metabolism, combining acetyl CoA with oxaloacetate and cycling through seven intermediates to generate oxaloacetate again (Fig. 13).
- The CAC is channeled within mitochondria, directly generating ATP or substrates such as reduced nicotinamide-NADH or flavin adenine ($FADH_2$) dinucleotides that are converted to ATP by ox-phos.

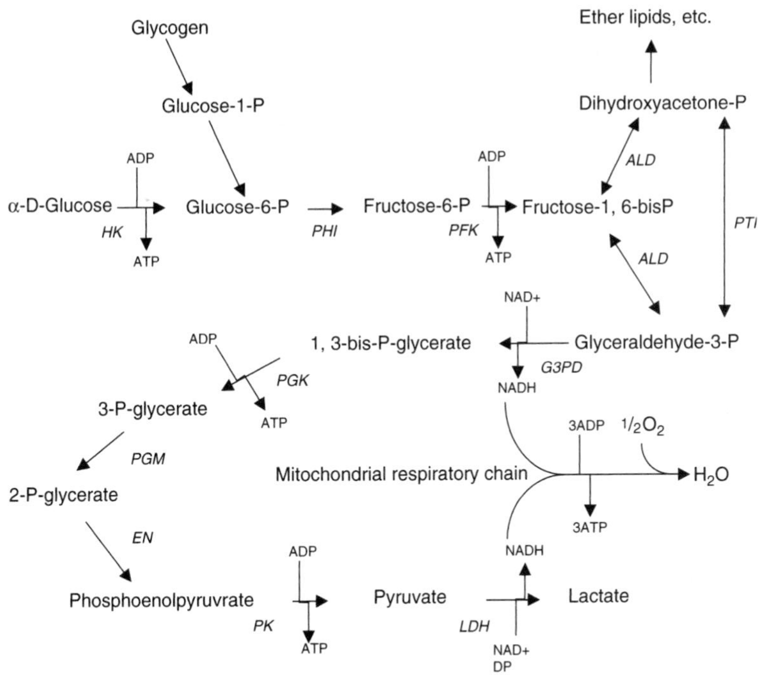

Figure 12

Pathway of glycolysis showing steps yielding ATP (adenosine triphosphate) and NADH (nicotinamide dinucleotide), which is subsequently oxidized in the mitochondrial respiratory chain. P, phosphoro- or phosphate; enzymes in italics: HK, hexokinase; PHI, phosphohexose isomerase; PFK, phosphofructokinase; ALD, aldolase; PTI, phosphotriose isomerase, G3PD, glyceraldehyde-3-phosphate dehydrogenase; PGK, phosphoglycerate kinase; PGM, phosphoglycerate mutase; EN, enolase; PK, pyruvate kinase; LDH, lactate dehydrogenase.

(Modified, with permission, from Murray RK, Granner DK, Mayes PA, Rodwell VW: Harper's Biochemistry. 26/e. New York, McGraw-Hill, 2003: 138.)

- The CAC is amphibolic, involved in catabolism to yield ATP energy and anabolism through gluconeogenesis and fatty acid synthesis.
- The CAC is under respiratory control, being tightly coupled to ox-phos by levels of oxidized cofactors (like NAD^+) and by end-product inhibition of PDH (acetyl CoA, NADH).

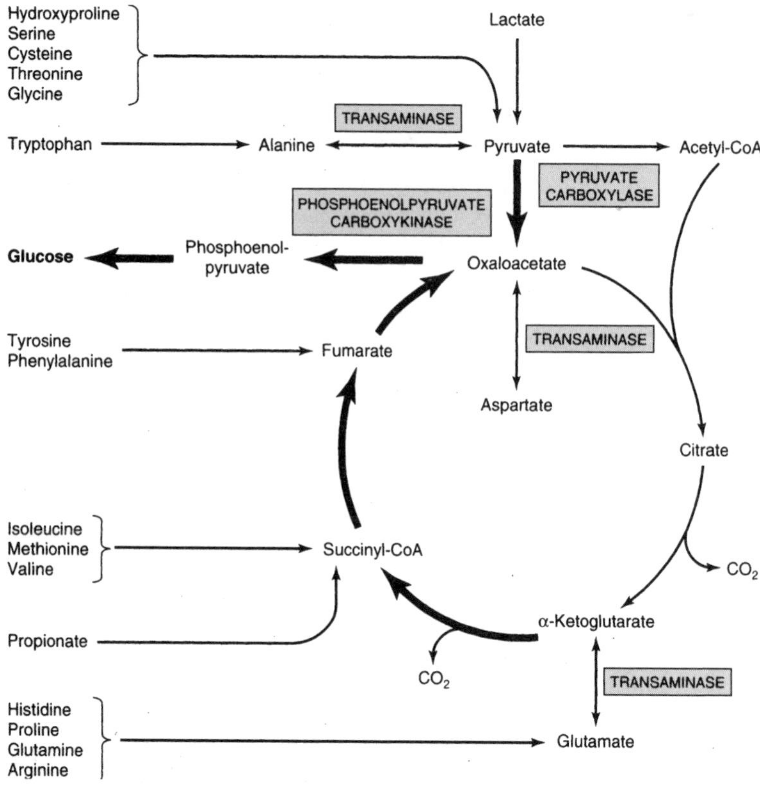

Figure 13
Involvement of the citric acid cycle in transamination and gluconeogenesis. Bold arrows indicate the main pathway of gluconeogenesis.
(Reproduced, with permission, from Murray RK, Granner DK, Mayes PA, Rodwell VW: Harper's Biochemistry. 26/e. New York, McGraw-Hill, 2003: 134.)

Key concepts: Glycogen metabolism and gluconeogenesis (Murray, pp 145–162. Scriver, pp 1521–1552.)

- Glycogen is stored glucose in the form of a branched polysaccharide analogous to starch in plants; it accounts for 6% of liver mass and 1% of muscle mass in fed states.

- Glycogenesis utilizes high energy uridine diphosphate glucose (UDPGlc) formed from glucose-1-phosphate and UTP, forming 1 → 4 links with a synthase and 1 → 6 links with branching enzymes.
- Glycogen synthase adds glucose units to preexisting glucose chains on the primer protein glycogenin; the primer glucose chain is attached to the hydroxyl of a tyrosine residue.
- Glycogenolysis is very different from glycogen synthesis, requiring multiple enzymes such as glycogen phosphorylase that employs phosphate to hydrolyze 1 → 4 links and debranching enzymes that hydrolyze 1 → 6 links. Liberated glucose-1-phosphate is converted to glucose-6-phosphate and (in liver) to glucose by glucose-6-phosphatase (thus increasing blood glucose—Fig. 14).
- Phosphorylases differ between liver and muscle, activated by phosphorylation of their serine hydroxyl groups (via phosphorylase kinase and protein phosphatase) and by allosteric interactions with cyclic AMP or AMP.
- Cyclic AMP is formed from ATP by adenyl cyclase in response to hormones such as epinephrine, norepinephrine, and glucagon; it is hydrolyzed by phosphodiesterase to produce 5′-AMP, an activator of muscle phosphorylase during fatigue (Fig. 14).
- Insulin slows glycogenolysis by direct stimulation of liver phosphodiesterase (to decrease cAMP) and inhibition of liver glycogen phosphorylase through glucose uptake, increased formation of glucose-6-P, and reduced activity of phosphorylase kinase.
- Inherited enzyme deficiencies produce glycogen storage in liver or muscle according to enzyme location (Table 4); failure of liver glycogenolysis and blood glucose supply cause recurrent hypoglycemia, lactic acidemia, and shift to fatty acid metabolism with hypercholesterolemia and hyperuricemia.

BIOENERGETICS, ENERGY METABOLISM, AND BIOLOGICAL OXIDATION

Key concepts: Bioenergetics and Energy Metabolism (Murray, pp 80–101. Scriver, pp 2261–2296.)

- Bioenergetics is the study of energy changes that accompany metabolism; biological systems use chemical energy, taking fuel from food.
- Food and micronutrient (vitamins, minerals) availability determine the rate of energy release, modulated by thyroid hormones.

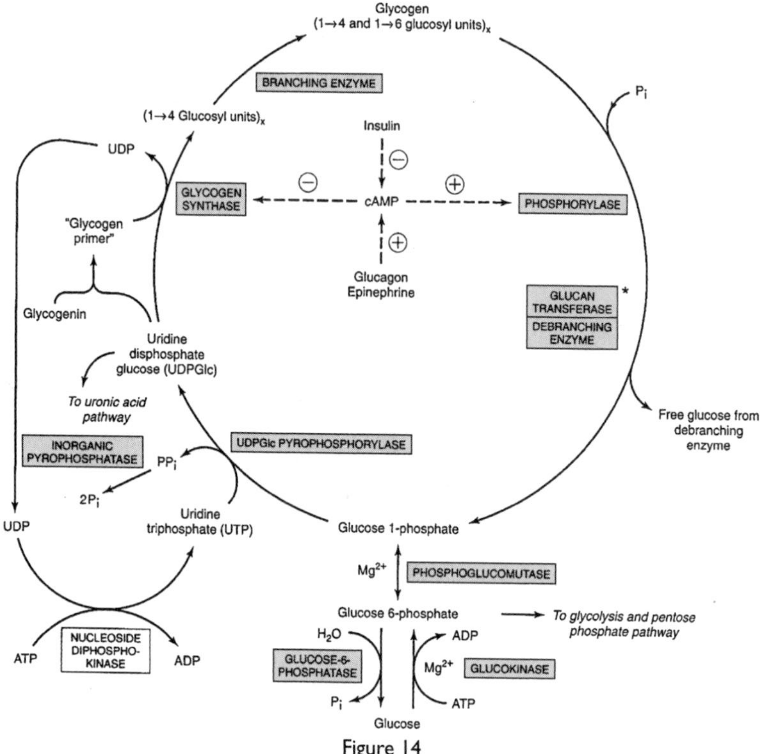

Figure 14

Pathway of glycogenesis and glycogenolysis in the liver. Two high energy phosphates are used in the incorporation of 1 mol of glucose into glycogen. + refers to simulation, - to inhibition. Insulin decreases the level of cAMP only after it has been raised by glucagons or epinephrine—that is, it antagonizes their action. Glucagon is active in heart muscle but not in skeletal muscle. At asterisk; Glucan transferase and debranching enzyme appear to be two separate activities of the same enzyme.

(Reproduced, with permission, from Murray RK, Granner DK, Mayes PA, Rodwell VW: Harper's Biochemistry. 26/e. New York, McGraw-Hill, 2003: 146.)

- States of energy depletion (starvation, marasmus) or excess (obesity) are powerful influences in medicine and disease.
- Biochemical reactions are of two types—exergonic (catabolic) that yield energy and endergonic (anabolic); exergonic reaction products (e.g., NADH, ATP) are often coupled to endergonic (synthetic) reactions.

TABLE 4. GLYCOGEN STORAGE DISEASES

Glycogenosis (% patients)	Type-Name	Cause of Disorder	Characteristics
Type I (a–c) (25%)	L-von Gierke disease (232200)	Deficiency of glucose-6-phosphatase catalytic subunit (a), microsomal glucose-6-phosphatase (b) or phosphate (c) transport	Liver cells and renal tubule cells loaded with glycogen. Hypoglycemia, lacticacidemia, ketosis, hyperlipemia
Type II (15%)	M-Pompe disease (232300)	Deficiency of lysosomal glucosidase (acid maltase)	Fatal, accumulation of glycogen in lysosomes, heart failure.
Type III (24%)	L- Forbes or Cori disease (232400) (limit dextrinosis)	Absence of debranching enzyme	Accumulation of branched polysaccharide
Type IV (3.3%)	L- Andersen disease (amylopectinosis—232500)	Absence of branching enzyme	Accumulation of unbranched polysaccharide. Death due to cardiac or liver failure in first year of life
Type V (2%)	M- McArdle syndrome (myophosphorylase deficiency—232300)	Absence of muscle phosphorylase	Diminished exercise tolerance; muscles have abnormally high glycogen content (2.5–4.1%). Little or no lactate in blood after exercise

(Continued)

TABLE 4. GLYCOGEN STORAGE DISEASES (Continued)

Glycogenosis (% patients)	Type-Name	Cause of Disorder	Characteristics
Type VI (30% with IX)	L-Hers disease (232700)	Deficiency of liver phosphorylase	High glycogen content in liver, tendency toward hypoglycemia.
Type VII (0.2%)	M—Tarui disease (232800)	Phosphofructokinase deficiency in muscle and erythrocytes	As for type V but also possibility of hemolytic anemia
Type IX (a–f) (30% with VI)	L-Phosphorylase kinase deficiencies (306000)	Phosphorylase kinase deficiencies in liver, skeletal, and/or heart muscle; various subunit deficiencies account for subtypes (a–f)	Similar to type VI. Type IXa was formerly called type VIII and is the only X-linked recessive disorder

- High energy phosphates are the currency of cellular energy exchange, including ATP and GTP; glycolytic compounds 1,3-bisphosphoglycerate and phosphoenolpyruvate; and creatine phosphate in muscle.
- Other high energy compounds include coenzyme A derivatives, S-adenosylmethionine, and UDP-glucose.
- The ratio of ATP to ADP reflects cellular energy potential and coordinates various processes like oxidative-phosphorylation, glycolysis, and the citric acid cycle.
- Enzymes such as myokinase or adenyl kinase catalyze ATP-ADP-AMP interconversions in response to cellular energy supplies.

Key concepts: Biological oxidation (Murray, pp 86–91. Scriver, pp 2261–2296.)

- Chemical oxidation of a substrate involves removal of electrons while chemical reduction involves a gain in electrons.
- Oxygen provided by animal respiration provides direct oxidation (addition of oxygen to substrates by oxidases, cytochromes P450, etc.) or indirect oxidation (removal of hydrogens from substrates to form water by dehydrogenases, etc.).
- The generation of energy by oxidation-reduction reactions is proportionate to their Redox potential (analogous to battery voltage); the conversion of oxygen to water (last step of the respiratory chain) has the greatest (most positive) Redox potential.
- The high Redox potential of oxygen to water conversion drives the intermediate reactions of food oxidation/metabolism, generating reducing equivalents that are converted to fuel (ATP, high energy phosphates) by oxidative phosphorylation.
- Several classes of enzymes catalyze oxidative reactions, using the Redox potential to generate high energy compounds or to detoxify drugs or environmental agents (see Table 5).

LIPID, AMINO ACID, AND NUCLEOTIDE METABOLISM

Key concepts: Significant lipids and lipid synthesis (lipogenesis—Murray, pp 111–121, 173–179. Scriver, pp 2705–2716.)

- Lipids, including fats, oils, steroids, and waxes, are related by their insolubility in water and function in energy storage, membrane barriers, and neural insulation.

TABLE 5. CLASSES OF ENZYMES USED IN OXIDATION REACTIONS

Enzyme Class	Example	Function	Cofactors/Inhibitors
Copper oxidases	Cytochrome oxidase	Last step of mitochondrial respiratory chain	Heme iron, copper/CO, CN
Flavoprotein oxidases	L-Amino acid oxidase	Oxidizes amino acids	FMN, FAD (riboflavin)
NAD^+ dehydrogenases	Respiratory chain carriers	Oxidation of substrates to water	NAD^+ $NADP^+$ (niacin)
FMN, FAD dehydrogenases	Succinate dehydrogenase	Transfer reducing equivalents from CAC to respiratory chain	FMN, FAD (riboflavin)
	Dihydrolipoyl dehydrogenase	Reduces lipoic acid during oxidative decarboxylation of pyruvate, α -ketoglutarate	
	Electron transfer flavoprotein	Acyl CoA intermediates and respiratory chain	
Hydroperoxidases	Glutathione peroxidase	Protects against peroxides	Reduced glutathione, selenium
	Catalase	Protects by removal hydrogen peroxide	Heme iron
Oxygenases	Cytochromes P450 (>100 enzymes)	Direct incorporation of oxygen into substrates; detoxification	
Free radical oxidation	Superoxide dismutase	Protects by removal superoxide radical	Works in concert with antioxidants like vitamin E

(Data from Murray RK, Granner DK, Mayes PA, Rodwell VW. Harper's Biochemistry. 26/e. New York, McGraw-Hill, 2003: 80–91.)

- Simple lipids are fatty acids linked with alcohols to form esters, including fats (solid glycerol esters), oils (liquid glycerol esters), and waxes (fatty acids linked to long chain alcohols).
- Complex lipids include links to phosphoric acid (phospholipids), the 18-carbon aminoalcohol sphingosine (sphingophospholipids), carbohydrate (glycosphingolipids), and proteins (including lipoproteins).
- Derived lipids include saturated (no double bonds) or polyunsaturated fatty acids (multiple double bonds), polyunsaturated fatty acids with rings (eicosanoids including prostaglandins and leukotrienes, vitamins including E and K), steroids derived from cholesterol including hormones (aldosterone, estrogen, testosterone) or vitamins (vitamin D), and polymers containing ceramide (a sphingosine derivative), carbohydrates (generating cerebrosides), or carbohydrates with sialic acid (gangliosides).
- Amphipathic lipids (e.g., glycerophospholipids) contain hydrophobic (water-repelling) and hydrophilic (water-soluble) regions; they form water-lipid interfaces such as bilayer membranes or multilamellar sheaths, micelles (droplets with oil inside), and liposomes (water inside).
- Fatty acid synthesis begins in the cytoplasm with biotin-mediated carboxylation of acetyl CoA to form malonyl CoA by acetyl CoA carboxylase (Fig. 15). Initial fatty acyl synthesis is sequestered within a dimeric, 14-enzyme fatty acid synthase complex that transfers the CoA molecules onto pantothenic acid sulfydryl groups before condensing them to form enzyme-bound acetoacetyl groups.
- A microsomal fatty acid elongase extends C10 and longer fatty acids through direct condensation of fatty acyl and acetyl CoA. Fatty acids are thus made using acetyl CoA building blocks, with similar steps of 2-carbon addition for the synthase or elongation pathways (Fig. 15).
- Linoleic (C18 with two double bonds), α-linolenic (C18 with three double bonds), and arachidonic acids (C20 with four double bonds and precursor to prostaglandins) cannot be synthesized in humans and must be supplied in the diet (essential fatty acids); essential fatty acid deficiencies can occur with intestinal malabsorption (cystic fibrosis, Crohn disease) or liver disease (cirrhosis, alcoholism, immature neonatal liver) while excess trans-unsaturated fatty acids are associated with atherosclerosis.
- Glycerophospholipids (i.e., lung surfactant, cholines, inositol second messengers) are synthesized from acyl CoAs (activated by acyl CoA synthetase) and glycerol-3-phosphate, while glycerol-ether lipids (platelet activating factor) are analogously synthesized from dihydroxyacetone phosphates.

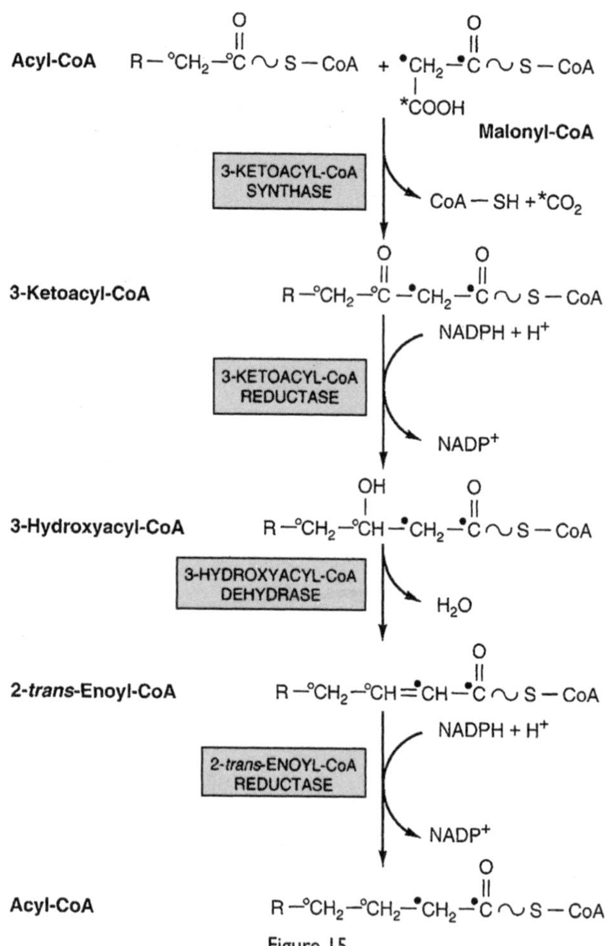

Figure 15

Synthesis and elongation of fatty acids. Initial synthesis of a fatty acid occurs within a fatty acid synthase complex composed of two symmetrical dimmers, each with 7 enzymes plus pantothenic acid. Acetyl CoA is carboxylated using biotin to yield malonyl CoA, and each molecule is transferred to apposing pantothenic acid sulfhydryl groups within the synthase followed by condensation to make acetoacetyl CoA (R = H in diagram). Elongation of fatty acids above 10 carbons is performed by a microsomal fatty acid elongase that condenses malonyl and acetyl CoA directly, followed by similar steps of reduction to hydroxyacyl CoA, enoyl CoA, and acyl CoA. Each cycle of this reaction sequence adds two carbons to the fatty acyl chain, occurring within the synthase complex for C4-C16 and/or within microsomes for C10 and above

(Reproduced, with permission, from Murray RK, Granner DK, Mayes PA, Rodwell VW: Harper's Biochemistry. 26/e. New York, McGraw-Hill, 2003: 177.)

- Fatty acid synthesis (lipogenesis) is promoted in fed states through supplies of NADPH from the pentose phosphate pathway, allosteric activation of acetyl CoA carboxylase by citrate (high concentrations when acetyl CoA is abundant), and inhibition of acetyl CoA carboxylase and pyruvate dehydrogenase by the products of lipogenesis, long-chain fatty acyl CoAs.
- Insulin increases lipogenesis by inhibiting phosphorylation and inactivation of acetyl CoA carboxylase, while epinephrine and glucagon inhibit lipogenesis and promote lipolysis; insulin also decreases cellular cAMP, reducing lipolysis in adipose tissue and decreasing plasma concentrations of free fatty acids.

Key concepts: Lipid catabolism (lipolysis) and transport (Murray, pp 205–218. Scriver, pp 2705–2716.)

- Glycosphingolipid polymers such as ceramides or gangliosides are degraded by lysosomal enzymes that, when deficient, cause lipid storage diseases affecting brain, bones, and the reticuloendothelial system (Tay-Sachs, Gaucher, Niemann-Pick diseases).
- Glycerophospholipids are degraded by phospholipases, some of which occur in snake venom; the combined action of phospholipases with fatty acyl activation and transfer allows remodeling of glycerol lipids through exchange of fatty acid groups.
- Fatty acid oxidation occurs in mitochondria, utilizing NAD^+, FAD, and oxygen to remove 2-carbon blocks and generate ATP (Fig. 16)
- Fatty acid oxidation produces ketone bodies (acetoacetate, 3-hydroxybutyrate, acetone) in the liver through mitochondrial formation of hydroxymethylglutaryl (HMG) CoA; ketone bodies provide energy for extrahepatic tissues through conversion to acetyl CoA and accumulate during starvation (ketosis) or insulin deficiency (ketoacidosis in diabetes mellitus).
- "Free" fatty acids are in fact bound to albumin in plasma and binding proteins in the cell, requiring activation to fatty acyl CoA molecules before oxidation; longer chain fatty acyl CoAs must be converted to acylcarnitines by carnitine palmitoyltransferase-1 (CPT-1) and transferred into mitochondria for oxidation by carnitine-acylcarnitine translocase.
- CPT-1 activity, the gateway into mitochondria, is an important regulator of fatty acid oxidation that is inhibited by malonyl CoA; starvation increases levels of free fatty acids and fatty acyl CoAs that inhibit acetyl CoA carboxylase and levels of its product, malonyl CoA.

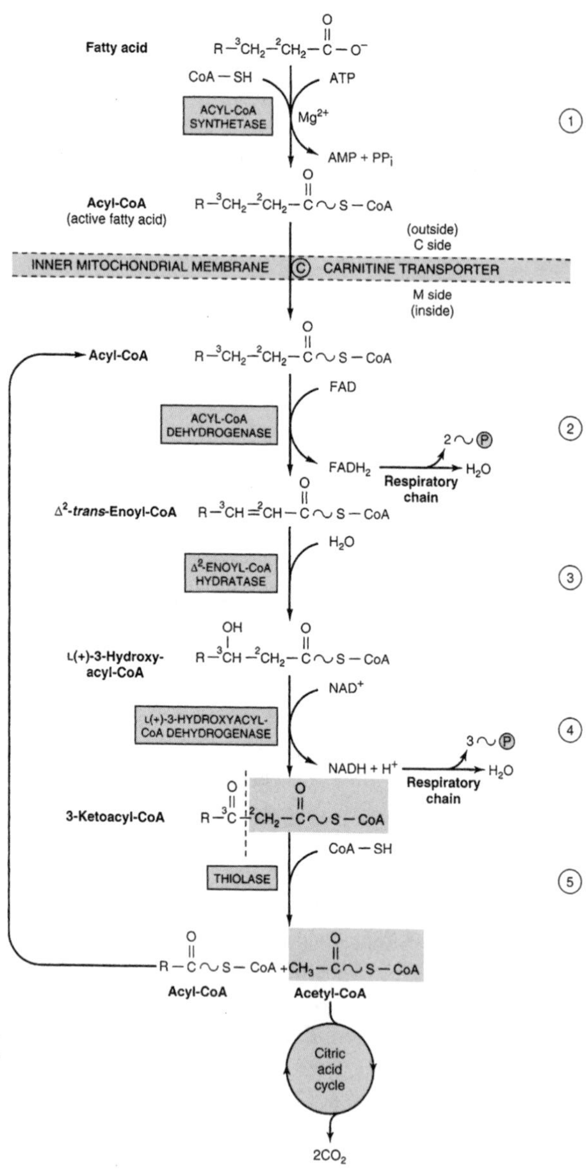

Figure 16

β-oxidation of fatty acids. Long-chain acylCoA is cycled through reactions 2 through 5, and one acetyl CoA moiety is removed with each cycle.

(Reproduced, with permission, from Murray RK, Granner DK, Mayes PA, Rodwell VW: Harper's Biochemistry. 26/e. New York, McGraw-Hill, 2003: 182.)

- Inherited defects of fatty acid oxidation include defects of carnitine transport, CPT deficiencies, and several enzyme deficiencies grouped as long, medium, or short chain disorders with differing symptoms; environmental insults include toxins such as hypoglycin in Jamaican vomiting sickness and nutritional deficiencies of carnitine with prematurity or renal disease.
- Lipid transport involves complexing of amphipathic lipids and proteins to form water-soluble lipoproteins, including chylomicrons (from intestine), very low density lipoprotein (VLDL) from liver, high density lipoproteins (HDLs), and free fatty acid-albumin from adipose tissue.
- Major plasma lipoproteins can be separated by density or lipoprotein electrophoresis, each including specific apolipoproteins as listed in Table 6.
- Plasma free fatty acids are released from adipose tissue during starvation, stored as triacylglycerol (particularly in heart and muscle), or rapidly metabolized; fatty acid oxidation provides 25–50% of energy requirements during fasting.
- Absorbed triacylglycerols are transported as chylomicrons in intestinal lymph and cleaved by lipoprotein lipase within capillary linings to form chylomicron remnants; the liberated fatty acids go to fat or heart and muscle while liver receptors (apo E and LDL) take up the remnant lipoproteins.
- Liver has key roles in lipid transport/metabolism including bile synthesis to promote digestion/absorption, oxidation/synthesis of fatty acids and glycerophospholipids, secretion of VLDL for use by other tissues, conversion of fatty acids to ketone bodies (ketogenesis), and the uptake/metabolism of lipoproteins.
- Free or esterified cholesterol is present in most tissues, derived in about equal parts from diet or biosynthesis; all cholesterol carbons are derived from acetyl CoA, first as the 5-carbon mevalonic acid (by hydroxymethylglutaryl CoA reductase that is inhibited by statins—Fig. 17), then as successive joining of 5-carbon isoprene units to generate geranyl phosphate (10 carbons), farnesyl phosphate (15 carbons), and squalene (30 carbons) that is oxidized and cyclized to form the four rings of cholesterol.
- The isoprenoid signal transducer dolichol and the respiratory constituent ubiquinone are derived from farnesyl diphosphate, while cholesterol is modified to form steroid hormones or vitamins and excreted as bile acids (cholic acid) and bilirubin.

TABLE 6. HUMAN PLASMA LIPOPROTEINS

Lipoprotein	Source	Density (g/mL)	Main Lipid Components (% as lipid)#	Apolipoproteins
Chylomicrons	Intestine	<0.95	Triacylglycerols (98–99%)	A-I, A-II, A-IV, B-48 C-I, C-II, C-III, E
Chylomicron remnants	Chylomicrons	<1.006	Triacylglycerols phospholipids cholesterol (92–94%)	B-48, E
VLDL	Liver (intestine)	0.95–1.006	Triacylglycerol (90–93%)	B-100, C-I, C-II, C-III
IDL	VLDL	1.006–1.019	Triacylglycerol cholesterol (89%)	B-100, E
LDL	VLDL	1.019–1.063	Cholesterol (79%)	B-100
HDLs*	Liver, intestine, VLDL Chylomicrons	1.063->1.210*	Phospholipids cholesterol (43–68%)	A-I, A-II, A-IV, C-I, C-II, C-III, D, E
Albumin-FFA	Adipose tissue	>1.281	FFA (1%)	

VL, very low; H, high; I, intermediate; DL, density lipoprotein; FFA, free fatty acids; # the remainder is protein; *several HDL classes including HDL_1 of density similar to LDL and pre β-HDL with very high density >1.21 (sometimes called VHDL).

(Modified, with permission, from Murray RK, Granner DK, Mayes PA, Rodwell VW: Harper's Biochemistry. 26/e. New York, McGraw-Hill, 2003: 206.)

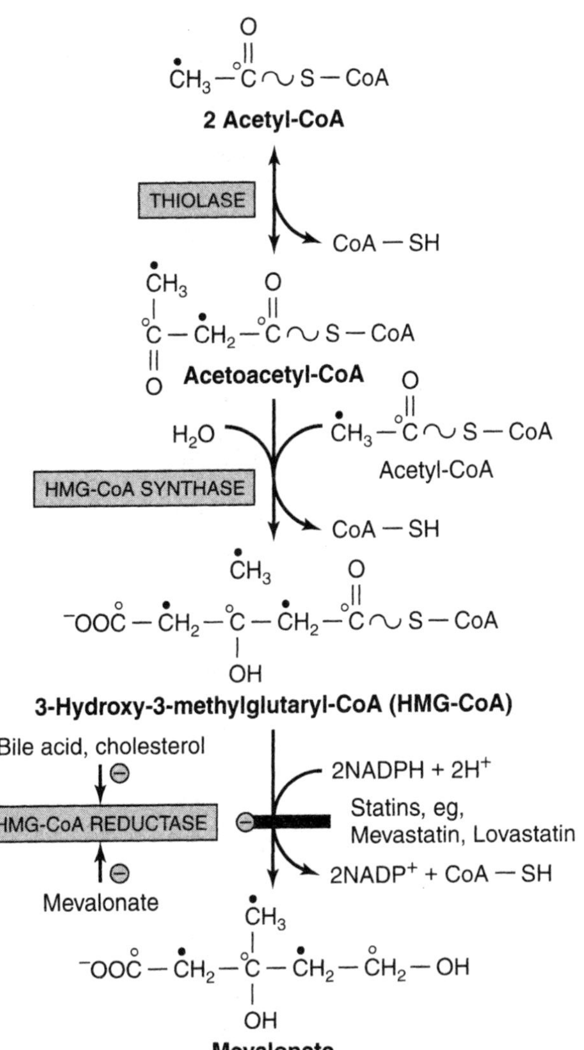

Figure 17

Biosynthesis of mevalonate, showing the critical step of HMG-CoA reductase that is inhibited by statins. The open and solid circles indicate the fates of carbons in acetyl CoA. *(Reproduced, with permission, from Murray RK, Granner DK, Mayes PA, Rodwell VW: Harper's Biochemistry. 26/e. New York, McGraw-Hill, 2003: 220.)*

- Diseases of lipoprotein metabolism include fatty liver due to triacylglycerol accumulation (alcoholism, toxins, diabetes), abetalipoproteinemia (apo B deficiency), several causes of atherosclerosis (hypercholesterolemia due to LDL receptor deficiency), high HDL, lipoprotein lipase deficiency), and apo A (HDL) deficiency (Tangier disease).

Key concepts: Amino acid metabolism (Murray, pp 237–263. Scriver, pp 1667–2108.)

- Of 20 amino acids in proteins, humans can synthesize 12 including 3 (cysteine, tyrosine, hydroxylysine) from the 8 nutritionally essential amino acids.
- Nonessential amino acids include glutamate/glutamine from α-ketoglutarate, alanine from pyruvate, aspartate/asparagines from oxaloacetate, serine from 3-phosphoglycerate, glycine from glyoxylate/serine/choline, proline from glutamate, cysteine from methionine, and tyrosine from phenylalanine.
- Hydroxylysine and hydroxyproline are hydroxylated after incorporation into protein (mostly collagens); vitamin C and iron-requiring oxygenases add the hydroxyl groups, and ascorbate deficiency causes bone and gum disease (scurvy).
- Normal but aged proteins are cleaved internally by proteases (including lysosomal cathepsins) and the peptides cleaved to amino acids by peptidases; abnormal proteins are targeted by ubiquitin (binding its carboxyl group to amino side groups using ATP) and degraded by a protease complex known as the proteasome.
- Amino acid nitrogen is catabolized to ammonia, which is neurotoxic, and to urea, which is excreted by the kidney.
- Ammonia is converted to glutamine (from glutamate), alanine (from pyruvate), and glutamate (from α-ketoglutarate) in the liver; cirrhosis produces collateral circulation with bypass of portal blood, causing hyperammonemia and neurologic symptoms including cognitive dysfunction, slurred speech, blurred vision, rapid breathing, coma, and death.
- Urea is the major end product of nitrogen metabolism in humans and is synthesized through the urea cycle (Fig. 18); carbamoyl synthetase is rate-limiting for urea synthesis and its activity is determined by acetyl-CoA levels through its conversion to *N*-acetylglutamate cofactor.
- Inherited enzyme deficiencies are associated with each enzyme of the urea cycle, producing severe hyperammonemia, neurotoxicity, and

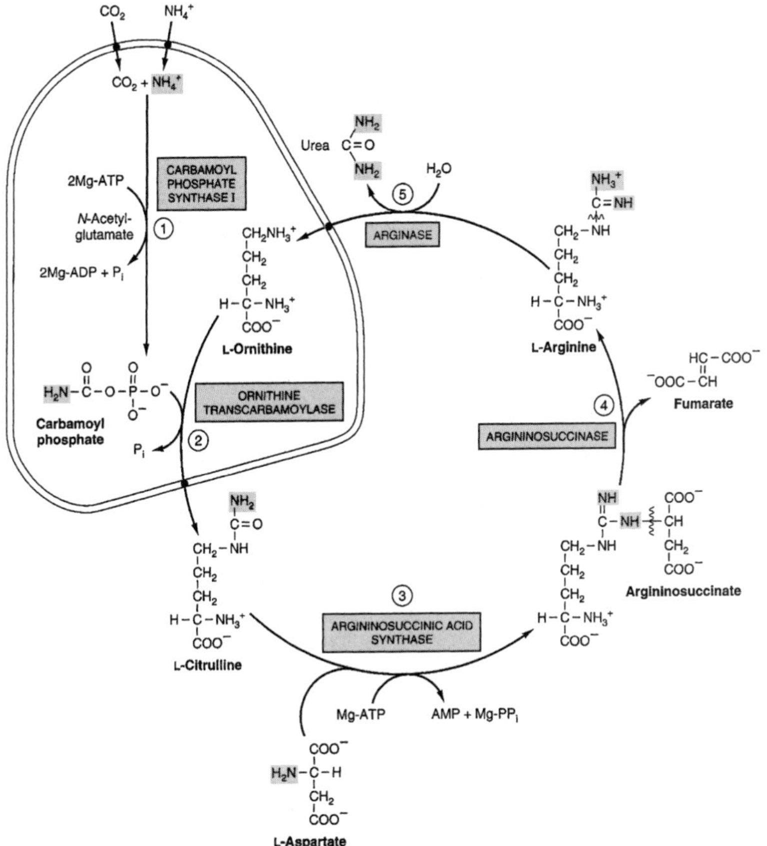

Figure 18

Reactions and intermediates of urea biosynthesis. The nitrogen-containing groups that contribute to the formation of urea are shaded. Reactions 1 and 2 occur in the matrix of liver mitochondria and reactions 3, 4, and 5 in liver cytosol. CO_2 (as bicarbonate), ammonium ion, ornithine, and citrulline enter the mitochondrial matrix via specific carriers (see heavy dots) present in the inner membrane of liver mitochondria. *(Reproduced with permission, from Murray RK, Granner DK, Mayes PA, Rodwell VW: Harper's Biochemistry. 26/e. New York, McGraw-Hill, 2003: 246.)*

death if the ammonia is not removed by dialysis or salvage agents (e.g., glutamate derivatives).

- Catabolism of amino acid carbon chains often yields acetyl CoA; enzyme deficiencies in the degradation pathways for phenylalanine (phenylketonuria), tyrosine (tyrosinemia, alkaptonuria), branched chain amino acids (maple syrup urine disease), and tryptophan (Hartnup disease) cause specific metabolic diseases.

Key concepts: Porphyrin and nucleotide metabolism (Murray, pp 270–302. Scriver, pp 2961–3104.)

- Porphyrins consist of four pyrrole rings containing a nitrogen and four carbons; porphyrins are synthesized from the condensate of succinyl CoA and glycine to form aminolevulinic acid, porphobilinogen, protoporphyrin, and (after incorporation of iron), heme.
- Porphyrias result from deficiencies of the enzymes responsible for porphyrin synthesis; deficiencies of hepatic enzymes (acute intermittent porphyria, porphyria cutanea tarda, variegate porphyria) produce abdominal pain, photosensitivity, and neuropsychiatric symptoms while those of erythrocyte enzymes (X-linked sideroblastic anemia, congenital erythropoietic porphyria, protoporphyria) produce anemia and skin changes with or without photosensitivity.
- Catabolism of heme removes iron and produces bilirubin, which is conjugated with glucuronide in liver, secreted into bile and then the intestine, and converted into urobilinogen by fecal flora; a fraction of urobilinogen is reabsorbed to produce an enterohepatic cycle that can be disrupted by liver disease or immaturity to produce hyperbilirubinemia (jaundice).
- Neonatal jaundice due to liver immaturity produces unconjugated (water insoluble or indirect-reacting) hyperbilirubinemia, while obstruction of the bile duct (gallstones, cancer, biliary atresia) produces conjugated (water soluble or direct-reacting) hyperbilirubinemia; excess unconjugated bilirubin can cross the blood-brain barrier and cause neurotoxicity (kernicterus).
- Rare enzyme deficiencies can affect liver secretion or conjugation of bilirubin (Crigler-Najjar, Gilbert syndromes with indirect hyperbilirubinemia) or bile excretion (Dubin-Johnson, Rotor syndromes with direct hyperbilirubinemia).

- Purine and pyrimidine nucleotides are not essential nutrients but require considerable energy to synthesize; nucleosides from the diet or cell cycles are often salvaged by conversion to nucleoside phosphates (nucleotides).
- Purine nucleotide synthesis begins with placement of a high energy pyrophosphate at the C1 position of ribose-5-phosphate; phosphoribosylpyrophosphate (PRPP) is the pyrophosphate donor and PRPP synthase catalyzes the rate-limiting initial reaction that is feedback inhibited by the end-products AMP, ADP, GMP, GTP (Fig. 19).

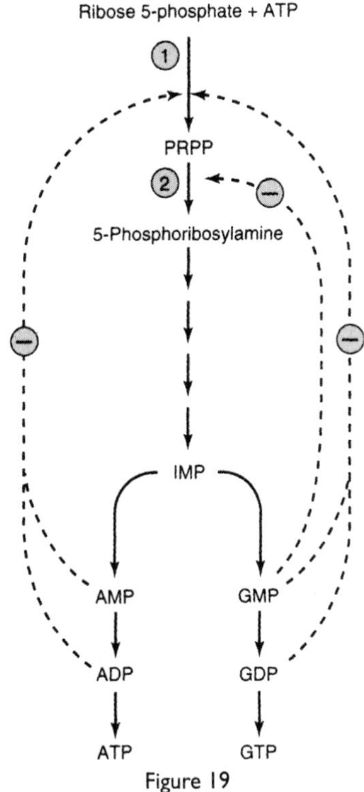

Figure 19

Control of the rate of de novo purine nucleotide synthesis. Solid lines represent metabolite flow, and dashed lines show feedback inhibition (0) by end-products of the pathway. Reactions 1 and 2 are catalyzed by PRPP synthase and PPRP glytamylamido-transferase respectively.

(Reproduced, with permission, from Murray RK, Granner DK, Mayes PA, Rodwell VW: Harper's Biochemistry. 25/e. New York, McGraw-Hill, 2000: 391.)

- Inosine monophosphate is the product of purine synthesis, converted to adenosine and guanine nucleotides that occur in nucleic acids; the amino acids aspartate, glycine, and glutamate contribute nitrogens to the purine ring, while folate derivatives contribute two carbons.
- Purines are catabolized to uric acid, increased in purine imbalance disorders (e.g., mutations increasing PRPP synthase activity), renal disorders (with decreased urate excretion), glycogen storage disorders (that produce increased ribose-5-phosphate), and Lesch-Nyhan syndrome with defects in hypoxanthine-guanine phosphoribosyl transferase (HGPRT—diminishing its role in purine salvage and increasing levels of PRPP); inborn errors or folate antagonists that inhibit purine synthesis impair DNA synthesis and disproportionately impact rapidly dividing cells, illustrated by the immune deficiencies adenosine deaminase or purine nucleoside phosphorylase deficiencies and the use of folate antagonists (e.g., methotrexate) in anticancer therapy.
- Pyrimidine synthesis begins with a cytosolic carbamoyl phosphate synthase II that is different from the mitochondrial carbamoyl synthase I of the urea cycle; enzyme complexes (including aspartate transcarbamoylase and orotic acid phosphoribosyl transferase) channel the first steps of pyrimidine synthesis.
- PRPP and folic acid derivatives are also important in pyrimidine synthesis, emphasizing the coordination of purine and pyrimidine synthesis appropriate for their use in nucleic acid; carbamoyl transferase (by UTP) and aspartate transcarbamoylase (by CTP) are inhibited by their product pyrimidines (analogous to purine feedback inhibition shown in Fig. 19).
- Ribonucleoside reductase (using thioredoxin) converts nucleoside diphosphates to deoxyribonucleoside diphosphates and is another step where pyrimidine and purine nucleotide levels are coordinated by cross-inhibition (GDP inhibits reduction of UDP and CDP, dTTP inhibits reduction of UDP but stimulates reduction of GDP, etc.); salvage reactions generating nucleotides by phosphoribosylation of nucleosides are also cross-regulated to ensure equal supplies of purine and pyrimidine nucleotides for nucleic acid synthesis.
- Pyrimidine catabolism yields water-soluble products like β-aminoisobutyrate with few consequences for disease (except for a rare anemia due to orotic aciduria); pyrimidine synthetic enzymes do convert analogues like allopurinol (lowers uric acid in treatment of gout) or 5-fluorouracil (anticancer drug) to nucleotides, and thymidylate synthase

that converts dUMP to TMP (using methylene tetrahydrofolate) is a prime target for anticancer folate antagonists.

NUTRITION

Key concepts: Nutrition (Murray, pp 474–480. Scriver, pp 155–166, 3897–3964.)

- Nutrition [including food availability (diet), ingestion, digestion, and intestinal absorption] provides carbohydrates and lipids as metabolic fuels, proteins for growth and tissue repletion, and the vitamins or minerals that are needed in small amounts for selected metabolic reactions.
- Abnormal diets, with over- or undernutrition, cause or contribute to the majority of human ills; diseases affecting dietary intake (neuromuscular swallowing problems), digestion (deficiency of bile acids in gall bladder disease, intestinal enzymes in cystic fibrosis), or absorption (lactose intolerance, celiac disease, vitamin B_{12} deficiency) are also common.
- Disorders of under-nutrition present as "failure to thrive" in infancy and at later stages with feeding or nutritional challenges (puberty, pregnancy, old age).
- Digestion begins with chewing as illustrated by salivary and pancreatic amylases that degrade starch; lipases, peptidases like pepsin and trypsin (secreted as inactive zymogens), and disaccharidases complete digestion and absorption using specific transporters in the intestinal brush border.
- Bile acids are essential for lipid emulsification and absorption, vitamin D for induction of calbindin and calcium absorption, intrinsic factor for vitamin B_{12} absorption, and vitamin C for promoting the limited human iron absorption through binding to mucosal cell ferritin and plasma transferring.
- The basal metabolic rate (BMR) measures body energy requirements at rest, assessed at 12 hours after feeding (morning); charts accounting for weight, age, and gender allow calculation of BMR rather than direct measurement.
- Vigorous activity, hypermetabolic states (AIDS, cancer), and protein catabolism after trauma or inflammatory illnesses can increase the BMR up to eightfold (with skiing, stair climbing, jogging); intake of calories above those needed to maintain the BMR causes obesity, defined by a body mass index (weight in kilograms divided by height in meters squared) over 25–30.

- Poor nutrition can produce specific deficiency diseases (e.g., the fragile/misshapen bones of rickets) or more general phenotypes such as marasmus (muscle and tissue wasting, resigned affect), kwashiorkor (reddish hair, swollen liver, subcutaneous swelling = edema), and cachexia (exaggerated symptoms of marasmus with greater protein deficiency) from eating disorders (anorexia nervosa), chronic diseases (AIDS, lupus), or cancers.

VITAMINS AND MINERALS

Key concepts: Vitamins and minerals (Murray, pp 481–497. Scriver, pp 155–166, 3897–3964.)

- Vitamins and minerals are micronutrients that generally cannot be synthesized by the body; their dietary intake must be between the extremes of low (causing clinical deficiency disease or high (causing overdose toxicity as with hypervitaminosis A or iron tablet ingestion).
- The lipid-soluble vitamins A, D, E, and K are absorbed with fat, so maintenance of adequate levels require normal intestinal fat absorption; disorders causing bile acid/gut enzyme deficiencies (cystic fibrosis) or intestinal transit/brush border dysfunction (inflammatory bowel disease, chronic diarrheas causing fatty stools = steatorrhea).
- A vitamin is defined as an organic compound needed in small amounts to foster metabolic integrity, usually as a cofactor in enzyme reactions; this definition highlights the illogical use of high-dose vitamin mixtures (megavitamin therapy) for various chronic illnesses (e.g., autism, Down syndrome, cancers).
- Vitamin deficiency diseases are listed in Table 7 along with scientific uses of high-dose vitamin therapy (to overcome altered enzyme/cofactor binding in specific genetic disorders or to lower risks for birth defects).
- Essential minerals (Table 8) include those with significant tissue concentrations and dietary requirements (e.g., sodium, potassium, calcium chloride) and trace metals required in small amounts that are analogous to vitamins (e.g., zinc, iron, copper).

HORMONES AND INTEGRATED METABOLISM

Key concepts: Types of hormones and hormone action (Murray, pp 434-473. Scriver, pp 3965–4292.)

- Integrated actions of the endocrine and neural systems produce hormones, acting on distant cells (endocrine), adjacent cells (paracine), or the same cell (autocrine) as agonists (stimulants) or antagonists (inhibitors) of various cell functions.

TABLE 7. VITAMIN FUNCTIONS, DEFICIENCY DISEASES, AND HIGH-DOSE THERAPIES

	Vitamin	Functions	Deficiency Disease	High-Dose Therapy
A	Retinols, β-carotene	Retinal pigment, signal transduction, antioxidant	Night blindness, dry eyes (xerophthalmia) with corneal ulcers and blindness, hyperkeratosis (scaly skin)	Contraindicated—causes increased intracranial pressure
D	Calciferol	Calcium absorption, bone formation	Rickets: poor bone mineralization (osteomalacia) and formation (bowed legs)	Vitamin D-resistant rickets
E	Tocopherols	Antioxidant	Neurologic symptoms (rare)	Common in skin care but not proven effective
K	Phylloquinone	Blood clotting and bone formation	Normal newborns; bleeding and bone changes (stippled epiphyses, short nose)	Routine nursery administration, rare inborn errors
B_1	Thiamin	Coenzyme for pyruvate dehydrogenase (PDH), other enzymes	Beriberi: burning sensory neuropathy, cardiac failure, edema; Wernicke-Korsakoff dementia in alcoholics	Leigh's disease and other mitochondrial disorders with PDH deficiency*
B_2	Riboflavin	Coenzyme in Redox reactions; precursor to flavoproteins FMN, FAD	Photophobia, stomatitis (irritation at corners of mouth, lips, and tongue), anemia	Mitochondrial enzyme deficiencies having flavin cofactors*
	Niacin	Coenzyme in Redox reactions as part of NAD(P)/NAD(P)H	Pellagra—photosensitive dermatitis, psychosis	Hartnup disease—defect in tryptophan transport

(Continued)

TABLE 7. VITAMIN FUNCTIONS, DEFICIENCY DISEASES, AND HIGH-DOSE THERAPIES (Continued)

	Vitamin	Functions	Deficiency Disease	High-Dose Therapy
B_6	Pyridoxine	Coenzyme for amino acid, glycogen, steroid metabolism	Convulsions; peripheral nerve pain in "slow metabolizers with P450 variants and alcoholics	Infantile convulsions of unknown cause; homocystinuria
	Folic acid	Coenzyme for one-carbon transfer as in nucleotide synthesis	Megaloblastic anemia	Megaloblastic anemia; preconceptional therapy to lower risk for neural tube defects
B_{12}	Cobalamin	Coenzyme for one-carbon transfer and in folate metabolism	Pernicious anemia with neuromuscular symptoms	Methylmalonic academia, folate metabolism defects
	Pantothenic acid	Part of fatty acyl synthase comples, fatty acid synthesis	Rare, usually with other vitamin deficiencies—irritability, depression, cramps	
H	Biotin	Coenzyme for carboxylation reactions in gluconeogenesis, fatty acid synthesis	Metabolic acidosis, hair loss, skin rashes, failure to thrive	Biotinidase deficiency, propionic acidemia
C	Ascorbic acid	Collagen proline, lysine hydroxylation, antioxidant, enhances iron absorption	Scurvy—poor wound healing, bone tenderness with rib swelling (rachitic rosary), gum disease with tooth loss, hemorrhage with bruising, nosebleeds	Wound healing after surgery; not effective for URI in controlled trials

*not highly effective; P450, cytochromes P450s responsible for drug detoxification; URI, upper respiratory infections.

TABLE 8. ESSENTIAL MACRO- AND MICROMINERALS

	Mineral	Functions	Deficiency and *Toxicity* Diseases	Dietary Sources
Essential macrominerals				
Na	Sodium	Main cation of extracellular fluid; water/salt balance; neuromuscular functions	Hypotonic dehydration in children; renal disorders; salt-wasting in chronic illness; *hypertension*	Table salt
K	Potassium	Main cation of intracellular fluid; water/base balance, neuromuscular functions	Muscle weakness, confusion, metabolic alkalosis; cardiac *arrest, intestinal ulcers*	Vegetables, fruits (bananas), nuts
Cl	Chloride	Fluid/electrolyte balance; gastric fluid;	Prolonged vomiting (as with pyloric stenosis), causing hyperchloremic alkalosis;	Table salt
Ca	Calcium	Constituent of bones, teeth; regulates neuromuscular function	Rickets (soft, fragile bones—osteomalacia—and bony deformities) in children; bone pain and osteoporosis in adults; muscle contractions (tetany); *renal disease*	Dairy products, beans, leafy vegetables
P	Phosphorus	Constituent of bones, teeth; high energy intermediates and nucleic acid at cellular level	Rickets in children, osteomalacia in adults; *bone loss by stimulating secondary hyperparathyroidism*	Phosphate food additives
Mg	Magnesium	Constituent of bones, teeth; enzyme co-factor (kinases, etc.)	Muscle contractions; muscle dysfunction with decreased reflexes and respiratory depression	Leafy green vegetables

(Continued)

TABLE 8. ESSENTIAL MACRO- AND MICROMINERALS (Continued)

	Mineral	Functions	Deficiency and *Toxicity* Diseases	Dietary Sources
Selected essential microminerals (silicon, vanadium, nickel, tin, manganese, lithium also thought to be essential)*				
Cr	Chromium	Potentiates insulin	Impaired glucose tolerance	Meat, liver, grains, nuts, cheese
Co	Cobalt	Constituent of vitamin B_{12}		
Cu	Copper	Constituent of oxidases, promotes iron absorption	Similar to scurvy; hair and connective tissue defects in Menke disease; *cerebral and liver toxicity in Wilson disease*	Liver
I	Iodine	Constituent of thyroid hormones	Hypothyroidism, producing low muscle tone, porcine features, and developmental retardation in children (cretinism), enlarged thyroid (goiter), lethargy, myopathy, and lower leg swelling (myxedema) in adults; *hyperthyroidism with protruding eyes (exophthalmos), tachycardia, goiter*	Iodized table salt, seafood
Fe	Iron	Constituent of heme cofactor for hemoglobins, cytochromes	Anemia (hypochromic, microcytic) with pallor, fatigue, and heart failure; *iron overload (hemosiderosis in cells) with liver and heart failure; those with hereditary hemochromatosis more susceptible*	

Se	Selenium	Constituent of glutathione peroxidase	Subtle protein-energy malnutrition; *hair loss, dermatitis, irritability*	Plants, meat
Zn	Zinc	Cofactor for diverse enzymes, constituent of zinc finger DNA-binding motifs of signal transduction proteins	Acrodermatitis enterohepatica with hair loss, skin rashes, bowel malabsorption; decreased taste and smell acuity; *gastrointestinal irritation, vomiting*	
F	Flouride	Can be incorporated into bones and teeth for increased hardness	Dental caries; ?osteoporosis; dental *fluorosis (spotting)*	Drinking water where added

*Aluminum, arsenic, antimony, boron, bromine, cadmium, cesium, germanium, lead, mercury, silver, and strontium are known to be toxic in excess.

- Group I hormones are fat soluble (lipophilic), freely entering cells, and binding to receptors in the cytosol or nucleus (e.g., androgens, estrogens, gluco- and mineralocorticoids, retinoic acid, and thyroid hormones); group II hormones are water soluble (hydrophilic), binding to the cell membrane as first messenger, and communicating by generating cytoplasmic "second messengers."
- Various second messengers employed by group II hormones include cAMP (e.g., adrenergic catecholamines, ACTH, FSH, glucagon, TSH), cGMP (e.g., atrial natriuretic factor, nitric oxide), calcium and/or phosphatidylinositols (e.g., acetylcholine, angiotensin II, oxytocin), and protein kinase/phosphatase cascades (e.g., epidermal growth factor, erythropoietin, fibroblast growth factor, growth hormone, insulin)
- Chemical types of hormone include cholesterol derivatives (steroid hormones—e.g., testosterone, cortisol), tyrosine derivatives (e.g., thyroxine, epinephrine), peptides (e.g., ACTH), and glycoproteins (e.g., TSH, FSH).
- Group I hormones act by diffusing into the cytoplasm or nucleus to form a ligand-receptor complex that interacts with (1) modifying proteins, (2) hormone response elements (HRE) in DNA, and (3) transcription factors to alter cell function.
- Group II hormones often interact with characteristic 7-membrane-spanning domain receptors that interact with G protein complexes: GTP is exchanged with GDP on the α-subunit, which activates the effector (adenyl cyclase, potassium/calcium channels, phospholipase, etc.).
- Group II hormones may also activate protein kinases through phosphorylation at serine or threonine or deactivate them with phosphodiesterases; activation-deactivation of over 300 kinases/phosphod esterases (including kinase cascades) by second messengers (cAMP, cGMP, calcium, phosphatidyl inositols) provides diverse and multifaceted regulation mechanisms.

Key concepts: Integrated metabolism (Murray, pp 122–129, 231–236. Scriver, pp 1327–1406.)

- Many metabolic fuels are interconvertible, with an equilibrium between oxidation/catabolism for energy and reduction/anabolism for synthesis and reserve; an imperative affecting this equilibrium is the need to maintain blood glucose levels to fuel central nervous system and erythrocyte functions.

- Fatty acids and their generated ketones or acetyl CoA cannot be used for gluconeogenesis (except for odd-carbon chains that generate propionic acid); certain (glucogenic) amino acids can enter the citric acid cycle with net synthesis of oxaloacetate (and thus of glucose through phosphoenolpyruvate phosphokinase, etc.) but others (ketogenic amino acids) yield acetyl CoA.
- The catabolic/anabolic equilibrium is precisely regulated by hormones controlling the level of blood fuels and their delivery to tissues; the primary control hormones of metabolism are insulin and glucagon, with antagonizing effects on blood glucose levels (see Table 9).
- After a meal, fuels are abundant with glucose being the principal substrate for oxidation; insulin released from pancreatic β-islet cells allows glucose uptake in muscle and adipose cells and promotes glycogen synthesis in liver and muscle.
- Blood levels of glucose, amino acids, fatty acids, and ketone bodies are maintained by the ratio of insulin/glucagon concentrations; high blood sugars increase this ratio, signaling the fed state and promoting anabolic

TABLE 9. ACTIVITIES OF METABOLIC PATHWAYS IN FED OR FASTED STATES

	Fed	Fasted	Diabetes
Glycogen synthesis	+	−	−
Glycolysis (liver)	+	−	−
Triacylglyceride synthesis	+	−	−
Fatty acid synthesis	+	−	−
Protein synthesis	+	−	−
Cholesterol synthesis	+	−	−
Glycogenolysis	−	+	+
Gluconeogenesis (liver)	−	+	+
Lipolysis	−	+	+
Fatty acid oxidation	−	+	+
Protein breakdown	−	±	±
Ketogenesis (liver)	−	+	+
Ketone body utilization (non-hepatic tissues)	−	+	+

activities; the ratio decreases as glucagon is secreted from pancreatic α-cells in response to falling blood glucose (between meals, during fasting or starvation).

- Glucagon inhibits liver glycogen synthase and activates its glycogen phosphorylase, releasing glucose-6-phosphate that is converted to glucose; falling insulin levels act to preserve blood glucose by diminishing adipose and muscle uptake.
- Glucagon inhibits lipogenesis and stimulates lipase in adipose tissue, causing increased lipid catabolism with increased ketone bodies, free fatty acids, and glycerol; glycerol is an effective substrate for gluconeogenesis in liver.
- Muscle lacks a glucose-6-phosphatase to produce glucose from glycogen catabolism (using glucose-6-phosphate for energy instead); its increased fatty acid oxidation increases acetyl CoA and citrate levels, inhibits glycolysis (to spare glucose), and yields pyruvate and alanine that travel to liver for gluconeogenesis.
- Epinephrine has effects similar to those of glucagon, except that glucagon has a greater effect on the liver, whereas epinephrine has a greater effect on muscle; epinephrine or norepinephrine is released during exercise to promote catabolism of glucose and fat that supports muscular activity.
- Glucagon inhibits lipogenesis in adipose cells. Fat is catabolized during fasting or starvation to supply energy, causing increases in ketone bodies and free fatty acids.
- Uncontrolled diabetes causes blood glucose levels to rise due to lack of insulin, decreased glucose uptake by adipose/muscle tissue, and increased liver gluconeogenesis from amino acids; increased lipolysis in adipose tissue produces fatty acids for liver ketogenesis (distributing ketone bodies as fuel) with progressive ketosis and acidosis (acetoacetic acid and β-hydroxybutyrate are strong acids).
- The increased osmolarity of hyperglycemic blood plus increased lipids and cholesterol produce chronic vascular damage in diabetes (leading to hypertension, coronary artery disease, and retinal hemorrhage with blindness); acute hyperosmolarity, exacerbated by polyuria/dehydration) and ketoacidosis can lead to fatal diabetic coma unless insulin is provided.

INHERITANCE MECHANISMS AND BIOCHEMICAL GENETICS

Key concepts: Inheritance mechanisms/Risk calculations (Lewis, pp 47–134, 241–266, 377–396. Scriver, pp 3–45. Murray, pp 396–414.)

- Human gametes have 23 chromosomes (haploid chromosome number n = 23), while most somatic cells have 46 chromosomes (diploid chromosome number 2n = 46).
- Genes occupy sites on chromosomes (loci) and occur in alternative forms (alleles); interaction of these alleles determine inheritance patterns of disease that can be recognized using standard family history (pedigree) symbols (Fig. 20).
- Rarer Mendelian diseases exhibit autosomal dominant, autosomal recessive, or X-linked inheritance, while more common disorders like birth defects (spina bifida), diabetes mellitus, schizophrenia, or hypertension are caused by multiple genes plus environmental factors (multifactorial determination).
- Characteristics of autosomal dominant diseases include a vertical pattern of affected individuals in the pedigree, affliction of both males and females, variable expressivity (variable severity among affected individuals), frequent new mutations, and a 50% recurrence risk for offspring of affected individuals (see pedigree A of Fig. 20). Corollary: germ-line mosaicism may produce affected siblings with autosomal dominant disease when neither parent is affected.
- Characteristics of autosomal recessive diseases include a horizontal pedigree pattern, affliction of males and females, frequent consanguinity (inbreeding), frequent carriers (heterozygotes without manifestations of disease), and a 25% recurrence risk for carrier parents (see pedigree B of Fig. 20). Corollary: normal siblings of individuals with autosomal recessive disease have a two-thirds chance of being carriers.
- Characteristics of X-linked recessive diseases include an oblique pedigree pattern, affliction of males only, frequent female carriers, and a 25% recurrence risk for carrier females (see pedigree C of Fig. 20). Corollary: Haldane's law predicts a two-thirds chance that the mother of an affected male with X-linked recessive disease is a carrier (and a one-third chance the affected male represents a new mutation).

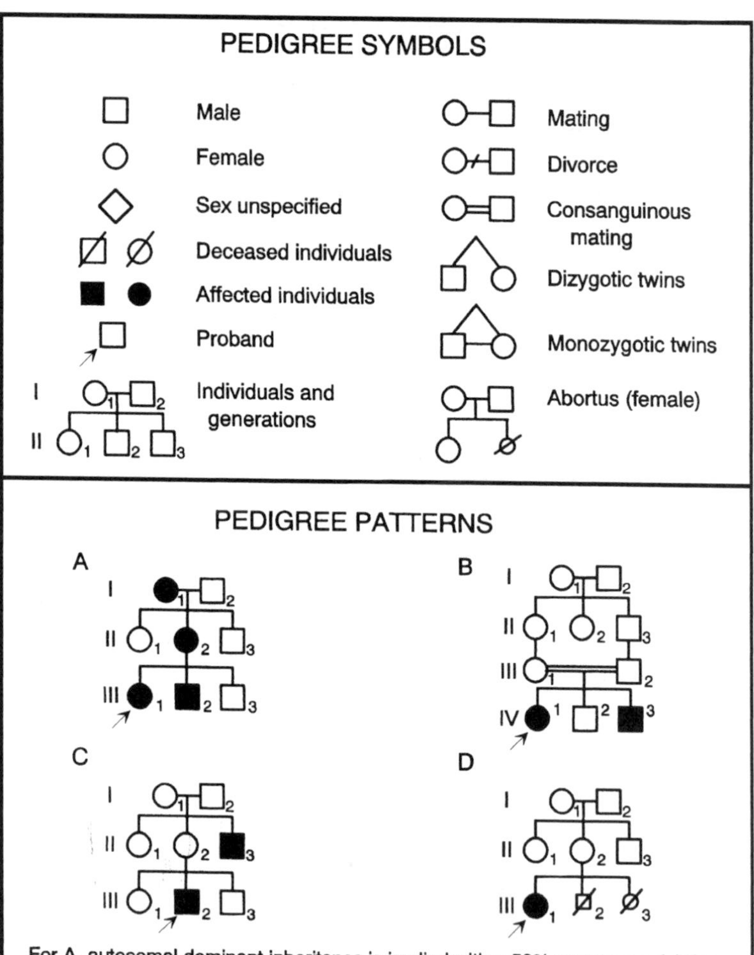

For A, autosomal dominant inheritance is implied with a 50% recurrence risk for individuals III-1 and III-2

For B, autosomal recessive inheritance is implied with a 25% recurrence risk for individuals III-1 and III-2

For C, X-linked recessive inheritance is implied with a 25% recurrence risk for individuals I-1 and II-2

For D, chromosomal inheritance is implied with individual II-2 being a translocation carrier

Figure 20
Pedigree symbols and pedigree patterns.

Key concepts: Genetic and biochemical diagnosis (Lewis, pp 331–442. Scriver, pp 3–45. Murray, pp 396–414.)

- Ethnic correlations with Mendelian disorders include higher frequencies of cystic fibrosis in whites, sickle cell anemia in blacks, β-thalassemia in Italians and Greeks, α-thalassemia in Asians, and Tay-Sachs disease in Jews.
- Advanced maternal age is associated with higher risks for chromosomal disorders (e.g., Down syndrome, trisomy 13), while advanced paternal age is associated with higher risks for new mutations (e.g., those producing achondroplasia or Marfan syndrome).
- The Hardy-Weinberg law predicts allele frequencies in an idealized population according to the formula $p^2 + 2pq + q^2 = 1$. Applied to cystic fibrosis, the law predicts that homozygotes (q^2) have a frequency of 1 in 1600, predicting that carriers (2pq) have a frequency of 1 in 20.
- A karyotype is an ordered arrangement of chromosomes that is described by cytogenetic notation. A karyotype can be obtained from dividing cells (blood leukocytes, bone marrow, fibroblasts, amniocytes), but not from frozen or formalin-fixed cells.
- Cytogenetic notation includes the chromosome number (usually 46), description of the sex chromosomes (usually XX or XY), and indication of missing, extra, or rearranged chromosomes. Examples include 47,XY,+21 (male with Down syndrome); 47,XX,13 (female with trisomy +13); 45,X (female with monosomy X or Turner syndrome); 46,XX,del(5p) (female with deletion of the chromosome 5 short arm).
- DNA diagnosis examines specific regions of genes for altered nucleotide sequences or deletions that affect gene expression and function; techniques include Southern blotting, gene amplification with the polymerase chain reaction (PCR), and mutant allele detection by hybridization with allele-specific oligonucleotides (ASOs). Chromosome microdeletions encompass several genes and are detected by fluorescent in situ hybridization (FISH).
- Non-Mendelian inheritance mechanisms include mitochondrial inheritance (exhibiting maternal transmission), expansion of triplet repeats (exhibiting anticipation in pedigrees as in the fragile X syndrome), and genomic imprinting (exhibiting different phenotypes according to maternal or paternal origin of the aberrant genes).
- Prenatal diagnosis can include fetal ultrasound, maternal serum studies, or sampling of cells from the fetoplacental unit by chorionic villus sampling [CVS at 8–10 weeks, amniocentesis at 12–18 weeks, or percutaneous umbilical sampling (PUBS) from 16 weeks to term].

Storage and Expression of Genetic Information

DNA Structure, Replication, and Repair

Questions

DIRECTIONS: Each item below contains a question or incomplete statement followed by suggested responses. Select the **one best** response to each question.

1. Fragile X syndrome (309550) and Huntington chorea (143100) exemplify a new category of genetic disease that involves triplet repeat instability. Boys with fragile X syndrome have over 500–1000 triplet repeats in a region proximal to the fragile X gene coding sequence, while normal males have repeat numbers of less than 60. The figure below diagrams the results of genetic analysis of a fragile X syndrome family as conducted by which of the following techniques?

a. Immunoblotting
b. Northern blotting
c. Southern blotting
d. Western blotting
e. Reverse transcriptase-PCR amplication

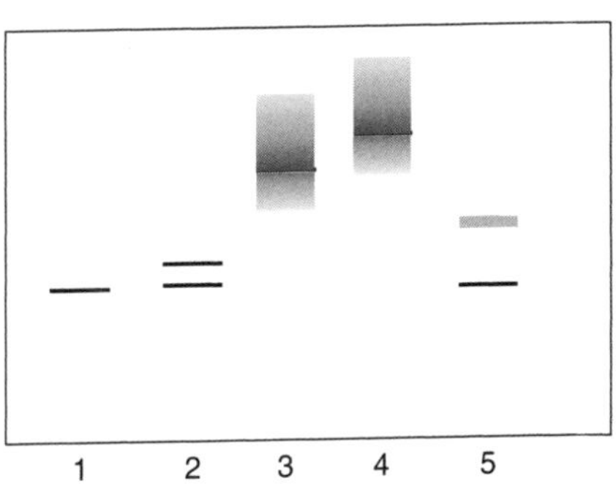

2. A child presents with deeply pigmented and scarred skin despite her Caucasian heritage, and her growth is delayed. Her dermatologist obtains a skin biopsy, suspecting the xeroderma pigmentosum group of diseases (278730); these have decreased ability to repair thymine-thymine dimers in DNA that are caused by ultraviolet light (sunlight exposure). Which of the following strategies would best measure unscheduled DNA synthesis (DNA repair) in the patient's skin fibroblasts?

a. Cell synchrony, then incubation with labelled iodine in G phase to complex with newly created hydroxyl groups in deoxyribose residues
b. Incubation with labelled purines to replace newly synthesized bases on the outside of the DNA duplex
c. Cell synchrony, then incubation with labelled deoxyribonucleotides in G phase to measure extension of single DNA strands in the 3′ to 5′ direction
d. Incubation with labelled deoxyribonucleotide triphosphates to measure extension of both strands in the 5′ to 3′ direction
e. Incubation with labelled deoxyribonucleotide triphosphates to measure extension of both strands in the 3′ to 5′ direction

3. The most common mutation causing cystic fibrosis (219700) in Caucasions is ΔF508, accounting for 70% of mutations. The terminology ΔF508 refers to deletion of a phenylalanine residue (F in the abbreviated amino acid code) at the 508th amino acid from the amino terminus of the cystic fibrosis transmembrane regulator (CFTR) protein. Which of the following would best describe DNA diagnosis of cystic fibrosis patients who are homozygous for the ΔF508 mutation?

a. Polymerase chain reaction using primers surrounding nucleotide #1522 of the normal cystic fibrosis DNA coding sequence; positive hybridization only with an oligonucleotide specific for the ΔF508 allele
b. Northern blotting of sputum RNA samples developed with CFTR gene probes, yielding two abnormally sized RNA transcripts
c. Southern blotting using restriction endonucleases that yield 100 bp fragments containing nucleotide #508 of the normal cystic fibrosis DNA coding sequence; hybridization with a DNA probe for this region yields two CFTR gene fragment sizes
d. Western blotting of sputum proteins developed with antibody to CFTR protein, yeilding two abnormally sized bands
e. Polymerase chain reaction using primers that amplify a 100 bp fragment surrounding nucleotide #508 of the normal cystic fibrosis DNA coding sequence, agarose gel electrophoresis demonstrates a single, abnormal fragment size using ultraviolet light

4. A research project examines multiple chromosome regions in Italian families selected because several individuals are affected with insulin-dependent diabetes mellitus (IDDM—222100). The results reveal a single nucleotide change from A to G in a noncoding region of chromosome 10 that is present in 9 of 10 diabetics and only 6 of 30 nondiabetics. The conclusion is best described by which of the following statements?

a. Mutations in a gene on chromosome 10 cause diabetes in Italians, allowing DNA diagnosis by Southern blot with a 90% sensitivity
b. Mutations in a gene on chromosome 10 cause diabetes in Italians, allowing DNA diagnosis by PCR amplification and DNA sequencing with a 60% positive predictive value
c. A single nucleotide polymorphism on chromosome 10, detected by PCR amplification and DNA sequencing, is associated with IDDM in Italian families (sensitivity is 90%).
d. A single nucleotide polymorphism on chromosome 10, detected by PCR amplification and DNA sequencing, is now available for worldwide screening of diabetes susceptibility.
e. Association of a chromosome 10 gene mutation with IDDM in Italian families suggests that HLA loci may exist outside of chromosome 6

5. It is recognized now that all cancers involve genetic changes, even though few are hereditary. An early example was the discovery of a Philadelphia chromosome (terminally deleted chromosome 22) in chronic myeloid leukemia. Which of the following results would be most diagnostic of chromosome 22 deletion in chronic myeloid leukemia (608232)?

a. Increased incorporation of labelled acetate into histones of chromatin regions on 22
b. Altered DNA restriction patterns of chromosome 22 regions with methylation-sensitive endonucleases
c. Altered pattern of small RNAs along leukemic chromatin
d. Altered DNA sequence for at least one chromosome 22 locus
e. Decreased transcription from loci on chromosome 22

6. Disorders like Prader-Willi syndrome (176270) can involve changes in gene structure or modification. Which of the following processes occurs at the 5 position of cytidine and often correlates with gene inactivation?

a. Gene conversion
b. Sister chromatid exchange
c. Pseudogene
d. Gene rearrangement
e. DNA methylation

7. A patient with the autosomal dominant Gardner syndrome (175100—tooth changes, bony tumors, and high rates of colonic polyps/colon cancer) was found to have a nucleotide substitution within the causative adenomatous polyposis coli (APC) gene. This mutation changed the DNA sequence from CAGAGGT to CAGGGGT and ablated the splice junction at the border of exon 7 and its adjacent intron. A partial sequencing result using the Sanger method is shown in the figure below, and supports which of the following conclusions about the child's APC genotype and expression?

a. Homozygous for the normal Gardner allele, some smaller mRNA molecules
b. Heterozygous for normal and mutant Gardner allele, some larger mRNA molecules
c. Heterozygous for normal and mutant Gardner allele, some smaller mRNA molecules
d. Homozygous for mutant Gardner allele, no change in mRNA molecules
e. Homozygous for mutant Gardner allele, some larger mRNA molecules

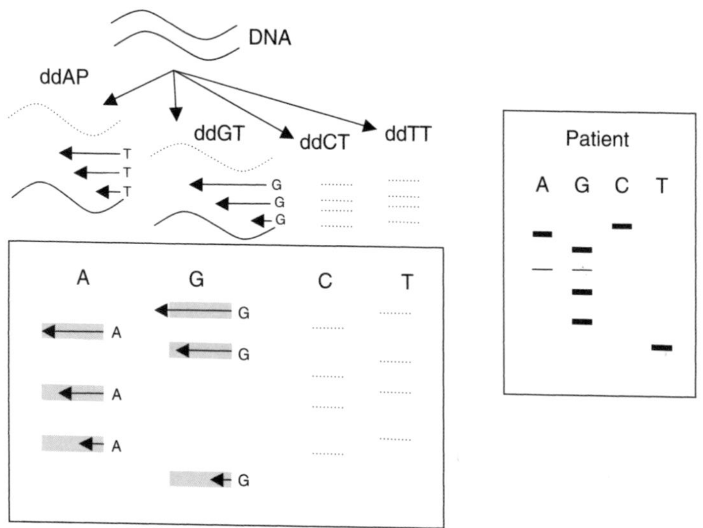

8. Restriction fragment length polymorphism (RFLP) analysis can only be used to follow the inheritance of a genetic disease in which of the following circumstances?

a. If mRNA probes are used in combination with antibodies
b. If the disease-causing mutation is at or closely linked to an altered restriction site
c. If proteins of mutated and normal genes migrate differently upon gel electrophoresis
d. If mutations are outside of restriction sites so that cleaving still occurs
e. If restriction fragments remain the same size but their charge changes

9. It is well known that DNA polymerases synthesize DNA only in the 5′ to 3′ direction. Yet, at the replication fork, both strands of parental DNA are being replicated with the synthesis of new DNA. An experiment examines incorporation of radiolabelled nucleotide triphosphates in unsynchronized cells, and finds a small amount of incorporated label in DNA fragments of small size. Which of the following best explains why experiment is compatible with new DNA from both strands being added in the 5′ to 3′ direction?

a. A different DNA polymerase replicates the complementary DNA strand as a series of small fragments
b. A 3′ to 5′ DNA polymerase is active in cells with high rates of DNA replication
c. DNA synthesis on complementary strand produces small 5′ to 3′ fragments that are continously ligated together
d. DNA replication switches strands every 100 nucleotides, a detail not resolved by microscopy.
e. DNA synthesis on the complementary strand does not use RNA primers

10. Over 200 disorders with complex phenotypes derive from changes in human chromosomes. Given that the chromosomes of mammalian cells may be 20 times as large as those of *Escherichia coli*, how can replication of mammalian chromosomes be carried out in just a few minutes?

a. Eukaryotic DNA polymerases are extraordinarily fast compared with prokaryotic polymerases
b. The higher temperature of mammalian cells allows for an exponentially higher replication rate
c. Hundreds of replication forks work simultaneously on each piece of chromosomal DNA
d. A great many different RNA polymerases carry out replication simultaneously on chromosomal DNA
e. The presence of histones speeds up the rate of chromosomal DNA replication

11. The fragile X DNA analysis shown in the figure below examines amplification of a 3 bp (triplet) repeat adjacent to the fragile X mental retardation-1 (FMR-1) gene (309550) on the X chromosome. Which of the descriptions of family members 1–5 shown on the analysis would be most consistent with the results (recall that females can be carriers for X-linked conditions with one normal and one abnormal allele on their two X chromosomes)?

a. 1-normal mother 2-normal father 3 and 4-sons with fragile X syndrome, 5-carrier daughter
b. 1-normal father 2-normal mother 3 and 4-sons with fragile X syndrome, 5-carrier daughter
c. 1-normal mother 2-normal father 3 and 4-carrier daughters, 5-son with fragile X syndrome
d. 1-carrier mother 2-normal father 3 and 4-sons with fragile X syndrome, 5-normal daughter
e. 1-normal father 2-carrier mother 3 and 4-normal sons, 5-carrier daughter

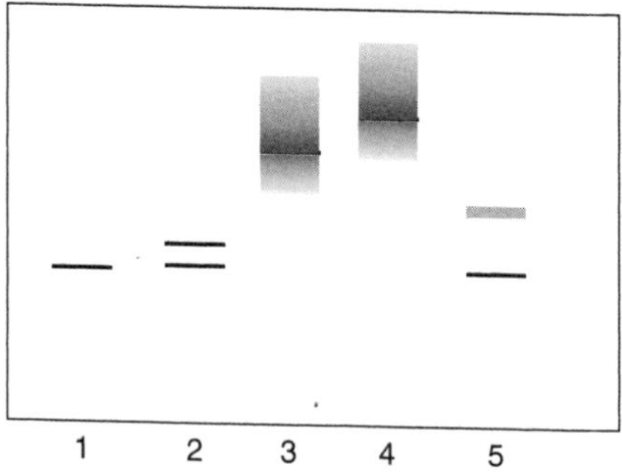

12. Children with Cockayne syndrome (216400) may appear normal at birth and during early childhood, but then display slowing growth and accelerated aging that produces adult complications such as diabetes and coronary artery disease. Adolescents may resemble nursing home residents, with aged skin, sparse hair, arthritis, mental deterioration, and degenerative disease. In vitro assay of labeled thymidine incorporation reveals decreased levels of DNA synthesis compared to controls, but normal-sized labeled DNA fragments. The addition of protein extract from normal cells gently heated to inactivate DNA polymerase restores DNA synthesis in Cockayne cells to normal. Which of the following enzymes used in DNA replication is most likely to be defective in Cockayne syndrome?

a. DNA-directed DNA polymerase
b. Unwinding proteins
c. DNA polymerase I
d. DNA-directed RNA polymerase
e. DNA ligase

13. Patients with hereditary nonpolyposis colon cancer (HNPCC—114500) have genes with microsatellite instability, that is, many regions containing abnormal, small loops of unpaired DNA. This is a result of a mutation affecting which of the following?

a. Mismatch repair
b. Chain break repair
c. Base excision repair
d. Depurination repair
e. Nucleotide excision repair

14. A recombinant viral DNA containing a 300 bp human gene sequence is replicated in vitro using media containing bromo-deoxyuridine triphosphate, completely saturating the DNA with bromo-deoxyuridine residues. The bromo-substituted viral DNA is then switched to media with regular deoxyuridine triphosphate, and allowed to undergo two rounds of DNA replication. The human DNA fragment is then cleaved by restriction enzyme digestion and subjected to ultracentrifugation in cesium chloride under conditions that will separate bromo-substituted DNA duplexes, hybrid bromo-substituted/normal duplexes, and normal duplexes. Which of the results depicted in the figure below (with their interpretations) should be obtained?

a. One DNA band of low density, meaning all DNA duplexes have two strands with normal uridine
b. One DNA band of intermediate density, meaning all DNA duplexes have one strand with uridine, one with bromouridine
c. One DNA band of high density, meaning all DNA duplexes have two strands with bromo-uridine
d. One DNA band of high density, one of intermediate density indicating the corresponding types of DNA duplexes
e. One DNA band of intermediate density, one of low density indicating the corresponding types of DNA duplexes

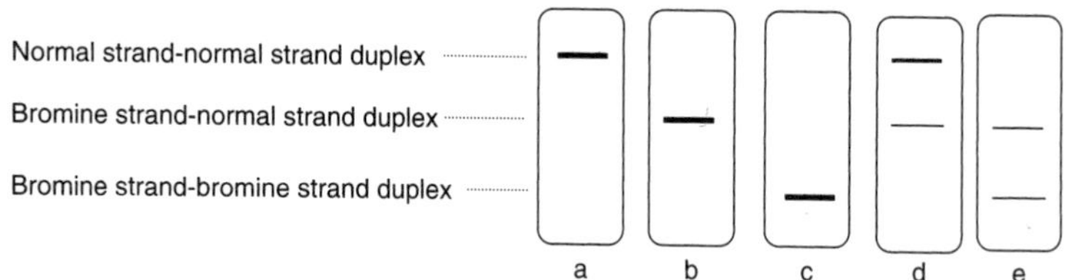

15. Sickle cell anemia (141900) is caused by a specific mutation in the gene for β-globin, one of the two globin proteins that complex with heme to form hemoglobin. The sickle cell anemia mutation is known to produce a single amino acid change, glutamic acid to valine, at position 6 of the β-globin peptide chain. Which of the following is the most likely mechanism for this mutation?

a. Crossing over
b. Two-base insertion
c. Three-base deletion
d. Single base insertion
e. Single-base substitution (point mutation)

16. Parents with normal pigmentation bring their newborn daughter to you for consultation about diagnosis and management. Their first two children, a boy and a girl, have a complete form of albinism (203100) with pink irides, blond hair, and pale skin. Which of the following represents the best advice concerning the newborn child?

a. A one-eighth risk for albinism and skin cancer from DNA deletions
b. A one-eighth risk for albinism and skin cancer from DNA cross-linkage
c. A one-fourth risk for albinism and skin cancer from DNA point mutations
d. A one-fourth risk for albinism and skin cancer from DNA deletions
e. A one-fourth risk for albinism and skin cancer from DNA cross-linkage

17. A parent is correcting his child's photograph for red eye and notes one of the child's pupils reflects the flash as white rather than red. An ophthalmologist confirms the presence of a tumor in the back of the white-reflecting eye, telling the parents about the possibility of retinoblastoma (180200). The parents return to their pediatrician, confused about the relation of retinoblastoma (Rb) and B-cell lymphoma (bcl) genes they saw on the Internet and the possibility their child's tumor is inherited. Which of the following is the most appropriate response?

a. Rb and bcl proteins are polymerases that prevent oncogenesis by stringent DNA repair; the parents are therefore carriers for autosomal recessive Rb deficiency with a 1 in 4 recurrence risk.
b. Rb protein binds transcription factors needed for cell division and bcl protein (cyclin D1) stimulates it; Rb is a tumor suppressor gene requiring homozygous mutations (two hits) that are likely sporadic in a child with unilateral tumor
c. Rb and bcl proteins are DNA-binding factors that suppress promoters near oncogenes and act as tumor suppressors; the child represents a new, dominant-acting mutation and the parents have a minimal recurrence risk.
d. Rb protein stimulates cyclins specific for retinal tissue and bcl does the same for lymphatic cyclins; the child represents a new mutation with excess Rb activity.
e. Rb protein forms complexes with bcl protein that promotes cell division in rapidly proliferating tissues; the child represents a new mutation with excess Rb-bcl complex activity.

18. A couple have a child with pigmented skin that becomes bright red after sunlight exposure and leaves scars after healing. A skin biopsy is obtained and the cultured fibroblasts tested for xeroderma pigmentosum (XP-278700). The laboratory reports positive testing with assignment to complementation group A. Which of the following is the most likely information in this report?

a. The fibroblasts had low amounts of thymine dimers after ultraviolet light exposure, but these were increased by extracts from another XP cell line
b. The fibroblasts had low exogenous nucleotide-excision repair that was restored to normal levels by transformation with viruses from XP cells.
c. The fibroblasts had low levels of DNA polymerase that was augmented by XP cell extracts
d. The fibroblast had low exogenous nucleotide-excision repair that was restored to normal levels by fusion with another XP cell line.
e. The fibroblast had high amounts of thymine dimers after x-ray exposure that were reduced by introduction of XP cell extracts

19. Children with the Roberts syndrome (268300) of cleft palate and absence of one to all limbs have abnormal centromere structures visualized by routine chromosome studies. This observation highlights the complexity of animal DNA as compared to that of experimental models like *E. coli* bacteria. Which of the following statements best describes the differences?

a. Animal nuclear DNA is discontinuous, with pieces (chromosomes) that are each the same size as a bacterial genome
b. Animal nuclear DNA has transcription factors that replace the histones and operons of bacterial DNAs
c. Animal nuclear DNA is so large that it cannot be replicated semiconservatively
d. Animal nuclear DNA is associated with many more histone and nonhistone proteins than bacterial DNA, producing a "second code" for genetic regulation
e. Animal nuclear DNA is divided into nucleosomes that allow different transcription regulators to occupy specific nuclear compartments

20. A large family has many individuals with colon cancer, affecting males and females in a manner compatible with autosomal dominant inheritance. The patients do not have multiple polyps as in Gardner syndrome or adenomatosis polyposis coli (APC), so that colonoscopy screening has not been helpful. The family is thought most compatible with hereditary nonpolyposis colon cancer (HNPCC-114500), and the diagnosis is confirmed by skin biopsy and fibroblast studies. Which of the following best describes the diagnostic results?

a. Defect in mismatch repair with accumulation of nucleotide repeats by replication slippage
b. Defect in double-strand break repair with accumulation of multiple small DNA fragments
c. Defect in base-excision repair with accumulation of depurinated DNA
d. Defect in nucleotide excision repair with accumulation of thymine dimers
e. Defect in nucleotide excision repair with defects in an *MSH* protein that is homologous to an *E. coli* muts gene

21. Double-stranded DNA replication is unidirectional in all organisms despite the antiparallel orientation of complementary strands. This is best explained by which of the following?

a. Use of helicase, single-strand binding proteins (SSBs), and DNA polymerase to effect continuous synthesis on the lagging strand
→b. Use of helicase, single-strand binding proteins (SSBs), and DNA polymerase to effect continuous synthesis on the leading strand.
c. Use of helicase, single-strand binding proteins (SSBs), and DNA polymerase effect continuous synthesis on the leading and lagging strands
d. Use of primase, RNA primers, and ligase to effect discontinuous synthesis on the leading strand
e. Use of primase, RNA primers, and ligase to effect continuous synthesis on the lagging strand

22. Which of the following descriptions of DNA replication is not common to the synthesis of both leading and lagging strands?

a. RNA primer is synthesized
b. DNA polymerase III synthesizes DNA
c. Helicase (rep protein) continuously unwinds duplex DNA at the replication fork during synthesis
d. Nucleoside monophosphates are added in a 5′ to 3′ direction along the growing DNA chain
e. DNA ligase repeatedly joins the ends of DNA along the growing strand

23. A teenage boy notices decreased performance in basketball and drooping of his eyelids when tired. He complains to his pediatrician that his leg muscles seem smaller despite consistent weight training, and he has trouble keeping his balance with his eyes closed or when not concentrating. The physician suspects Kearns-Sayre syndrome (530000), and confirms the diagnosis by demonstrating a deletion of mitochondrial DNA in tissue obtained by muscle biopsy. Unique properties of mitochondrial DNA are best summarized as which of the following?

a. Circular, single-stranded, comprising 1% of cellular DNA with high mutation rates
b. Linear duplex DNA with a length similar to that of one nuclear chromosome, present as 50–100 copies per cell
c. Circular duplex DNA of about 16,000 bp that encodes unique tRNAs and all mitochondrial proteins
d. Circular, single-stranded DNA with low mutation rate that encodes a minority of mitochondrial peptides
e. Linear duplex DNA that encodes over 70 proteins of the respiratory chain and has a mutation rate 5–10 times higher than nuclear DNA

24. DNA fingerprinting is used for paternity testing and forensic identification of suspects. Which of the following is the most accurate description of DNA fingerprinting?

a. DNA can be isolated from blood, skin, or sperm and analyzed for variable patterns of restriction fragments arising from tandemly repeated sequences (microsatellites)
b. DNA is copied from blood, skin, or sperm RNA using reverse transcriptase and analyzed for the pattern of complementary DNAs
c. DNA is isolated from blood, skin, or sperm and its fragment size distribution is analyzed by gel electrophoresis
d. DNA is isolated from blood, skin, or sperm and hybridized with probes from the HLA locus to visualize HLA gene patterns
e. DNA is isolated from blood, skin, or sperm, centrifuged to separate satellite DNA fractions, and analyzed by gel electrophoresis

25. The first drug to be effective against AIDS (609432), including the reduction of maternal-to-child AIDS transmission by 30%, was AIDS drug azidothymidine (AZT). Which of the following describes its mechanism of action?

a. It inhibits viral protein synthesis
b. It inhibits RNA synthesis
c. It inhibits viral DNA polymerase
d. It stimulates DNA provirus production
e. It inhibits viral reverse transcriptase

26. A 2-year-old girl is the product of a normal pregnancy and delivery and developed normally until age 12 months. After learning many words, crawling, and walking, she becomes progressively unsteady and stops walking, also refusing to speak. She begins wringing her hands frequently, has staring spells, and seems to be regressing in performance and memory. Her physician suspects a disorder called Rett syndrome (312750), and orders a diagnostic test that is based on increased DNA methylation around the MECP gene on the X chromosome. Which of the results below would be consistent with a positive diagnosis?

a. Increased expression of the MECP protein
b. Increased size of MECP mRNA
c. Loss of methylated sites as detected by methylation-sensitive restriction endonucleases
d. Gain of methylated sites as detected by methylation-sensitive restriction endonucleases
e. Amplification of triplet repeats surrounding the MECP gene promotor region.

27. Recombinant cloning of a human gene may involve several of the steps numbered below. Which of the following represents the correct sequence of these steps?

1. Digestion of human genomic and plasmid DNA with the appropriate restriction endonuclease
2. Transformation of bacteria with the recombinant DNA library
3. Characterization of a restriction fragment that contains the desired human gene
4. Mixing and ligation of restricted plasmid and human genomic DNA to form an assembly of recombinant molecules (recombinant DNA library).
5. Selection of a colony showing positive hybridization, culture, and isolation of the recombinant DNA
6. Screening of the recombinant DNA library by plating on agar, nitrocellulose transfer, and hybridization with a probe for the desired gene

a. Steps 1-2-3-4-5-6
b. Steps 3-1-4-2-6-5
c. Steps 1-4-2-3-6-5
d. Steps 4-2-6-5-3-1
e. Steps 3-4-2-6-5-1

28. Which of the following characteristics distinguishes most RNA molecules from DNA?

a. A purine or pyrimidine base linked to a pentose sugar
b. A 3′-phosphate group linked to a pentose sugar
c. A 5′-phosphate group linked to a pentose sugar
d. Susceptibility to alkaline hydrolysis because of neighboring pentose hydroxyl groups
e. A terminal triphosphate on newly synthesized strands

29. Which of the following is the correct sequence of events in gene repair mechanisms in patients without a mutated repair process?

a. Nicking, excision, replacement, sealing, recognition
b. Nicking, recognition, excision, sealing, replacement
c. Nicking, sealing, recognition, excision, replacement
d. Recognition, nicking, excision, replacement, sealing
e. Sealing, recognition, nicking, excision, replacement

30. Which of the following indicates the correct sequence of chromosome constituents, going from smaller to larger?

a. Chromatin fibril, nucleosome, histone octamer, chromosome loop
b. Nucleosome, chromatin fibril, chromosome loop, histone octamer
c. Chromatin fibril, histone octamer, nucleosome, chromosome loop
d. Nucleosome, histone octamer, chromosome loop, chromosome fibril
e. Histone octamer, nucleosome, chromatin fibril, chromosome loop

31. Radiation therapy is employed for many cancers, including irradiation of the central nervous system to destroy lymphoblasts in leukemia. Which of the following accounts for the destruction of rapidly growing cells?

a. Cross-linking of DNA
b. Demethylation of DNA
c. Cleavage of DNA double strands
d. Disruption of DNA-RNA transcription complexes
e. Disruption of purine rings in DNA

32. Mammalian chromosomes have specialized structures with highly repetitive DNA at their ends (telomeres). Which of the following aspects of telomeric DNA replication is different from that of other chromosomal regions?

a. A special DNA polymerase called telomerase contains a template RNA primer
b. DNA polymerase contains a unique telomeric oligonucleotide used on chromosome ends
c. DNA polymerase has a special activity that cross-links DNA ends
d. DNA polymerase has a subunit that facilitates binding to repetitive DNA
e. A special DNA polymerase called telomerase can reverse direction of replication at DNA termini

33. A child with developmental delay and unusual features has had routine chromosome analysis that was normal. The physician then considers a "telomere FISH"—analysis of the child's chromosomes using fluorescent DNA probes specific for repetitive DNA sequences near telomeres. The laboratory provides a summary of abnormal FISH results. Which of the following would be the best conclusion from that summary?

a. Longer telomeres in older patients and those with subtle chromosome change
b. Shorter telomeres in cancer tissue and longer telomeres in patients with subtle chromosome change
c. Shorter telomeres in aging patients and a single, specific telomere rearrangement in patients with subtle chromosome change
d. Longer telomeres in cancer tissue and a single, specific telomere rearrangement in patients with subtle chromosome change
e. Shorter telomeres in cancer tissue and a single, specific telomere rearrangement in patients with subtle chromosome change

34. A 9-month-old girl presents to hematology clinic after her 9-month checkup showed anemia. Her serum iron and transferring levels were normal, and her hemoglobin electrophoresis demonstrated an abnormal hemoglobin in addition to A and A2. Which of the following represents the most likely change at her β-globin locus and the genetic process that produced it? (Recall that the normal β-globin locus has the gene order Gγ-Aγ-δ-β.)

a. Gγ-Aγ-deletion-β, gene conversion
b. Gγ-Aγ-δ-deletion, gene conversion
c. Gγ-Aγ-fusion-δ-β, unequal recombination
d. Gγ-Aγ-δ-β fusion, unequal recombination
e. Gγ-Aγ-δ-β-Gγ-Aγ-δ-β, equal recombination

DNA Structure, Replication, and Repair

Answers

1. The answer is c. *(Lewis, pp 231–232, 274–279. Murray, pp 403–407. Scriver, pp 11–18, 1257–1290.)* DNA diagnosis of genetic disease requires characterization of the responsible gene, then detection of size or sequence changes in at-risk patients. When changes like triplet repeat amplifications produce dramatic size differences in gene (DNA) fragments, they can be displayed by Southern blotting (Dr Ed Southern derived the technique). The patient's genomic DNA (from blood, skin biopsy, amniocentesis, etc.) is extracted, digested with the appropriate restriction enzymes, size-fractionated on agarose gels, blotted (transferred onto a membrane using capillary pressure), stabilized by heat/drying, hybridized with radioactive DNA probes, and exposed to x-ray film. Those fragments of size-fractionated DNA that are complementary to the probe are highlighted as dark bands on the autoradiogram. In severely affected males with fragile X syndrome, amplifications are so great that restriction enzymes bracketing the triplet repeat region yield 500–2000 bp fragments that are easily distinguished from normal sizes of 15–60 bp (as illustrated in the figure accompanying this question). Analogous blotting techniques were named as puns on the name of Southern, including "Northern" blotting to detect RNA molecules and "Western" blotting to detect proteins. Immunoblotting is one version of the "Western" blot technique where proteins are separated by electrophoresis and transferred to a membrane for probing with antibody to the proteins of interest. Reverse transcription of RNA into single, then double-stranded DNA, followed by polymerase chain reaction amplification (RT-PCR), is a more sensitive method for RNA measurement. RT-PCR could demonstrate altered levels of fragile X mRNA but would not measure triplet repeats because these are outside of the fragile X coding region.

2. The answer is d. *(Murray, pp 335–339. Scriver, pp 677–704. Lewis, pp 234–237.)* In the classic double-helical model of DNA proposed by Watson and Crick, the purine (adenosine and guanine) and pyrimidine (cytosine and thymine) bases (see Fig. 2) attached to the sugar backbone are perpendicular to the axis and parallel to each other. They are paired (A to G or T to C) and held together by hydrogen bonds. The DNA strands (nucleotide polymers) are joined by linkages between the 3′-hydroxyl of each pentose (deoxyribose) and the 5′-phosphate of its deoxyribose neighbor. Each strand composing the double helix is different and antiparallel. The 3′ end of one strand is opposite the 5′ end of its complement and vice versa (see Fig. 2). DNA replication occurs in the 5′ to 3′ direction on both strands of DNA during the S phase of the cell cycle. It consists of five steps—unwinding by helicases, priming by short RNAs, 5′ to 3′ addition of deoxyribonucleotides via their triphosphates and DNA polymerase in elongation of the "leading" strand (discontinuously using Okazaki fragments for the "lag" strand), replacement of RNA primers with newly synthesized DNA, and sealing of gaps (on the lag strand) with DNA ligase. DNA repair occurs at all cell cycle phases, and among the types is excision repair that uses endonuclease to nick strands adjacent to thymine dimers, DNA polymerase to degrade and replace damaged nucleotides, ligase to restore integrity. All types of DNA synthesis will incorporate deoxyribonucleotide triphosphates rather than isolated bases or deoxyribose residues, and the new nucleotides are synthesized in the 5′ to 3′ direction using both strands of the DNA helix as templates.

3. The answer is a. *(Murray, pp 335–339. Scriver, pp 677–704. Lewis, pp 217–240.)* An individual homozygous for the ΔF508 cystic fibrosis mutation would have a 3 bp deletion beginning at nucleotide #1522 on both versions (alleles) of the cystic fibrosis gene, and such small changes are best detected by PCR followed by allele-specific-oligonucleotide (ASO) hybridization (answer a) or direct nucleotide sequencing. Note that the 3 bp genetic code predicts that amino acid #508 will correspond to nucleotides #1522–1524 of the coding sequence (excluding introns); this eliminates answers c and e. Homozygous individuals will have identical mutant alleles, meaning that molecular analyses would demonstrate a single size or band rather than two (normal and mutant) seen with a carrier (eliminating answers b, c, and d). Blotting techniques would not be sensitive enough to detect a 3 bp difference in DNA or RNA, and the effects on protein conformation could not be predicted. Acrylamide electrophoresis with direct visualization of DNA fragments could be performed as in answer e, but only one band corresponding to the two ΔF508 alleles (each 3 bp shorter than normal) would be detected.

4. The answer is c. *(Murray, pp 405–406. Lewis, pp 183–186. Scriver, pp 3–45.)* The result described in answer c is correct, emphasizing that the nucleotide change is a polymorphism associated with IDDM in Italian families, not a causative mutation and not necessarily associated with IDDM in other ethnic groups. PCR allows rapid amplification of target DNA sequences using heat-stable DNA polymerases and multiple denaturation, annealing, and extension cycles. Multiple PCR reactions coupled with DNA sequencing of amplified fragments has allowed systematic identification of single nucleotide polymorphisms (SNPs), occurring at an average 1 in every 600 nucleotides in the human genome. Genes that contribute to multifactorial diseases like diabetes mellitus, schizophrenia, and the like can be identified by scanning affected families with SNPs from all chromosome regions, using SNPs that cotransmit (are "associated") with the disease. The polymorphic HLA locus on chromosome 6 provided the first allele associations ≡ linkage disequilibria, but the implicated genes near SNPs will not necessarily encode surface antigens as implied in answer e—they could influence insulin uptake, degradation, conformation, and the like.

5. The answer is d. *(Lewis, pp 176–178. Murray, p 305.)* Chromosome deletion involves a breakage of DNA, with loss of the distal chromosome. The primary change in chronic myelogenous leukemia with chromosome 22 deletion would be a break in the chromosomal DNA that deletes certain sequences, joining DNA before the deletion point with telomeric sequences that foster chromosome replication (answer d). The other answers refer to changes in gene expression that could occur as a result of chromosome alteration, and do occur in various cancers—altered primary transcription (answer e), altered "second" code of epigenesis through histone modification (answer a), altered DNA methylation (answer b), or altered decoration patterns of small RNAs that influence chromatin transcription (answer c). In fact, most patients with the Philadelphia chromosome (22 deletion) actually have a chromosome 9:22 translocation that joins the Abelson ABL oncogene on chromosome 9 to a BCR (breakpoint cluster region) on chromosome 22. These discoveries follow a trend in cancer genetics where chromosomal abnormalities identify underlying cancer genes, in this case an ABL oncogene know from viral carcinogenesis and a BCR region known to be interrupted in other chonic myelogenous leukemias. Current research focuses on how altered expression of BCR-ABL gene products lead to chronic myelogenous leukemia.

6. The answer is e. *(Murray, pp 303–313. Scriver, pp 3–45. Lewis pp 241–266.)* DNA methylation occurs mainly at CpG dinucleotides that often cluster in at the upstream promoter regions of genes (CpG islands). While these are generally correlated with gene inactivation, there are many exceptions. Double crossovers at meiosis can substitute a normal allele for a mutant allele (conversion), and reverse transcriptases can copy intronless mRNA into complementary DNAs (cDNAs) that integrate into the genome as pseudogenes. Immunoglobulin genes undergo gene rearrangement to unite variable, joining, and constant regions for expression of a unique antibody. Unequal crossing over between sister chromatids is thought to be an important mechanism for variation in copy number within gene clusters.

7. The answer is b. *(Murray, pp 404–405. Lewis, pp 446–447. Scriver, pp 3–45.)* The Sanger method of DNA sequencing primes DNA synthesis of key gene regions in the presence of the usual deoxynucleotides (dNTPs) plus low concentrations of one dideoxynucleotides (ddNTPs). Incorporation of a ddNTP terminates synthesis of the DNA strand as there is no free 3′ OH group for addition of the next nucleotide. Four reactions with A, C, T, and G ddNTPs are run, then applied to adjacent lanes on a gel to separate the labelled, synthesized strands by size. The sequence of the DNA is determined by reading the order of the terminated chains going up the gel. The DNA sequencing gel for the patient indicates some bands at heavier density and others at lighter density, compatible with the autosomal APC alleles having identical sequence (homozygous) for the heavier bands and different sequences for the lighter bands (heterozygous). The gel can be read from top to bottom as CAG A/G GGT, where A/G represents comigrating DNA fragments of lighter density. The patient has one allele with CAGAGGT sequence (normal) and another with CAGGGGT (mutant), making them heterozygous and at increased risk for colon cancer in this autosomal dominant syndrome. Interruption of a splice site for one copy of the gene will yield some larger mRNA molecules with failure of the intron to be removed.

8. The answer is b. *(Murray, pp 409–411. Scriver, pp 3–45. Lewis, pp 41–45, 151–186.)* A variety of genetic diseases, such as sickle cell anemia (141900), Huntington chorea (143100), and cystic fibrosis (219700), can be detected by restriction fragment length polymorphism (RFLP) analysis. In order for

RFLP to be able to detect and follow the inheritance of these genes, the detected mutation must be at or closely linked to an altered restriction site. Mutations within the restriction sites change the size of restriction fragments. The differently sized fragments migrate at speeds inversely proportional to their weights during electrophoresis through a porous agarose gel. Specific gene fragments can be detected amidst background DNA fragments after Southern transfer, hybridization with fluorescent or radiolabeled DNA probes, and visualization by fluorescence or autoradiography.

9. The answer is c. *(Murray, pp 326–333. Scriver, pp 3–45.)* Since both strands of parental DNA serve as templates for the synthesis of new DNA, it appears that DNA synthesis must be 5′ to 3′ for one daughter strand and 3′ to 5′ for the other daughter strand at the replication fork. Despite the apparent need for 3′ to 5′ synthesis, all DNA polymerases and repair enzymes can only synthesize DNA in the 5′ to 3′ direction. The apparent contradiction is solved by understanding that one strand of DNA is synthesized continuously in the 5′ to 3′ direction, and the other strand is made up of small fragments known as Okazaki fragments. The small Okazaki fragments are, in fact, synthesized in a 5′ to 3′ direction and then joined together by DNA ligase. Each Okazaki fragment is about 1000 nucleotides long. Thus, while the overall direction of growth of the lagging strand that is made up of small fragments is in fact in the 3′ to 5′ direction, the actual polymerization of individual nucleotides is in the 5′ to 3′ direction. Crossing over of the DNA strands does not occur during replication.

10. The answer is c. *(Murray, pp 326–333. Scriver, pp 3–45. Lewis, 241–266.)* Despite the great length of the chromosomes of eukaryotic DNA, the actual replication time is only minutes. This is because eukaryotic DNA is replicated bidirectionally from many points of origin. The hundreds of initiation sites for DNA replication on chromosomes share a consensus sequence called an autonomous replication sequence (ARS). Thus, while the process of DNA replication in mammals is similar to that in bacteria, with DNA polymerases of similar optimal temperatures and speed, the many replication forks allow for a rapid synthesis of chromosomal DNA. Proteins such as histones, which are bound to mammalian chromosomes, inhibit DNA replication or transcription. Dissociation of the protein-DNA complex (chromatin) and unwinding of DNA supercoils (followed by chromatin reassembly) is part of the replication process.

11. The answer is c. *(Murray, pp 401–402. Lewis, pp 373–376. Scriver, pp 262–264.)* Females have two X chromosomes and males one X plus a small Y chromosome that does little besides initiate male sex determination. Women will thus have minimal or no symptoms of recessive diseases caused by mutant X chromosomal genes, while males with their single X are often severely affected. The variable expansion of triplet repeats upstream of the fragile X syndrome (FMR-1) gene produces differently sized DNA fragments if restriction sites (Southern blot) or amplifying primers (PCR) are chosen that bracket the expandable region. Normal women will have two DNA fragment sizes within the normal size range (less than 60 repeats), normal men one such fragment. Female carriers of fragile X syndrome will have one normally sized and one expanded DNA fragment, while affected males will have a single expanded fragment. An intriguing feature of expanding repeat disease is progressive instability of amplified repeat regions. The moderately expanded abnormal alleles of female carriers (60–200 repeats) can expand dramatically during meiosis to 500–2000 repeats in their affected sons. These large repeat regions are highly unstable during development, producing variable numbers of repeats in the different male tissues, explaining the smear (range of fragment sizes) for individuals 3 and 4, as shown in Fig. 1.

12. The answer is b. *(Murray, pp 326–333. Scriver, pp 3–45. Lewis, pp 171–184.)* Before DNA replication can actually begin, unwinding protein must open segments along the DNA double helix. A defective unwinding protein slows the overall rate of DNA synthesis, but does not alter the size of replicated DNA fragments. Defects in DNA synthesis or transcription may produce a phenotype of accelerated aging, as in Cockayne syndrome [216400 (usually defective in a transcription factor)]. After unwinding, DNA-directed RNA polymerase (primase) catalyzes the synthesis of a complementary RNA primer of approximately 50–100 bases on each DNA strand. Then DNA-directed DNA polymerase III adds deoxyribonucleotides to the 3′ end of the primer RNA, which replicates a segment of DNA, the Okazaki fragment. DNA polymerase I then removes the primer RNA and adds deoxyribonucleotides to fill the gaps between adjacent Okazaki fragments. The fragments are finally joined together by DNA ligase to create a continuous DNA chain.

13. The answer is a. *(Murray, pp 334–340. Scriver, pp 769–784. Lewis, pp 171–184.)* One of the most common types of inherited cancers is nonpolyposis colon cancer [HNPCC-(114500)]. Most cases are associated with mutations of either of two genes that encode proteins critical in the surveillance of mismatches. Mismatches are due to copying errors leading to one- to five-base unmatched pieces of DNA. Two- to five-base-long unmatched bases form miniloops. Normally, specific proteins survey newly formed DNA between adenine methylated bases within a GATC sequence. Mismatches are removed and replaced. First, a GATC endonuclease nicks the faulty strand at a site complementary to GATC; then an exonuclease digests the strand from the GATC site beyond the mutation. Finally, the excised faulty DNA is replaced. In HNPCC, the unrecognized mismatches accumulate, leading to malignant growth of colon epithelium. The other forms of DNA repair are important for rectifying damage from ultraviolet light.

14. The answer is d. *(Murray, pp 326–333. Scriver, pp 3–45. Lewis, pp 171–184.)* The replication of double-stranded DNA is semiconservative, meaning that each strand separates and serves as a template for synthesis of a new complementary strand. The first round of replication of a bromodeoxyuridine (dU)-labeled DNA helix in a solution with normal dU will yield two daughter duplexes, each with one bromo-dU and one dU strand. The second round of replication will yield four daughter duplexes, two with one bromo-dU and one dU strand (intermediate density, middle of tube in the figure accompany Question 14) and two with both strands containing dU (low density, top of tube). Centrifugation to equilibrium in cesium chloride causes a density gradient to form in the centrifuge tube with banding of DNA duplex molecules at their corresponding density.

15. The answer is e. *(Murray, pp 326–340. Scriver, pp 3–45. Lewis, pp 185–204.)* A change from one DNA codon to another is required to cause a replacement of amino acids such as the valine to glutamic acid change in the β-globin peptide chain of hemoglobin S (141900). A single nucleotide substitution (point mutation) could effect such an codon change, and involves a thymine to adenine substitution at the second position of the codon 6. The other answers would not change one DNA/RNA codon and its translated amino acid. Equal exchange (crossing over) among homologous β-globin genes could exchange alleles, replacing normal alleles with mutant partners or vice-versa (converting heterozygosity to homozygosity). Unequal crossing over could generate mutant alleles with duplicated or deficient nucleotides. One or two-base insertions would change the reading frame of the genetic code (frame-shift mutation) and produce a nonsense peptide or termination codon (chain-terminating mutation) after the point of insertion. Three-base deletions could also cause frame shifts if out of codon phase, or remove one codon and delete its corresponding amino acid from the peptide product.

16. The answer is e. *(Murray, pp 326–340. Scriver, pp 5587–5628. Lewis, pp 171–184.)* Normal parents having two affected children, male and female, is suggestive of autosomal recessive inheritance. This interpretation fits with the usual inheritance of oculocutaneous albinism (203100), implying a one-fourth risk for a newborn in whom signs and symptoms of albinism are not yet evident. The defect in melanin synthesis in albinism decreases the amount of this protective pigment in skin and increases the exposure of DNA in skin cells to sunlight. Ultraviolet rays from sunlight cause DNA cross-linkage between at least two bases in the same or opposite strands of DNA. Cross-linking occurs through the formation of thymine-thymine dimers. The DNA cross-links cause higher rates of mutation and skin cancer in albinism, mandating the wearing of protective clothing, sunglasses, and sunscreens by affected individuals. DNA deletions and point mutations are less common than DNA cross-links after sunlight exposure.

17. The answer is b. *(Scriver, pp 3–45. Murray, pp 333–335. Lewis, pp 171–184.)* DNA synthesis occurs only in the S phase of the cell cycle, a process regulated by numerous proteins called cyclins. A key cyclin (cyclin D) is phosphorylated as the cell commits from gap 1 (G1) quiescent phase to the S phase of DNA synthesis, and a cascade of secondary phosphorylations by cyclin-dependent kinases (CDK) activates cyclins, transcription factors, and the DNA synthesis machinery. The Rb protein, discovered as the product of the gene causing hereditary retinoblastoma, undergoes phosphorylation early in S phase and releases its inhibition (binding) of E2F transcription factor, promoting gene activation and DNA synthesis. Rb, like the genes for neurofibromatosis (neurofibromin) or breast cancer (BRCA1), acts as a tumor supressor gene requiring mutation of both Rb alleles to inactivate Rb protein and foster continuous E2F action and cell proliferation. Individuals with germ-line Rb mutations are more likely to incur a "second hit" in several retinal cells and present with retinoblastomas in both eyes. Individuals without germline Rb mutations are much less likely to incur two Rb mutations in the same retinal cell, having unilateral tumors if they occur at all. The bcl protein, discovered by its excess in B-cell lymphomas, was then identified as a stimulator of cell division called cyclin D1. Bcl is thus an oncogene, requiring one abnormal allele or "one hit" to be genetically activated in a cell and stimulate proliferation (oncogenesis). Several proteins of cancer-causing viruses (v-onc) have been adapted from putative cellular oncogenes (c-onc), while others inactivate the Rb protein and promote cell proliferation. Despite characterization of many tumor suppressor and oncogene proteins, the tissue specificity and variable ages of onset of different tumors speak for multifactorial, polygenic pathways to cancer.

18. The answer is d. *(Murray, pp 335–340. Scriver, pp 3–45. Lewis, pp 171–184.)* Defective DNA repair and accumulation of abnormal DNA structures inhibits cell division and may program the cell for death (apoptosis). A group of DNA repair enzymes act continuously to correct errors in DNA copying (mismatch repair), spontaneous loss of purines (base excision-repair), or cross-links and base modifications such as thymine-thymine dimers (Nucleotide-excision repair). Xeroderma pigmentosum is an autosomal recessive disorder with enhanced DNA damage from ultraviolet irradiation, manifest by photosensitivity (reddening of skin and eyes from sunlight), pigmentation, blistering and scarring, and a 1000-fold greater risk for skin cancer. The thymine-thymine dimers produced by sunlight are normally removed by excision-repair. A UV-specific exinuclease nicks the dimer on its 5′ side, DNA polymerase I replicates the damaged sequence, the damaged piece is hydrolyzed by the 5′ to 3′ exonuclease activity of DNA polymerase I, and DNA ligase joins the patched and original DNA. Cultured skin cells (fibroblasts) from patients with XP are deficient in nucleotide excision-repair, but it was surprising to find that fusion with cells from a different XP patients could restore excision-repair activity, that is, complemented the repair deficiency. Systematic testing of various XP fibroblast lines demonstrated there were seven groups of XP cells—fusion of cells within a group would not correct mutual repair deficiencies but fusion of those in different groups would restore (complement) repair deficiency. These results indicate that XP is actually an end-point phenotype caused by seven different genes, identified as a DNA recognition protein (XP group A), exinuclease (XP group C), or helicase/transcription factor components (XP groups B, D-G).

19. The answer is d. *(Murray, pp 314–340. Scriver, pp 3–45. Lewis, pp 171–184.)* Like bacterial DNA, eukaryotic DNA is replicated in a semiconservative manner. However, in contrast to most bacterial DNA, which is circular in structure, nuclear chromosomal DNA is a single, uninterrupted molecule that is linear and unbranched. A eukaryotic chromosome contains a strand of DNA at least 100 times as large as the DNA molecules found in prokaryotes. The animal DNA is thousands of times as long as its nuclear diameter, and is condensed with proteins to form chromatin. Chromatin consists of fundamental 146 bp DNA-histone octamer units called nucleosomes, with many nucleosomes per gene. The chromatin histones can be modified covalently through attachment of acetyl, methyl, phosphate, or ubiquitin groups and the DNA bases can be variously opened to nucleoplasm by nonhistone proteins and subjected to methylation or other modifications. Chromatin modifications and protein interactions produce tremendous variation in DNA structure, visualized by karyotyping (centromeres, satellites, etc.) and in DNA expression, visualized by "puffs" of transcription in the fruit fly or by imprinted (DNA methylation) regions in mammals. The chromatin interactions comprise a "second code" for gene regulation that, with vastly more genes and gene families, far transcends the simple operon models of bacteria. The significance of many animal DNA variations, like the premature centromere condensation in Roberts syndrome, is not yet understood.

20. The answer is a. *(Murray, pp 335–340. Scriver, pp 3–45. Lewis, pp 171–184.)* Hereditary nonpolyposis colon cancer (114500) is caused by defects in *hMLH1* or *hMSH2* genes that cause faulty mismatch repair. Mismatch repair corrects errors in newly synthesized DNA that arise from abnormal base-pairing or slippage at the replication fork that introduces point mutations or small nucleotide repeats (microsatellites). The mismatch repair apparatus, first characterized as Mut S, Mut C, and Mut H proteins in *E. coli*, match newly synthesized DNA strands with their templates relative to adenine-methylated GATC sequence sites. New strands have unmethylated GATC sites, and mismatched sequences are excised by exonuclease and restored correctly by polymerase and ligase. Human *hMLH* genes are homologous to *E. coli* Mut genes, but the way in which accumulated point mutations and microsatellites in colon cell DNA lead to cancer is not yet clear. It is known that accumulation of abnormal DNA inhibits the cell cycle, so perhaps the continuous demand for high-turnover intestinal cells drives some colon cells to aberrant and unregulated pathways of proliferation.

21. The answer is d. *(Murray, pp 326–333. Lewis, pp 178–184. Scriver, pp 3–45.)* DNA polymerase moves along the DNA in one direction and synthesizes new DNA from both antiparallel strands at one replication fork. Since DNA is always synthesized 5′ to 3′, one of the strands (the leading strand) is synthesized continuously, whereas the other (the lagging strand) is synthesized in short stretches called Okazaki fragments. The reinitiation of DNA synthesis for Okazaki fragments requires an RNA primer because DNA polymerase I, the major enzyme for DNA replication, can only add bases to an existing strand in the presence of template strand. A unique enzyme called primase synthesizes the short RNA molecules required to prime synthesis of Okazaki fragments and a ligase joins these fragments to elongate the lagging strand. Initiation of DNA replication occurs at specific sites with easily unwound AT-rich sequences characterized as autonomously replicating sequences (ARS) or origin recognition complexes (ORC) in *E. coli.* Formation and procession of the replication fork requires helicases for DNA unwinding, SSBs (single-strand binding proteins) to prevent premature reannealing, and DNA polymerase I for chain elongation.

22. The answer is e. *(Murray, pp 326–333. Scriver, pp 3–45. Lewis, pp 171–184.)* In the leading strand, DNA is synthesized continuously in the 5′ to 3′ direction by DNA polymerase. In contrast, in the lagging strand, which is in the 3′ to 5′ direction, DNA polymerase III synthesizes small (approximately 1000 nucleotides) Okazaki fragments. For the synthesis of these small fragments, all the same roles and steps apply except that additional enzymes are needed to fill the gap between the fragments and join the fragments. Consequently, DNA ligase is repeatedly needed to join the ends of the DNA fragments along the growing lagging strand. DNA ligase catalyzes the formation of a phosphodiester bond between the 3′ hydroxyl group at the end of one DNA chain and the 5′ DNA phosphate group at the end of the other. DNA ligase is only functional when double-helical DNA molecules are the substrate. It does not work on single-stranded DNA. DNA ligase affects the joining of strands of DNA not only during the normal synthesis of DNA, but during the splicing of DNA chains in genetic recombination as well as the repair of damaged DNA.

23. The answer is a. *(Murray, pp 322–323. Scriver, pp 2415–2512. Lewis, pp 178–180.)* Mitochondrial DNA is similar to bacterial DNA in structure as a circular, double-stranded molecule of 16,569 bp. Present in 500–1000 copies per cell, it comprises 1% of cellular DNA and encodes 13 peptides of the respiratory chain compared to 54 encoded by nuclear DNA. Mitochondrial DNA encodes unique ribosomal and transfer RNAs, has some unique coding properties (UGA stop codon read as tryptophan), and exhibits a 5- to 10-fold higher mutation rate than nuclear DNA. This fragility contributes to a dozen mitochondrial DNA diseases that range from optic atrophy to Kearns-Sayre syndrome (530000), not to be confused with similar disorders caused by mutation of nuclear-encoded peptides that are imported into mitochondria. Sperm heads contain few mitochondrial, so mitochondrial DNA diseases often exhibit maternal inheritance due to contribution of zygote mitochondria from oocyte cytoplasm. Mitochondrial DNA mutations may arise during oogenesis, causing appearance of new disease, and may affect only a portion of the cell's mitochondria, producing mutant-normal mitochondrial mixtures (heteroplasmy). Proportions of mutant mitochondia can differ with age and among tissues, accounting for worsening symptoms, variable ages of onset, and variable symptoms in disorders such as Kearns-Sayre syndrome.

24. The answer is a. *(Murray, pp 396–414. Scriver, pp 3–45.)* Restriction fragment length polymorphisms (RFLPs) arising from variable numbers of tandem repeats (VNTRs) are the basis of the DNA fingerprinting technique. The process is (1) isolation of DNA from parent/child or forensic specimens using blood, skin, or semen; (2) PCR amplification and radioactive labeling of DNA from variable regions in each sample; (3) separation of the variable DNA fragments by gel electrophoresis; and (4) comparison of the DNA fragment patterns among samples. Since numbers of arrays of repeats of 2, 3, or 4 bp (microsatellites) may vary from 5 to 100 at a particular chromosome locus, particular alleles may occur in less than 1% of the population. As a result, analysis of three loci, each with two alleles, can produce odds as high as $(100)^6$ that the pattern matches a putative father or suspect as compared to a random person from the general population. Reverse transcription based on RNA-directed DNA synthesis is not utilized in DNA fingerprinting, and the size distribution of undigested DNA reflects its integrity during isolation rather than individual identity. HLA typing uses antibodies to define the constellation of alleles from various loci in the HLA region on chromosome 6. The tendency for certain HLA alleles to occur together (associate) on the same chromosome as haplotypes greatly reduces their odds of identity when compared to DNA fingerprinting.

25. The answer is e. *(Murray, pp 303–313. Scriver, pp 3–45. Lewis, pp 171–184.)* The AIDS treatment drug azidothymidine (AZT) exerts its effect by inhibiting viral reverse transcriptase. Thus, it prevents replication of the human immunodeficiency virus. Reverse transcriptase is an RNA-directed DNA polymerase. The RNA of retroviruses utilizes reverse transcriptase to synthesize DNA provirus, which in turn synthesizes new viral RNA. AZT inhibits DNA provirus production, but does not directly inhibit synthesis of new viral RNA.

26. The answer is d. *(Murray, pp 326–333. Lewis, pp 178–184. Scriver, pp 3–45.)* The DNA of eucaryotes is associated with histone and nonhistone proteins and small RNAs. The DNA and its associated components are subject to chemical modifications that can alter gene expression, a process known as epigenesis or the "second code" to distinguish it from the primary code by which DNA codons are converted to protein amino acids. DNA methylation is an important mode of epigenesis that usually operates to shut genes down (inactivation). Diseases that involve methylation changes in a specific gene, like those of the MECP gene in Rett syndrome, are amenable to DNA diagnosis by demonstrating altered DNA methylation patterns. Primers are used to amplify characterized MECP gene fragments using the polymerase chain reaction, and their size distribution after methylation-sensitive endonuclease cleavage is determined by gel electrophoresis. Increased DNA methylation will modify cytosines within the gene sequence that are not normally methylated, causing insensitivity to endonuclease cleavage and larger fragment sizes on the appropriate size-separating gel.

27. The answer is b. *(Murray, pp 396–414. Scriver, pp 3–45. Lewis, pp 377–396.)* Plasmids are duplex DNA circles that may carry genes determining antibiotic resistance (R factors), sex (F factors), or toxin production (colicinogenic factors) in their bacterial hosts. Restriction of plasmid vector DNA and mammalian DNA with the same endonuclease produces cohesive ends that may be joined together with DNA ligase. The ligated molecules, which consist of one or more mammalian DNA segments inserted between plasmid DNA ends, are recombinant DNA molecules that can be replicated in the host bacteria. Plasmids can be used to clone particular human gene segments by determining a restriction endonuclease that liberates the desired human gene fragment, mixing the restricted plasmid and human DNA, screening the recombinant molecules for the gene fragment of interest by plating and hybridization, selecting the recombinant giving positive hybridization, and culturing it to yield recombinant plasmid DNA with the desired gene segment. The recombinant plasmid provides a pure and abundant sample of the human gene segment that is separated from all other DNA segments in the human genome. Plasmid vectors are useful for gene segments under about 10 kilobases (kb) in size, but bacteriophage and recently yeast artifical chromosomes (YACs) can incorporate DNA segments up to 1000 kb or 1 megabase (Mb) in size. These larger vectors allow genomes like those of humans or mice (3000 Mb in size) to be entirely represented in a collection (library) of about 3000 recombinant molecules.

28. The answer is d. *(Murray, pp 306–307.)* RNA and DNA are composed of nucleoside units where a purine or pyrimidine base is linked to a pentose sugar. The 1′ carbon of the pentose is linked to the nitrogen of the base. In DNA, 2′-deoxyribose sugars are used; in RNA, ribose sugars are used that contain 2′ and 3′-hydroxyls, allowing alkaline release of one proton and initiation of phosphate cleavage by oxide. The nitrogenous bases are adenine, thymine, guanine, and cytosine in DNA, with thymine replaced by uridine in RNA. Nucleotide polymers are chains of nucleotides with single phosphate groups, joined by bonds between the 3′-hydroxyl of the preceding pentose and the 5′-phosphate of the next pentose. Polymerization requires high-energy nucleotide triphosphate precursors that liberate pyrophosphate (broken down to phosphate) during joining. The polymerization reaction is given specificity by complementary RNA or DNA templates and rapidity by enzyme catalysts called polymerases.

29. The answer is d. *(Murray, pp 314–340. Scriver, pp 3–45. Lewis, pp 171–184.)* In all of the forms of DNA repair in normal cells, a common sequence of events occurs:

1. The single or multiple base abnormality is surveyed and detected by a specific protein or proteins.
2. The DNA is nicked on one side of the damaged DNA.

3. A specific enzyme excises the damaged portion (steps 2 and 3 can be combined if an exinuclease cuts on both sides of the damaged DNA).
4. The damaged portion of the strand is replaced by resynthesis catalyzed by DNA polymerase I.
5. A ligase seals the final gap.

With some variability, these general principles apply in nucleotide excision repair (segments of about 30 nucleotides), base excision repair of single bases, and mismatch repair of copying errors (1–5 bases).

30. The answer is e. *(Murray, pp 314–316. Lewis, pp 178–184; Scriver, pp 3–45.)* DNA does not exist naked in eucaryotic cells but as a complex with histones and nonhistone proteins. The four core histones are present as the dimers H2A-H2B and H3-H4, and these dimers in turn pair to produce a histone octamer. The histone octamer associates with DNA and histone H1 to form nucleosomes—arrayed like beads on a string to form a chromatin fibril of 30 nm width. Each histone octamer complexes with 146 base pairs of coiled (superhelical) DNA, and each of the core histones or histone H1 is susceptible to chemical modification by acetylation, methylation, phosphorylation, ribosylation, or ubiquination. Phosphorylation of histone H1 causes chromatin condensation, and the 10 nm fibril can condense to form successive 30 nm fibrils, chromosome loops or domains, and finally the highly condensed metaphase chromosomes that are analyzed in human cytogenetics. Chromatin upstream of active genes is typically less condensed, forming hypersensitive sites to nuclease. The modification of histones, along with methylation of DNA and changes in chromosome condensation, comprises a "second code" for regulation of gene expression. These changes are often distinguised as "epigenetic" in contrast to genetic changes in the primary code of DNA to RNA to protein.

31. The answer is e. *(Murray, pp 314–340. Scriver, pp 3–45. Lewis, pp 171–184.)* The major effects of radiation are to damage cellular DNA by opening purine rings and rupturing phosphodiester bonds. Chemical agents such as formaldehyde can cross-link DNA, and inhibitors of DNA methylation, such as methotrexate (an inhibitor of folic acid), were the first anticancer drugs. Experimental gene therapies for cancer include the inhibition of oncogene expression and the enhancement of tumor suppressor gene activity. These therapies target particular DNA-RNA transcription complexes or signal transduction cascades that are active in cancer cells.

32. The answer is a. *(Murray, pp 314–340. Scriver, pp 3–45. Lewis, pp 171–184.)* A special DNA polymerase called telomerase is responsible for replication of the telomeric DNA. Telomerase contains an RNA molecule that guides the synthesis of complementary DNA. Telomerase is therefore an RNA-dependent DNA polymerase in a category with reverse transcriptase. Telomerase does not require an RNA primer, initiating synthesis of the leading strands at 3′ ends within the telomeric DNA. Synthesis of the lagging strands uses primase, DNA polymerase III, and DNA polymerase I, as with the replication of other chromosomal regions.

33. The answer is c. *(Murray, pp 318–319. Lewis, pp 178–184. Scriver, pp 3–45.)* Special DNA structures at the end of chromosomes, called telomeres, consist of repetitive DNAs including a particular 6-base pair repeat (5′-TTAGGG-3′ at each chromosome terminus. A special DNA polymerase called telomerase replicates these terminal repeats using a complementary RNA primer that makes it analogous to the viral enzyme reverse transcriptase. The number of 6-base pair repeats is normally in the thousands, but has been noted to shorten in tumor tissues and in normal tissues as a function of aging. The adjacent repetitive DNAs in telomeres, like those comprising centromeres, can be generally distributed or unique to the particular chromosome. Multicolor, fluorescent DNA probes to these unique telomeric DNAs allow labelling of the various chromosome ends and can detect rearrangements by Flourescent *In Situ* Hybridization (FISH) showing a shift of signal from telomere to chromosome interior. Such rearrangements may not change the length or banding pattern of the chromosome arm and will not be obvious on routine karyotypes. Telomere array analysis is thus useful on children with mental disability and malformations who are suspected to have a chromosome aberration but prove to have a normal routine karyotype.

34. The answer is d. *(Murray, pp 322–325. Lewis, pp 178–184. Scriver, pp 3–45.)* Gene recombination during chromosome synapsis at the first and second meiotic divisions produces unique genetic constitutions in each gamete and derived conception. In the first meiotic division, the chromosomes are tetraploid and recombination occurs mostly between sister chromatids of the same chromosome. In the second meiotic division, recombination may occur between chromosome homologues. Recombination is normally "equal," meaning that the crossover of DNA strands is at the same base pair on each chromosome arm and produces no excess or deficient DNA. Among chromosome regions with repetitive DNAs, including gene families like the globins that are similar in sequence, it is common to have "unequal" crossovers with mismatched pairing. The child with anemia proved to have hemoglobin Lepore (141900), produced by unequal recombination between a δ-globin gene on one chromatid and a β-globin gene on the other. The child therefore had normal fetal hemoglobin produced from α- and γ-globin genes, but produced an abnormal hemoglobin due to δβ-globin gene fusion on one chromosome. The reciprocal anti-Lepore recombination would be lost at meiosis II, and the child would have a normal β-globin locus on the chromosome 11 received from the other parent. This produces a mild to moderate anemia once the switch occurs from fetal to adult hemoglobin at 3–6 months.

Gene Expression and Regulation

Questions

DIRECTIONS: Each item below contains a question or incomplete statement followed by suggested responses. Select the **one best** response to each question.

35. Which of the following statements about the "genetic code" is most accurate?

a. There are 64 codons, all of which code for amino acids
b. The code is degenerate
c. Information is stored as sets of dinucleotide repeats called codons
d. Information is stored as sets of trinucleotide repeats called codons
e. The sequence of codons that make up a gene exhibits an exact linear correspondence to the sequence of amino acids in the translated protein

36. Sickle cell anemia (141900) is caused by a point mutation in the hemoglobin gene, resulting in the substitution of a single amino acid in the β-globin peptides of hemoglobin. This mutation is best detected by which of the following?

a. Isolation of DNA from red blood cells followed by polymerase chain reaction (PCR) amplification and restriction enzyme digestion
b. Isolation of DNA from blood leukocytes followed by Southern blot analysis to detect globin gene exon sizes
c. Isolation of DNA from blood leukocytes followed by DNA sequencing of globin gene introns
d. Isolation of DNA from blood leukocytes followed by polymerase chain reaction (PCR) amplification and allele-specific oligonucleotide (ASO) hybridization
e. Western blot analysis of red blood cell extracts

37. Cystic fibrosis (219700) is caused by various types of mutations, most commonly (70% of mutant alleles in Caucasians) a 3 bp deletion that removes a codon for phenylalanine (ΔF508). The DNA sequence shown below is the sense strand from a coding region known to be a mutational "hot spot" for a gene. It encodes amino acids 21–25. Given the genetic and amino acid codes CCC = proline (P), GCC = alanine (A), TTC = phenylalanine (F), and TAG = stop codon, which of the following sequences is a frameshift mutation that causes termination of the encoded protein 5′-CCC-CCT-AGG-TTC-AGG-3′?

a. -CCA-CCT-AGG-TTC-AGG-
b. -GCC-CCT-AGG-TTC-AGG-
c. -CCA-CCC-TAG-GTT-CAG-
d. -CCC-CTA-GGT-TCA-GG-
e. -CCC-CCT-AGG-AGG-

38. A child returns from a mushroom hunt in Northern Michigan begins vomiting and by the next morning is hospitalized with jaundice, hyperammonemia, and delirium. A toxicologist is called, who suggests poisoning from Amanita phylloides, a mushroom containing the toxin α-amanitin that inhibits RNA polymerase II. She suggests that the child's liver failure is most likely due to which of the following?

a. Inhibition of tRNA and protein synthesis
b. Inhibition of mRNA synthesis
c. Inhibition of small RNA synthesis
d. Inhibition of ribosomal RNA synthesis
e. Inhibition of mitochondrial RNA synthesis

39. Numerous genetic diseases, including the thalassemias (141900), are caused by abnormalities in processing of messenger RNA. The hypothetical "stimulin" gene contains 2 exons that encode a protein of 100 amino acids. They are separated by an intron of 120 bp beginning after the codon for amino acid 10. Stimulin messenger RNA (mRNA) has 5′ and 3′ untranslated regions of 70 and 30 nucleotides, respectively. A complementary DNA (cDNA) made from mature stimulin RNA would have which of the following sizes?

a. 520 bp
b. 400 bp
c. 300 bp
d. 120 bp
e. 100 bp

40. A "factor" is studied that stimulates a gene controlling differentiation of human immune stem cells into B-cells that fight bacterial infection. Some diseases like Bruton agammaglobulinema (300300) involve an inability to produce B-cells. The factor can hybridize to DNA, is hydrolyzed by alkali treatment, and migrates as a 20–30 bp species on electrophoresis. The differentiation gene is not stimulated by the factor if a 10 bp promoter element near the initiation site for transcription is removed. Which of the following factors is most likely?

a. A transfer RNA that recognizes a codon within the promoter element
b. An mRNA that is translated to produce a stimulatory transcription factor
c. A small RNA that binds the promoter and enhances transcription
d. A transposon that recognizes the promoter element and inserts to activate the gene
e. An RNA catalyst that is essential for mRNA splicing

Questions 41, 43–47, 51, and 53. Refer to the figure below for these questions.

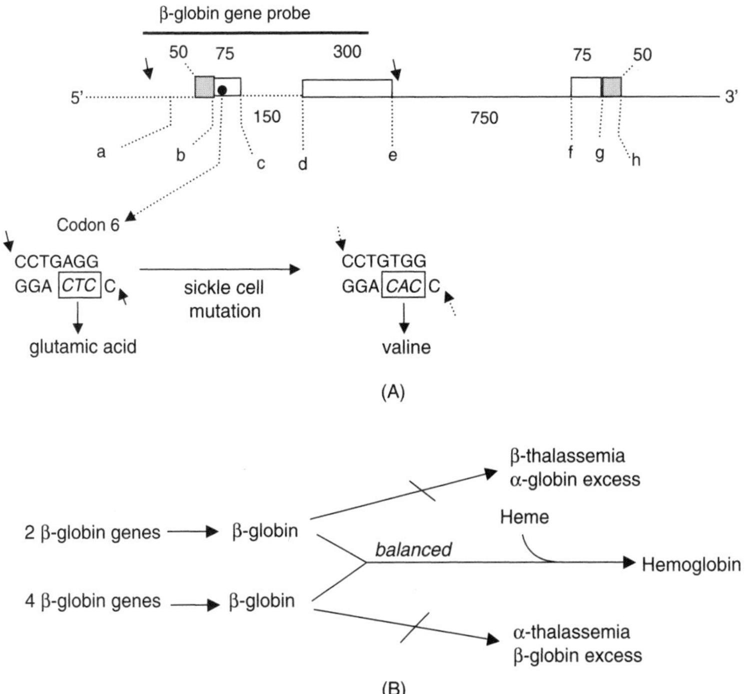

(A)

(B)

41. The β-globin gene is diagrammed in the figure A below, consisting of untranslated RNA regions, three exons, and two introns. DNA diagnosis for sickle cell anemia was facilitated by finding that a cleavage site for restriction endonuclease (MstII) included the sixth codon of β-globin gene exon 1 that is mutated to cause a glutamic to valine amino acid change (see Fig. A on the previous page). Recall that the β-globin gene is on chromosome 16, and that both copies are mutated (homozygous) in individuals with sickle cell anemia (603903). Analysis of β-globin gene structure and expression in an individual with sickle cell anemia would yield which of the following results? (Southern blotting is performed using MstII endonuclease cleavage and hybridization with the β-globin gene probe shown in the figure.)

a. MstII DNA cleavage segment of 515 and 165 bp by Southern blot, nucleic acid segment of ~700 bp by Northern blot, abnormal protein by hemoglobin electrophoresis
b. MstII DNA cleavage segments of 515 and 165 bp by Southern blot, no nucleic acid segment detected by Northern blot, abnormal protein by hemoglobin electrophoresis
c. MstII DNA cleavage segments of 515 and 165 bp by Southern blot, nucleic acid segment of ~1400 bp by Northern blot, abnormal protein by hemoglobin electrophoresis
d. MstII DNA cleavage segment of 680 bp by Southern blot, nucleic acid segment of ~700 bp by Northern blot, abnormal protein by hemoglobin electrophoresis
e. MstII DNA cleavage segments of 515 and 165 bp by Southern blot, nucleic acid segment of ~700 bp by Northern blot, abnormal protein by hemoglobin electrophoresis

42. The removal of introns and subsequent self-splicing of adjacent exons occurs in some portions of primary ribosomal RNA transcripts. The splicing of introns in messenger RNA precursors is which of the following?

a. RNA catalyzed in the absence of protein
b. Self-splicing
c. Carried out by spliceosomes
d. Controlled by RNA polymerase
e. Regulated by RNA helicase

43. During study of hemoglobinopathies affecting the β-globin gene, a mutation was detected just upstream (5′ to) the transcription initiation site (point a in the above figure). In homozygous individuals, this mutation decreased the amount of β-globin mRNA and subsequent β-globin protein and hemoglobin, producing anemia. Which of the following is most likely true regarding this mutation?

a. It affects a promoter sequence that codes for RNA polymerase
b. It affects a promoter sequence and the rate at which RNA polymerase II initiates transcription
c. it affects the termination site of an upstream gene
d. It alters a sequence encoding a subunit of RNA polymerase II (the sigma factor).
e. It affects a promoter sequence and the rate at which RNA polymerase II terminates transcription

44. A mountain climber in excellent physical condition suffers shortness of breath and low oxygen (hypoxia) at high altitude in Nepal. After transport to base camp and oxygen treatment, a family history reveals that his mother has sickle cell anemia. With reference to Fig. A above, laboratory studies of his β-globin gene structure and expression would be expected to show which of the following results? (Note that the same MstII restriction and β-globin probe in the above figure is used for Southern blotting).

a. MstII DNA cleavage segment of 515 and 165 bp by Southern blot, RNA segment of ~700 bp by Northern blot, normal and abnormal proteins by hemoglobin electrophoresis
b. MstII DNA cleavage segments of 680, 515, and 165 bp by Southern blot, RNA segment of ~700 bp by Northern blot, normal and abnormal proteins by hemoglobin electrophoresis
c. MstII DNA cleavage segments of 515 and 165 bp by Southern blot, RNA segment of ~1400 bp by Northern blot, single abnormal protein by hemoglobin electrophoresis
d. MstII DNA cleavage segment of 680 bp by Southern blot, RNA segment of ~700 bp by Northern blot, single normal protein band by hemoglobin electrophoresis
e. MstII DNA cleavage segments of 680, 515, and 165 bp by Southern blot, RNA segment of ~700 bp by Northern blot, single abnormal protein by hemoglobin electrophoresis

45. The Figure B on page 95 diagrams the consequences of unbalanced synthesis of α-globin and β-globin, producing deficient β-globin and α-globin excess in β-thalassemia and the reverse in α-thalassemia. An individual with severe anemia was suspected of having sickle cell anemia, but instead was found to have a mutation at the promoter site (point a in Fig. A above) on one β-globin gene and a sickle cell mutation on the other. Which of the following laboratory results would be expected in such an individual, using the same MstII restriction and β-globin probe (Fig. A) for Southern blotting described previously?

a. MstII DNA cleavage segment of 515 and 165 bp by Southern blot, normal amounts of ~700 bp RNA segment by Northern blot, normal and abnormal proteins by hemoglobin electrophoresis
b. MstII DNA cleavage segments of 680, 515, and 165 bp by Southern blot, decreased amounts of ~700 bp RNA segment by Northern blot, normal and abnormal proteins by hemoglobin electrophoresis
c. MstII DNA cleavage segments of 680, 515 and 165 bp by Southern blot, decreased amounts of a ~700 bp RNA segment by Northern blot, mostly abnormal protein by hemoglobin electrophoresis
d. MstII DNA cleavage segment of 680 bp by Southern blot, normal amounts of a ~700 bp RNA segment by Northern blot, mostly normal protein band by hemoglobin electrophoresis
e. MstII DNA cleavage segments of 680, 515, and 165 bp by Southern blot, lower amounts of 700 bp DNA segment by Northern blot, mostly abnormal protein by hemoglobin electrophoresis

46. Study of several patients with characteristics of β-thalassemia revealed a sequence 5′-TATAAAA-3′ at the 5′-end of the β-globin gene (site a in the above figure). This sequence was found at the 5′-boundary of other eukaryotic genes, and is quite similar to a consensus sequence observed in prokaryotes. It is important as which of the following?

a. Only site of binding of RNA polymerase III
b. Promoter for all RNA polymerases
c. Termination site for RNA polymerase II
d. Major binding site of RNA polymerase I
e. First site of binding of a transcription factor for RNA polymerase II

47. A homozygous mutation in the β-globin gene at the junction of exon 1 and intron 1 (site c in Fig. A on page 95) was found in an individual with severe anemia. Which of the following best describes the nature and clinical consequence of this mutation?

a. Altered splice donor site, absent mRNA by Northern blotting, β-globin protein deficiency presenting as α-thalassemia
b. Altered splice acceptor site, altered mRNA size by Northern blotting, β-globin protein deficiency presenting as β-thalassemia
c. Altered splice donor site, altered mRNA size by Northern blotting, β-globin protein deficiency presenting as β-thalassemia
d. Altered promoter site, altered mRNA size by Northern blotting, β-globin protein deficiency presenting as β-thalassemia
e. Altered promoter site, deficient β-globin mRNA by Northern blotting, β-globin protein deficiency presenting as α-thalassemia

48. Which of the following is true regarding the so-called caps of RNA molecules?

a. They allow correct translation of prokaryotic mRNA
b. They are unique to eukaryotic mRNA
c. They allow tRNA to be processed
d. They occur at the 3′ end of tRNA
e. They are composed of poly A

49. During study of human chromosome variations (cytogenetics), amplification of satellite regions on chromosomes 13–15 and 21–22 (acrocentric chromosomes) were noted. These amplified regions were found to be transcriptionally active in the nucleolus, and their associated molecules could be selectively stained with silver to distinguish them from other satellite regions. The molecules associated with these nucleolar organizing regions (NOR) would most likely be which of the following?

a. Messenger RNA used to synthesize histone proteins
b. Small silencing RNA (siRNA)
c. 5S RNA
d. Ribosomal RNA
e. Transfer RNA

50. Which one of the following statements correctly describes the synthesis of mammalian messenger RNA (mRNA)?

a. There is colinearity of the RNA sequence transcribed from a gene and the amino acid sequence of its encoded protein
b. Each mRNA often encodes several different proteins
c. Several different genes may produce identical mRNA molecules
d. The RNA sequence transcribed from a gene is virtually identical to the mRNA that exits from nucleus to cytoplasm
e. Mammalian mRNA undergoes minimal modification during its maturation

51. The α-globin genes are similar in structure to the β-globin gene diagrammed in the figure on page 95, but are present in duplicate copies on each chromosome 16 in humans. Which of the following best describes the consequences of mutations at the promoter sequence of α-globin genes?

a. Promoter mutations will always produce a mild α-thalassemia with minimal consequences because only one of four genes is affected
b. Promoter mutations will produce a mild form of α-thalassemia plus a more severe form when homozygous
c. Promoter mutations will alter the amino acid sequence of α-globin, producing a variant hemoglobin with minimal clinical consequences
d. Promoter mutations will not affect the amount of α-globin mRNA and thus should not cause α-thalassemia
e. Promoter mutations can produce four different varieties of α-thalassemia depending on how many of the four α-globin genes are affected

52. Which of the following binds to specific nucleotide sequences that are upstream of the start site of transcription?

a. Helicase
b. Histone protein
c. Primase
d. Restriction endonuclease
e. RNA polymerase

53. Eucaryotic mRNAs undergo several forms of post-transcriptional processing. Some forms of thalassemia are due to incorrect processing of the α- and β-globin mRNAs, causing deficiency of the corresponding α- or β-globin peptide with imbalance in hemoglobin. Referring to the β-globin gene structure shown in the figure below, which of the following homozygous mutations would most likely present as an altered hemoglobin (hemoglobinopathy) but not as a β-thalassemia?

a. Mutations changing the consensus AGGUAAGU splice donor sequence at exon-intron junctions
b. Missense mutations in exon 2
c. Mutations changing the AAUAA recognition sequence at the terminus (3′-end) of the gene
d. Mutations altering TATA or CAAT boxes
e. Mutations changing the consensus UACUAAC-30bp-CAGG splice acceptor sequence at intronexon junctions

54. During study of a family with early onset of heart attacks, an unusual pattern of expression was found for a gene encoding a serum lipoprotein. This apolipoprotein B (apoB) gene (200100) had identical DNA sequences at both alleles, produced apoB mRNAs of identical sizes and amounts in liver or intestine, and yielded a single apoB peptide of similar abundance in both tissues. Yet the apoB peptide in intestine was much smaller than that in liver, corresponding to translation of only the proximal portion of the apoB gene. Which of the following explanations is most likely?

a. ApoB mRNA undergoes alternative splicing in intestine
b. An exon of the ApoB gene is deleted in intestine
c. Intestinal apoB mRNA undergoes a codon alteration that causes termination of translation and a smaller peptide
d. Polyadenylation of apoB mRNA is deficient in intestine
e. Transcription of apoB mRNA occurs from a different plromoter in intestine

55. Which of the following is the best method to demonstrate yield of different apolipoprotein B (apoB) protein sizes through RNA editing?

a. Western blot using apoB DNA as probe
b. Northern blot using antibody to apoB protein as probe
c. Southern blot using the proximal apoB gene segment as probe
d. Western blot using apoB cDNA as probe
e. Western blot using antibody to the amino-terminal portion of apoB protein

56. Which of the following is the correct order of the following steps in protein synthesis?

1. A peptide bond is formed
2. The small ribosomal subunit is loaded with initiation factors, messenger RNA, and initiation aminoacyl-t RNA
3. The intact ribosome slides forward three bases to read a new codon
4. The primed small ribosomal subunit binds with the large ribosomal subunit
5. Elongation factors deliver aminoacyl-tRNA to bind to the A site

a. 1, 2, 5, 4, 3
b. 2, 3, 4, 5, 1
c. 4, 5, 1, 2, 3
d. 3, 2, 4, 5, 1
e. 2, 4, 5, 1, 3

57. Several disorders, like one form of α1-antitrypsin deficiency, can result from mistargeting of proteins into the wrong cellular compartments. New proteins destined for secretion are synthesized in which of the following?

a. Free polysomes
b. Golgi apparatus
c. Nucleus
d. Rough endoplasmic reticulum
e. Smooth endoplasmic reticulum

58. A form of β-thalassemia (141900) was found to have a promoter mutation on one copy of the β-globin gene and a mutation in the middle of exon 2 on the other copy. What is the most likely type of mutation in exon 2 that would lead to β-thalassemia (i.e., decreased production of β-globin peptide from both β-globin gene copies)?

a. Deletion of 3 bp
b. Insertion of 1 bp
c. Insertion of 3 bp
d. Missense mutation
e. Silent mutation

59. A disorder called primary oxalosis or hyperoxaluria (259900) is caused by abnormal location of enzyme in the endoplasmic reticulum, causing increased production of oxalic acid with consequent accumulation in kidney (urinary stones) and joints (arthritis). A potential cure for the disorder was pioneered by altering the mutant oxalate enzyme so its normal cytosolic location was restored. This alteration most likely consisted of which of the following?

a. Cleaving its carboxy-terminal segment
b. Changing its RNA splicing to include an extra exon
c. Proteolytic cleavage within the cytosol
d. Changing its protein processing to produce a smaller peptide
e. Ablating its amino-terminal signal recognition sequence

60. How many high-energy phosphate-bond equivalents are utilized in the process of activation of amino acids for protein synthesis?

a. Zero
b. One
c. Two
d. Three
e. Four

61. The hydrolytic step leading to the release of a polypeptide chain from a ribosome is catalyzed by which of the following?

a. Dissociation of ribosomes
b. Peptidyl transferase
c. Release factors
d. Stop codons
e. UAA

62. The sequence of the template DNA strand is 5′-GATATCCATTAGT-GAC-3′. What is the sequence of the RNA produced?

a. 5′-CAGUGAUUACCUAUAG-3′
b. 5′-CTATAGGTAATCACTG-3′
c. 5′-CUAUAGGUAAUCACUG-3′
d. 5′-GTCACTAATGGATATC-3′
e. 5′-GUCACUAAUGGAUAUC-3′

63. Which of the following statements about ribosomes is true?

a. They are composed of RNA, DNA, and protein
b. They are composed of three subunits of unequal size
c. They are bound together so tightly they cannot dissociate under physiologic conditions
d. They are found both free in the cytoplasm and bound to membranes
e. They are an integral part of transcription

64. Guanosine triphosphate (GTP) is required by which of the following steps in protein synthesis?

a. Aminoacyl-tRNA synthetase activation of amino acids
b. Attachment of ribosomes to endoplasmic reticulum
c. Translocation of tRNA-nascent protein complex from A to P sites
d. Attachment of mRNA to ribosomes
e. Attachment of signal recognition protein to ribosomes

65. Erythromycin is the antibiotic of choice when treating respiratory tract infections in Legionnaires' disease, whooping cough, and mycoplasma-based pneumonia because of its ability to inhibit protein synthesis in certain bacteria by doing which of the following?

a. Inhibiting translocation by binding to 50S ribosomal subunits
b. Acting as an analogue of mRNA
c. Causing premature chain termination
d. Inhibiting initiation
e. Mimicking mRNA binding

66. An immigrant family from rural Mexico brings their 3-month-old child to the emergency room because of whistling inspiration (stridor) and high fever. The child's physician is perplexed because the throat examination shows a gray membrane almost occluding the larynx. A senior physician recognizes diphtheria, now rare in immunized populations. The child is intubated, antitoxin is administered, and antibiotic therapy is initiated. Diphtheria toxin is often lethal in unimmunized persons because it does which of the following?

a. Inhibits initiation of protein synthesis by preventing the binding of GTP to the 40S ribosomal subunit
b. Binds to the signal recognition particle receptor on the cytoplasmic face of the endoplasmic reticulum receptor
c. Shuts off signal peptidase
d. Blocks elongation of proteins by inactivating elongation factor 2 (EF-2, or translocase)
e. Causes deletions of amino acid by speeding up the movement of peptidyl-tRNA from the A site to the P site

67. Aminoacyl-tRNA synthetases must be capable of recognizing which of the following?

a. A specific tRNA and a specific amino acid
b. A specific rRNA and a specific amino acid
c. A specific tRNA and the 40S ribosomal subunit
d. A specific amino acid and the 40S ribosomal subunit
e. A specific amino acid and the 60S ribosomal subunit

68. Ribosomes similar to those of bacteria are found in which of the following?

a. Cardiac muscle cytoplasm
b. Liver endoplasmic reticulum
c. Neuronal cytoplasm
d. Pancreatic mitochrondria
e. Plant nuclei

69. Insulin is ineffective in diabetes mellitus (222100), leading to high blood glucose levels (hyperglycemia) with gradual effects on blood vessels in eye, kidney, and skin. Pregnant women with diabetes mellitus present high glucose loads to their fetus; this stimulates production of fetal insulin (hyperinsulinemia) and causes rapid fetal growth with large birth weight. The stimulation of fetal growth by insulin may be correlated with its effect on gene expression, which is which of the following?

a. Stimulation of mRNA production by enhancing 5′-capping
b. Acceleration of protein synthesis by phosphorylating initiation inhibitors
c. Acceleration of protein synthesis by phosphorylating the 40S ribosomal subunit
d. Acceleration of protein synthesis by phosphorylating proteinase K
e. Stimulation of mRNA production by enhancing RNA splicing

70. Which of the following eukaryotic promoter/regulatory elements has the most variable position with respect to the start site of transcription?

a. Downstream promoter element (DPE)
b. Enhancer
c. Initiator sequence
d. Operator
e. TATA box

71. Which of the following is required for certain types of eukaryotic protein synthesis but not for prokaryotic protein synthesis?

a. GTP
b. Messenger RNA
c. Ribosomal RNA
d. Peptidyl transferase
e. Signal recognition particle

72. An older man with severe emphysema is found to have decreased amounts and abnormal mobility of α_1 antitrypsin (AAT) protein in his serum when analyzed by serum protein electrophoresis (α_1 antitrypsin deficiency—107400). Liver biopsy discloses mild scarring (cirrhosis) and demonstrates microscopic inclusions due to an engorged endoplasmic reticulum (ER). Which of the following is the most likely explanation for these findings?

a. Defective transport from hepatic ER to the plasma
b. A mutation affecting the N-terminal methionine and blocking initiation of protein synthesis
c. A mutation affecting the signal sequence
d. Defective structure of the signal recognition particles
e. Defective energy metabolism causing deficiency of GTP

73. A patient suffers from adenosine deaminase (ADA) deficiency (102700), an autosomal recessive immune deficiency in which bone marrow lymphoblasts cannot replicate to generate immunocompetent lymphocytes. This deficiency leads to defective B- and T-cells, with severe combined immune deficiency (SCID) and susceptibility to viral, fungal, and bacterial infections. Which of the following treatment options would permanently cure the patient?

a. Germ-line gene therapy to replace one ADA gene copy
b. Germ-line gene therapy to replace both ADA gene copies
c. Somatic cell gene therapy to replace one ADA gene copy in circulating lymphocytes
d. Somatic cell gene therapy to replace both ADA gene copies in circulating lymphocytes
e. Somatic cell gene therapy to replace one ADA gene copy in bone marrow lymphoblasts

74. A major obstacle to gene therapy involves the difficulty of homologous gene replacement. Which of the following strategies addresses this issue?

a. A recombinant vector contains complementary DNA sequences that will facilitate site-specific recombination
b. A recombinant vector expresses antisense nucleotides that will hybridize with the targeted mRNA
c. A recombinant vector replaces inessential viral genes with a functional human gene
d. A recombinant vector transfects patient cells, which are returned to the patient
e. A recombinant vector contains DNA sequences that target its expressed protein to lysosomes

75. A family in which several individuals have arthritis and detached retina is diagnosed with Stickler syndrome (108300), a collagen disease that results in short stature and retinal detachments. The locus for Stickler syndrome has been mapped near that for type II collagen on chromosome 12, and mutations in the COL2A1 gene have been described in Stickler syndrome. The family became interested in molecular diagnosis to distinguish normal from mildly affected individuals. Which of the following results would be expected in an individual with a promoter mutation at one COL2A1 gene locus?

a. Western blotting detects no type II collagen chains
b. Southern blotting using intronic restriction sites yields normal restriction fragment sizes
c. Reverse transcriptase-polymerase chain reaction (RT-PCR) detects one-half normal amounts of COL2A1 mRNA in affected individuals
d. Fluorescent in situ hybridization (FISH) analysis using a COL2A1 probe detects signals on only one chromosome 12
e. DNA sequencing reveals a single nucleotide difference between homologous COL2A1 exons

76. Gyrate atrophy (258870) is a rare autosomal recessive genetic disorder caused by a deficiency of ornithine aminotransferase. Affected individuals experience progressive chorioretinal degeneration with vision and neurologic defects. The gene for ornithine aminotransferase has been cloned, its structure has been determined, and mutations in affected individuals have been extensively studied. Which of the following mutations best fits with test results showing normal Southern blots with probes from all ornithine aminotransferase exons but absent enzymatic activity?

a. Duplication of entire gene
b. Two-kb deletion in coding region of gene
c. Two-kb insertion in coding region of gene
d. Deletion of entire gene
e. Missense mutation

77. A 5-year-old Egyptian boy receives a sulfonamide antibiotic as prophylaxis for recurrent urinary tract infections. Although he was previously healthy and well-nourished, he becomes progressively ill and presents to your office with pallor and irritability. A blood count shows that he is severely anemic with jaundice due to hemolysis of red blood cells. Which of the following is the simplest test for diagnosis?

a. Northern blotting of red blood cell mRNA
b. Enzyme assay of red blood cell hemolysate
c. Western blotting of red blood cell hemolysates
d. Amplification of red blood cell DNA and hybridization with allele-specific oligonucleotides (PCR-ASOs)
e. Southern blot analysis for gene deletions

78. Hurler syndrome (252800) is caused by a deficiency of L-iduronidase, an enzyme normally expressed in most human cell types. It was demonstrated by Neufeld that exogenous L-iduronidase could be taken up by deficient cells via a targeting signal that directed the enzyme to its normal lysosomal location. Which of the following therapeutic strategies is the most realistic and efficient mode of therapy?

a. Germ-line gene therapy
b. Heterologous bone marrow transplant
c. Infection with a disabled adenovirus vector that carries the L-iduronidase gene
d. Injection with L-iduronidase purified from human liver
e. Autologous bone marrow transplant after transfection with a virus carrying the L-iduronidase gene

79. It is now recognized that all cancers involve genetic changes, even though few are hereditary. An early example was the discovery of a Philadelphia chromosome (terminal deletion of chromosome 22) in leucocytes from patients with chronic myeloid leukemia (608232). Later work demonstrated that the deleted material was in fact translocated to the terminus of chromosome 9, being an example of a balanced translocation between 9 and 22. Of the following results, which would be most diagnostic of the 9;22 translocation in chronic myeloid leukemia?

a. All chromosome 22 genes show increased incorporation of labeled acetate into histones of chromatin regions
b. A particular gene near the terminus of chromosome 22 shows altered DNA restriction endonuclease patterns
c. The pattern of small RNA "decoration" along leukemic chromatin is changed
d. Increased transcription of mRNA from genes near the terminus for chromosome 9
e. Decreased transcription of mRNA from all loci on the chromosome 22 long arm

80. Gaucher disease (231000) causes accumulation of complex lipids in white cells, brain, liver, and spleen caused by deficiency of glucocerebrosidase enzyme. A developmentally delayed child presented with hepatosplenomegaly (enlarged spleen), his white blood cells showing the typical foamy appearance of cytoplasm due to lipid accumulation. Although unusual in children, Gaucher disease was considered and blood obtained for DNA testing so as to avoid liver or bone marrow biopsy. A homozygous glucocerebrosidase gene mutation was found that changed the mRNA sequence of codon 93 from UAC to the UAA depicted in the figure below. Which of the following best describes this result?

a. Missense mutation that may interfere with glucocerebrosidase function and could be diagnostic of Gaucher disease
b. Silent mutation that should not interfere with glucocerebrosidase function and is not diagnostic of Gaucher disease
c. Nonsense mutation that produces a truncated, nonfunctional glucocerebrosidase polypeptide and is diagnostic of Gaucher disease
d. Suppressor mutation that interferes with glucocerebrosidase mRNA transcription and is diagnostic of Gaucher disease
e. Frame shift mutation that produces a nonfunctional glucocerebrosidase and is diagnostic of Gaucher disease

88	89	90	91	92	93	94
GUC	GAC	CAG	UAC	GGC	UAA	CCG

81. Over 80 types of X-linked mental retardation (XLMR) have been described by recognition of characteristic transmission through females with severe affliction of males. At least half of the XLMR disorders have no defining medical characteristics such as the coarsened face and bone changes of Hunter syndrome (mucopolysaccharidosis type II—309900) or the kinky hair and severe hypotonia (low muscle tone) of Menkes disease (309400). These "nonspecific" XLMR syndromes without facial or organ system changes must be delineated by mapping to distinct regions of the X chromosome, then delineated by positional cloning of the gene and demonstration of mutations in affected families. The figure below shows a partial sequence of the coding strand of DNA from a hypothetical XLMR type 42, together with mutations detected in males from different candidate families. Which of the following studies would be most compatible with the mutation shown for Gordon?

a. Usual band of usual intensity on Northern and Western blots
b. Absent bands on Northern and Western blots
c. Usual band plus a second band of lower size on Northern, usual band on Western
d. Usual band on Northern, band of unusual size and reduced intensity on Western blot
e. Two unusual bands on Northern blot, usual bands on Western blot

---ACA-ATT-ATT-ATT | TAC-AAA-ATA—

met---phe---ala-

Met	Phe	Ala	Leu	stop
TAC	AAA	ATA	CTG	ATT

James --A*G*A-ATT-ATT-ATT-TAC-AAA-ATA—

Barney --ACA-ATT-ATT-ATT-TAC-AA*T*-ATA—

John -ACA-ATT-ATT-ATT-TAC-AAA-AT*T*—

Gordon -ACA-ATT-ATT-ATT-*G*AC-ATA-ATA—

82. Lipoproteins transport lipids from intestine and liver where they are absorbed and metabolized to peripheral tissues via the bloodstream. They contain core proteins (apo proteins) that bind various types of lipid, thus producing lipoprotein complexes of varying densities—very low density lipoproteins (VLDL), low density lipoproteins (LDL), and high density lipoproteins (HDL) after plasma lipoprotein electophoresis. A disorder called abetalipoproteinemia (200100) was distinguished by its deficiency of the bands for very low density lipoproteins (VLDL) and low density lipoproteins (LDL) after plasma electrophoresis. Affected patients have ataxia (wide gait, incoordination), retinopathy (retinal degeneration with blindness), and myopathy (muscle weakness). VLDL and LDL contain the same apoB core protein, their different densities produced by association with different lipids, and apoB became good candidate for mutation in the disorder. Initial characterization of the apoB gene together with its mRNA and protein products demonstrated identical mRNA sizes in all tissues. Western blotting using antibody specific for the amino-terminus of apoB protein showed a 100-kDa species in liver and a 48-kDa species in intestine, as did antibody specific for the C-terminus of the 48-kDa intestinal protein. Molecular study of a patient with abetalipoproteinemia showed normal mRNA sizes, but 100-kDa peptide species were identified in both liver and intestine using the amino or carboxy-terminus antibody probes. Which of the following processes is most likely deficient in this patient with apobetalipoproteinemia?

a. RNA splicing
b. DNA amplification
c. Transcription initiatiion
d. Transcription factor phosphorylation
e. RNA editing

83. During the analyses described in Question 82, another patient with abetalipoproteinemia was found to have negligible amounts of apoB protein in either liver or intestine. Analysis of the patient's DNA and RNA would most likely yield which of the following results?

a. Substitution of the last base of a codon near the middle of the first apoB exon
b. Insertion of two bases near the apoB amino terminus
d. Transversion producing a nonsense mutation within the first apoB intron
c. Transition affecting the thirtieth base of the first apoB intron
e. Base substitution changing glycine for alanine near the apoB carboxyl terminus

84. Cancers may be caused by mutations in two types of genes, those that affect cell proliferation (oncogenes, tumor suppressor genes) and those that control rates of mutation (caretaker genes—i.e., those altering DNA repair). A child develops a wide gait and is found to have different leg lengths. On examination, one leg is larger (hemihypertrophy) and a mass is found in the lower abdomen. Surgery reveals a Wilms tumor (194070), and the IGF2 (insulin-like growth factor 2) gene is known to be specifically overexpressed in Wilms tumor. Restriction analysis of the child's tumor DNA showed that both IGF2 alleles were undermethylated. It is known that normal adult tissues have one methylated and one undermethylated IGF2 allele, while the single IGF2 allele in sperm DNA is always undermethylated. The results are best summarized as which of the following?

a. A loss of imprinting (LOI) mutation that increased tumor IGF2 expression and identifies IGF2 as a caretaker gene
b. A loss of imprinting (LOI) mutation that increased tumor IGF2 expression and identifies IGF2 as an oncogene
c. A loss of imprinting (LOI) mutation that increased tumor IGF2 expression and identifies it as a tumor suppressor gene
d. A loss of imprinting (LOI) mutation that increased tumor IGF2 expression and causes Wilms tumor in females only
e. A loss of imprinting (LOI) mutation that increased tumor IGF2 expression and causes Wilms tumor in males only

85. Part of the triplet genetic code involving mRNA codon triplets that start with U is shown below. Using the portion of the genetic code shown, which of the following mutations in the 32 to 52 DNA template segments corresponds to a nonsense mutation?

a. ACGACGACG to ACAAACACG
b. AGGAATATG to AGGAATATT
c. AGAATAACA to AAAATAACA
d. AAAATGAGC to AAAATAAGC
e. AACAACAAC to AACAAGAAC

5′ End (Nucleotide I)		Middle		3′ End (Nucleotide 2)	(Nucleotide 3)
	U	C	A	G	
	phe	ser	tyr	cys	U
	phe	ser	tyr	cys	C
U	leu	ser	stop	stop	A
	leu	ser	stop	stop	G

86. A child with an abdominal mass was suspected of having Wilms tumor (194070), supported by blood and unusual cells in the urine sediment. The physicians suspected erosion of surrounding kidney with invasion of the renal pelvis, causing tumor cells to be excreted in urine. Because a version of the p57 gene is known to be silenced preferentially in Wilms tumor, analysis of p57 gene methylation and expression was performed on the urine tumor cells with the results shown below. Which of the following best summarizes these results?

a. Biallelic p57 gene methylation and with normal p57 gene expression making a diagnosis of Wilms tumor unlikely
b. Bi-allelic p57 gene methylation and with increased p57 gene expression making a diagnosis of Wilms tumor unlikely
c. Bi-allelic p57 gene methylation and with decreased p57 gene expression supporting the diagnosis of Wilms tumor
d. Undermethylation of both p57 alleles with increased p57 gene expression supporting the diagnosis of Wilms tumor
e. Methylation of one p57 allele with increased p57 gene expression supporting the diagnosis of Wilms tumor

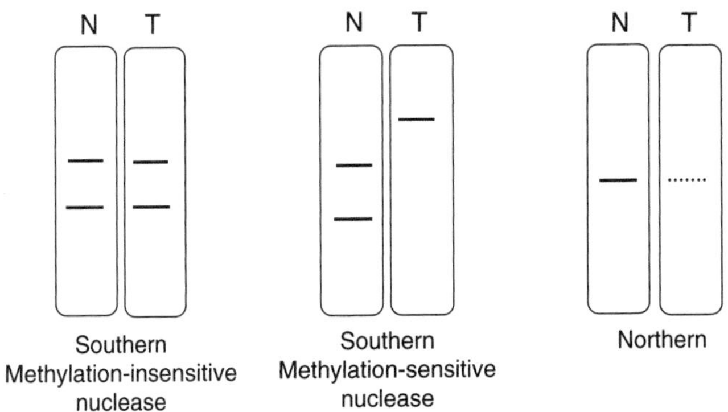

87. The lactose operon is negatively controlled by the lactose repressor and positively controlled by which of the following?

a. Increased concentrations of glucose and cyclic AMP (cAMP)
b. Decreased concentrations of glucose and cAMP
c. Increased concentrations of glucose, decreased concentration of cAMP
d. Decreased concentrations of glucose, increased concentration of cAMP
e. Increased concentrations of glucose and adenosine triphosphate (ATP)

88. Which of the following regulators are said to act in "cis"?

a. The lac repressor and the lac operator
b. The lac operator and mammalian transcription factors
c. The lac operator and mammalian enhancers
d. Mammalian transcription factors and enhancers
e. The lac repressor and mammalian transcription factors

89. A severe birth defect syndrome called retinoic acid embryopathy (243440) is caused by medications such as Accutane when taken by pregnant women for treatment of acne. Retinoic acid and steroid hormones are group I signals that cross the cell membrane to interact with cytosolic or nuclear receptors. Which of the structural domains of such receptors would interact with retinoic acid?

a. Response elements
b. Antirepressor domains
c. Transcription-activating domains
d. Ligand-binding domains
e. DNA-binding domains

90. The proopiomelanocortin (POMC—176830) gene encodes several regulatory proteins that affect pituitary function. Children with severe brain defects like holoprosencephaly (157170) often have abnormalities in the hypothalamic-pituitary axis. In different brain regions, proteins encoded by this gene have different carboxy-terminal peptides. Which of the following best explains the regulatory mechanism?

a. POMC transcription is regulated by different factors in different brain regions
b. POMC translation elongation is regulated by different factors in different brain regions
c. POMC transcription has different enhancers in different brain regions
d. POMC protein undergoes different protein processing in different brain regions
e. POMC protein forms different allosteric complexes in different brain regions

91. An Asian child has severe anemia with prominence of the forehead (frontal bossing) and cheeks. The red cell hemoglobin concentration is dramatically decreased, and it contains only β-globin chains with virtual deficiency of α-globin chains. Which of the following mechanisms is the most likely explanation?

a. A transcription factor regulating the α-globin gene is mutated
b. A regulatory sequence element has been mutated adjacent to an α-globin gene
c. A transcription factor regulating the β-globin gene is mutated
d. A transcription factor regulating the α- and β-globin genes is deficient
e. A deletion has occurred surrounding an α-globin gene

92. A mutation that results in a valine replacement for glutamic acid at position 6 of the β chain of hemoglobin S hinders normal hemoglobin function and results in sickle cell anemia (602903) when the patient is homozygous for this mutation. This is an example of which of the following types of mutation?

a. Deletion
b. Frameshift
c. Insertion
d. Missense
e. Nonsense

93. Two boys with mental disability are found to have mutations in a gene on the X chromosome that has no homology with globin genes. Both are also noted to have deficiency of α-globin synthesis, causing imbalance of globin chains and the severe anemia and skeletal changes of α-thalassemia plus mental retardation (301040). Which of the following is the best explanation for their phenotype?

a. The mutation disrupted an enhancer for an α-globin pseudogene
b. The mutation disrupted an X-encoded transcription factor that regulates the α-globin loci
c. There is a second mutation that disrupts an enhancer near the α-globin gene
d. There is a DNA rearrangement that joins the mutated X chromosome gene with an α-globin gene
e. There is a second mutation that disrupts the promoter of an α-globin gene

94. A middle-aged man presents with a markedly enlarged tonsil and recurrent infections with serum immunoglobulin deficiency. He has enlarged lymph nodes along his neck. Chromosome analysis demonstrates a translocation between the immunoglobulin heavy-chain locus on chromosome 14 and an unidentified gene on chromosome 8. Which of the following is the most likely cause of his phenotype?

a. The translocation has deleted constant chain exons on chromosome 14 and prevented heavy-chain class switching
b. The translocation has deleted the interval containing diversity (D) and joining (J) regions
c. The translocation has activated a tumor-promoting gene on chromosome 8
d. The translocation has deleted the heavy-chain constant chain Cμ so that virgin B cells cannot produce IgM on their membranes
e. The translocation has deleted an immunoglobulin transcription factor gene on chromosome 8

Gene Expression and Regulation

Answers

35. The answer is b. *(Murray, pp 358–373. Scriver, pp 3–45. Lewis, pp 205–240.)* The "genetic code" uses three-nucleotide "words," or codons, to specify the 20 different amino acids. There are 64 different three-base pair codons (three positions with four possible nucleotides at each). It follows that the genetic code must be degenerate, that is, different codons can specify the same amino acid. Three codons are reserved as "stop" signals that result in peptide chain termination. The linear correspondence of codons in DNA and of amino acids in protein domains is interrupted by the presence of introns in DNA. Codons differ from the dinucleotide tandem repeats that provide useful DNA polymorphisms, or the trinucleotide repeats that can be responsible for disease. The genetic code is universal in the sense that codon-amino acid relationships are the same in all organisms.

36. The answer is d. *(Murray, pp 358–373. Scriver, pp 3–45. Lewis, pp 205–240.)* Sickle cell anemia (141900) is an autosomal recessive hemoglobinopathy with an incidence of 1 in 500 African American births. It is caused by a single-nucleotide substitution in codon 6 of the β-globin gene. This mutation abolishes an enzyme site so that a larger DNA fragment is obtained after Southern blot analysis with the appropriate enzyme. Single-nucleotide substitutions do not change the length of coding regions (exons). The amplification of DNA segments using the polymerase chain reaction (PCR) allows more sensitive detection of restriction enzyme differences and can be followed by allele-specific oligonucleotide (ASO) hybridization to determine the presence of normal versus sickle alleles. The equivalence of DNA in most tissues (with the exception of red blood cells that extrude their nucleus) makes DNA diagnosis a powerful technique that is independent of gene or protein expression. Western blotting is a technique that uses antibodies to highlight the size and amount of mutant protein in cell extracts. Since single-nucleotide changes in the gene may not affect protein size or conformation, Western blotting is generally less sensitive and specific than DNA diagnosis.

37. The answer is c. *(Murray, pp 358–373. Scriver, pp 3–45. Lewis, pp 205–240.)* Insertion (choice c) or deletion (choice d) of nucleotides shifts the reading frame unless the change is a multiple of 3 (choice e). Frame shifts may create unintended stop codons as in choice c. Point mutations resulting in nucleotide or amino acid substitutions are conveniently named by their position in the protein, that is, $P_{21}A$ (choice b). The protein change $P_{21}A$ could also be denoted by the corresponding change in the DNA reading frame, that is, $C_{63}A$. Deletions may be prefixed by the letter delta, as with ΔF_{25} (choice e).

38. The answer is b. *(Murray, pp 396–414. Scriver, pp 3–45. Lewis, pp 205–240.)* Three RNA polymerases are responsible for RNA transcription in Mammalian cells, RNA polymerase I for ribosomal RNA, RNA polymerase II for messenger RNA, and RNA polymerase III for transfer and small RNAs (5s, microRNAs). Mammalian RNA polymerase II is highly sensitive to the mushroom toxin α-amanitin, and even experienced mushroom gatherers can confuse the toxic Amanita species with edible varieties. Inhibition of RNA polymerase II-catalyzed HnRNA transcription seems to have the most dramatic effects in liver, perhaps because of its active role in protein synthesis. The liver damage caused by α-amanitin ingestion cannot be treated, requiring regeneration in milder ingestions and transplant in severe ones.

39. The answer is b. *(Murray, pp 341–357. Scriver, pp 3–45. Lewis, pp 205–240.)* Exons are the coding portions of genes and consist of trinucleotide codons that guide the placement of specific amino acids into protein. Introns are the noncoding portions of genes that may function in evolution to provide "shuffling" of exons to produce new proteins. The primary RNA transcript contains both exons and introns, but the latter are removed by RNA splicing. The 5′ (upstream) and 3′ (downstream) untranslated RNA regions remain in the mature RNA and are thought to regulate RNA transport or translation. A poly(A) tail is added to the primary transcript after transcription, which facilitates transport and processing from the nucleus. The discovery of introns complicated Mendel's idea of the gene as the smallest hereditary unit; a modern definition might be the colinear sequence of exons, introns, and adjacent regulatory sequences that accomplish protein expression. Using these principles, one can determine the size of the stimulin gene. It contains a coding region of 300 bp (100 amino acids = 3 bp per amino acid), plus 120 bp in the intron, plus 70 + 30 = 100 bp in the untranslated regions (total = 520 bp). The mature RNA contains the same number of bp except for the 120 bp in the intron (520 – 120 = 400 bp). Transcription begins at the start of the 5′ untranslated region (70 bp) and the splice site occurs 30 bp (10 codons × 3 bp per codon) into the coding region at the beginning of the intron.

40. The answer is c. *(Murray, pp 286–290, 304–308. Scriver, 3-45. Lewis, pp 205–240.)* The ability of the factor to bind a DNA element suggests it is nucleic acid or protein, and its hydrolysis by alkali suggests it is an RNA. Its small size would exlude mRNA (>100 to thousands of bp) or tRNA (75–90 bp), suggesting it is a small RNA. Some simple RNAs can self-catalyze their own splicing, but such mechanisms are less important during the complex processing of mammalian mRNAs. A transposon is a mobile DNA element that usually inhibits gene expression.

Small RNAs ranging from 21 to 30 nucleotides in length are now recognized in all eucaryotes and include more than 1000 species in humans. Small RNAs may stimulate genes (microRNAs) or silence them (intefering or siRNAs), influencing gene transcription by binding to chromatin or DNA sequence elements. Regulation by small RNAs is complex since many have double-stranded or hairpin regions that are cleaved and activated by specific nucleases like *Dicer, Drosha,* or *Pasha* in flies. Small RNAs have been implicated in regulating the conversion of mouse hematopoetic stem cells to B-cells. Silencing or interfering RNAs have become an important tool for genetic analysis, allowing specific knockout of genes in animals or *in vitro* systems to define their effects.

41. The answer is d. *(Murray, pp 314–357. Scriver, pp 4571–4636. Lewis, pp 218–219.)* The single nucleotide transition from A to T on the sense strand in codon six of the β-globin gene causes the amino acid substitution glutamic acid to valine in the encoded β-globin protein. The valine lacks the negative charge of the glutamic acid carboxyl group, changing the shape of the β-globin protein and its subsequent complex with α-globin protein and heme to form hemoglobin. Correlation of this DNA change with its effect on hemoglobin and its resulting clinical symptoms earned Linus Pauling a Nobel Prize and initiated the era of molecular medicine. The lack of a negative charge and change in protein conformation also produced altered mobility of the hemoglobin, uniquely visualized by hemoglobin electrophoresis because of its red color. A search for revealing restriction sites allowed use of endonuclease MstII for DNA diagnosis of sickle cell anemia, since the A to T mutation ablated the restriction site and produced a single DNA fragment of 680 bp in sickle cell as opposed to the 515 bp and 165 bp fragments expected in normal individuals (see the figure accompanying this question). Southern blotting was devised by biochemist Ed Southern, allowing electrophoresis of restricted DNA, transfer to a nitrocellulose membrane, and detection of DNA fragments through hybridization with radioactive or fluorescent nucleic acid segments (probes). Northern blotting, a pun on Southern's name, is an analogous technique for detection of RNA fragments through transfer and hybridization. A nucleic acid species of about 700 bp representing β-globin mRNA would be expected upon Northern blotting of tissue extracts from normal or sickle cell individuals since the mutation should not change transcription or RNA processing.

42. The answer is c. *(Murray, pp 314–357. Scriver, pp 3–45. Lewis, pp 205–240.)* Self-splicing of the introns of some primary ribosomal RNA transcripts occurs because of the presence of catalytic RNAs (ribozymes) generated from the introns. This occurs in the absence of protein catalysis. In contrast, the splicing of messenger RNA is carried out by spliceosomes. Spliceosomes are large complexes of three kinds of small ribonucleoprotein particles (snRNPs) and the messenger RNA precursor. The snRNPs are involved in recognizing the 5′ splice site and the 3′ splice site and then binding to these sites. Once the spliceosome is bound, it mediates excision of the intron and splicing of the two adjacent exons. It is the RNA within the spliceosome that catalyzes intron excision.

43. The answer is b. *(Murray, pp 314–357. Scriver, pp 3–45. Lewis, 218–219.)* Promoter sites are initiation sites for transcription that are located just upstream (5′) of the transcription unit (site a in the figure for the β-globin gene). Transcription starts when RNA polymerase binds to the promoter. It then unwinds the closed promoter complex, where DNA is in the form of a double helix, to form the open promoter complex in which about 17 base pairs of template DNA are unwound. RNA synthesis then begins with either a pppA or a pppG inserted at the beginning 5′-terminus of the new RNA chain, which is synthesized in the 5′ to 3′ direction. The antiparallel DNA strand (coding or template strand) provides the sequence information for RNA polymerase to copy as nascent, single-stranded RNA (heterogenous or HnRNA). RNA polymerases in bacteria have special subunits that favor transcription to particular genes, but those in eucaryotes are guided by DNA sequence elements surrounding the gene—promoters, enhancers, and the like. These sequence elements in turn bind proteins called transcription factors, assembling a multiprotein RNA polymerase II aggregate that is more complex and variable than those in bacteria.

44. The answer is b. *(Murray, pp 314–357. Scriver, pp 4571–4636. Lewis, pp 205–240.)* The offspring of a woman with sickle cell anemia must receive one of her abnormal β-globin alleles and be a heterozygote or carrier known as sickle cell trait. Approximately 1 in 12 African Americans will have sickle trait, justifying its inclusion in American neonatal screening protocols. Caucasians, especially those of Mediterranean origin, can also be affected. Individuals with sickle trait will be asymptomatic under normal conditions, but may show symptoms under conditions of low oxygen tension (high altitudes, diving, etc.) due to the lower oxygen-binding capacity of their red blood cells (half normal, half sickle cell hemoglobin). Those with sickle trait will have one β-globin gene with a sickle mutation that ablates the sixth codon MstII site, yielding a 680 bp fragment by Southern blot in addition to the 515 and 165 bp fragments yielded by the normal β-globin gene. RNA transcription and processing willl not be affected, yielding a β-globin mRNA of about 700 bp. The sickle hemoglobin will have a different charge and conformation due to its glutamic acid to valine substitution, migrating differently by electrophoresis and yielding a second, abnormal hemoglobin band in addition to that of normal hemoglobin.

45. The answer is c. *(Murray, pp 341–357. Scriver, pp 4571–4636. Lewis, pp 190–196.)* A mutation affecting the transcription initiation or promoter site of the β-globin gene will decrease transcription of that allele and diminish the amount of ~700 bp β-globin mRNA detected by Northern blot. The minimal amount of β-globin mRNA will in turn yield minimal amounts of β-globin protein and normal hemoglobin detected by hemoglobin electrophoresis. The promoter mutation on one β-globin allele will not affect the 515 and 165 bp MstII cleavage fragments detected by Southern blotting, but the sickle cell mutation on the other allele will ablate the MstII site at the sixth codon and produce an additional 680 bp fragment. Because both β-thalassemia and sickle cell anemia are common in Mediterranean populations, compound heterozygotes with both mutations, known colloquially as "sickle-thal," are fairly common. Their symptoms will be as severe as those of sickle cell homozygotes, including anemia, strokes, and pain crises due to vascular occlusion from sickled red blood cells.

46. The answer is e. *(Murray, pp 341–357. Scriver, pp 4571–4636. Lewis, pp 218–219.)* The first event that occurs in mRNA synthesis is the binding of transcription factor TFIID to the TATA box. This consensus sequence portion of virtually all eukaryotic genes coding for mRNA is centered at about −25 and is similar to a 10-sequence promoter box found in prokaryotes. TFIID contains a TATA box-binding protein. The following sequence occurs in the initiation of mRNA synthesis:

1. TFIID binding to the TATA box
2. TFIIA binding
3. TFIIB binding
4. RNA polymerase II binding
5. TFIIE binding

When all these elements are bound to DNA, the basal transcription apparatus complex is formed and can transcribe DNA slowly. Other factors are required for fast, efficient mRNA synthesis.

47. The answer is c. *(Murray, pp 341–357. Scriver, pp 4571–4636. Lewis, pp 218–219.)* The primary RNA transcript produced by RNA polymerase is a heterogenous RNA containing introns and exons. RNA processing then occurs as the newly transcribed RNA is transported from nucleus to cytoplasm, and includes RNA splicing to remove intronic sequences in the transcript, methyl capping of the 5′-end, and polyadenylation (addition of 50–200 adenylate residues) to the 3′-end. RNA splicing is catalyzed by a spliceosome, using consensus donor sites at the proximal exon-intron junction and consensus acceptor sites at the distal intron-exon junction. Mutation of splice donor or acceptor sequences will disrupt normal splicing, yielding an aberrant mRNA that contains intronic sequences (if not degraded, a larger size by Northern blot). Decreased amounts of normal mRNA and production of an aberrant protein due to translation of nonsense intronic sequences will decrease the amounts of normal β-globin protein and produce β-thalassemia. Mutations at splice sites will not affect promoter sites or transcription initiation, producing a different category of β-thalassemia that is due to aberrant RNA processing.

48. The answer is b. *(Murray, pp 341–357. Scriver, pp 3–45. Lewis, 205–216.)* The primary transcripts of all eukaryotic mRNAs are capped at the 5′ end. Prokaryotic RNAs and eukaryotic tRNA and rRNA are not capped. The cap is composed of 7-methylguanylate attached by a pyrophosphate linkage to the 5′ end. This is known as cap 0. One of the adjacent riboses is methylated in cap 1, and both of the adjacent riboses are methylated in cap 2. The cap protects the 5′ ends of mRNAs from nucleases and phosphatases and is essential for the recognition of eukaryotic mRNAs in the protein-synthesizing system. When prokaryotic monocistronic mRNAs are artificially capped, translation occurs in a eukaryotic, in vitro translation system.

49. The answer is d. *(Murray, pp 307–308, 341–357. Scriver, pp 3–45. Lewis, 241–266.)* The nucleolus, an organelle unique to eukaryotic cells, is the site where RNA polymerase I transcribes the hundreds of copies of tandemly repeated genes for three of the four ribosomal RNAs to give 45S primary transcripts. The ribosomal RNA gene clusters can undergo amplification through unequal crossing over, accounting for individual variability in the size of these clusters, located at the ends of the five pairs of acrocentric chromosomes (numbers 13–15, 21–22). These variably sized clusters form stalks and "satellites" on the acrocentric chromosomes when visualized at metaphase by karyotyping, and their associated ribosomal RNA gives a distinctive dark color when incubated with silver stain.

Enzymatic modification and cleavage remove spacer regions to yield 28S, 18S, and 5.8S ribosomal RNA. The 5S subunit is synthesized by RNA polymerase III in the nucleoplasm rather than in the nucleolus. Ribosomal proteins combine with the ribosomal subunits to assemble into a 60S subunit containing the 5S, 5.8S, and 28S RNAs and a 40S subunit containing the 18S RNA. Combined, the two subunits produce a functional eukaryotic ribosome with a sedimentation coefficient of 80S. Messenger RNAs are synthesized by RNA polymerase II in the nucleoplasm, while 5S, tRNA, and small RNAs are synthesized by RNA polymerase III in the cytoplasm.

50. The answer is c. *(Murray, pp 341–357. Scriver, pp 3–45. Lewis, 205–216.)* About 30% of the DNA of humans and other mammals consists of repeated sequences. Repetitive DNA includes numerous families of genes like those for histones. Some families of repeated genes make identical mRNA molecules, suggesting that their multiple gene copies are needed to make adequate amounts of protein. Although many genes in bacteria produce a polycistronic mRNA that encodes several different peptides, all mRNAs in mammals encode a single peptide and are monocistronic. In addition, RNA is initially transcribed from protein-encoding genes as larger molecules called heterogenous nuclear RNA (hnRNA). These immature hnRNA molecules must be spliced to remove introns and chemically modified with 5′ caps and 3′-poly(A) sequences before reaching the cytoplasm as functional mRNA. The initial hnRNA transcript is colinear with its encoded protein within exons but not within introns. Mature mRNAs also have 5′ and 3′ untranslated regions that are not colinear with the encoded peptide.

51. The answer is e. *(Murray, pp 341–357. Scriver, pp 4571–4636. Lewis, pp 218–219.)* The globin genes exist in two clusters in mammals, one containing the α-globin genes (chromosome 16 in humans) and another containing β-globin genes (chromosome 11 in humans). The globin genes are highly similar to one another, suggesting that their clusters evolved by unequal crossing over to generate duplicate genes with later diversion in function. Both clusters have globin genes that are expressed during embryonic or fetal life, exemplified by the switch from the fetal γ-globin to adult β-globin expression in the β-globin cluster at about 6 months of infancy. The result of this evolution is that γ-globin and α-globin genes are present in duplicate within their respective clusters, while β-globin is present in a single copy. Promoter mutations that disrupt transcription initiation or splicing mutations decrease globin mRNA with resulting imbalance of α-globin or β-globin peptides, causing aberrant hemoglobins with four α-globin or β-globin chains rather than the normal two of each. The β-globin mutations that decrease β-globin mRNA can be heterozygous (thal trait) or homozygous (β-thalassemia), but the corresponding α-globin mutations can be present in one, two, three, or four α-globin genes. Only patients with mutations in three α-globin genes or in all four have significant α-thalassemia, distinguished by the type of aberrant hemoglobin produced (hemoglobin H or Bart's hemoglobin, respectively).

52. The answer is e. *(Murray, pp 341–357. Scriver, pp 3–45. Lewis, pp 205–216.)* In mammals, RNA polymerase binds to promoter sites upstream from the start site. These include the TATA box (TATAAT), the CAAT box, and the GC box. DNA primase and helicase are involved in DNA replication and do not bind specifically to sequences upstream of genes. Restriction endonucleases recognize specific sequences in double-helical DNA and cleave both strands. Histones nonspecifically bind to chromosomal DNA and constitute about half the mass of mammalian chromosomes.

53. The answer is b. *(Murray, pp 341–357. Scriver, pp 4571–4636. Lewis, pp 218–219.)* Homozygous mutations that decrease β-globin mRNA synthesis will decrease β-globin peptide and hemoglobin synthesis, causing the aberrant red blood cells and severe anemia of β-thalassemia. Mutations can decrease mRNA amounts by interfering with sequence elements (promoters, enhancers) that promote gene transcription or sequence elements (consensus splice donor and acceptor sites, consensus polyadenylation sites) that interfere with mRNA processing. Eukaryotic mRNAs are polyadenylated at the 3′ end to protect it from exonuclease attack. The polyadenylation signal AAUAA is found 10–30 bp upstream of the polyadenylation site. Homozygous mutations affecting the β-globin gene polyadenylation signal can reduce β-globin mRNA synthesis by 95–97%, producing β-thalassemia. Single-base substitutions within exons should not change mRNA transcription or processing, but may produce amino acid changes (missense mutations) and yeild an aberrant protein with defective function (e.g., a hemoglobinopathy).

54. The answer is c. *(Murray, pp 341–357. Scriver, pp 2717–2752. Lewis, pp 205–216.)* Though unanticipated, the apoB mRNA was found to undergo RNA editing wherein a cytidine deaminase in intestine changed a CAA codon to UAA. The UAA is a termination codon and caused a truncated 48 kilodalton apoB mRNA peptide to be synthesized in intestine compared to the full-length 100 kb peptide synthesized in liver. The other explanations (alternative splicing, exon deletion, polyadenylation, different promoter) would not produce mRNA of similar size and abundance, and the exon deletion is additionally excluded by finding identical apoB gene sequences for both alleles. The serum lipoproteins are concerned with transporting lipids absorbed from intestine to other organs, and inherited abnormalities in their peptides (apolipoproteins) can predispose to heart attacks by releasing excess lipids to the coronary artery endothelium.

55. The answer is e. *(Murray, pp 341–357. Scriver, pp 2717–2752. Lewis, pp 205–216.)* Northern blotting to detect RNA and Western blotting to detect protein were named as puns on the name of Ed Southern who developed his cognate method for electrophoretic separation and hybridization probe detection of DNA segments. Complementary DNA or RNA probes, like the complementary DNA (cDNA) made using oligo-dT primed DNA synthesis from mRNA, provide the specificity of DNA/RNA segment detection in Southern and Northern analysis. Detection of proteins requires the raising of specific antibody through injection into rabbits, purification of antibody from rabbit serum, labeling with radioactive iodine or fluorescent dyes, and floating the antibody over the Western blot membrane to bind and identify specific peptides.

Once a specific antibody is raised to a protein, it can be used to screen expression libraries for gene segments that direct synthesis of the desired protein in bacteria. Mammalian tissue mRNAs are extracted, copied into cDNAs, rendered double-stranded, and ligated with excess bacterial DNAs (vectors) so as to make a collection of cDNA-vector DNA reccombinant clones (expression library). Then the bacteria, each containing a different mammalian cDNA segment, are arrayed on plates, transferred to a membrane in a manner similar to Western blotting, and reacted with labeled antibody probe to determine which bacterial harbor the desired cDNA. The ability to construct DNA or expression (mRNA to cDNA) libaries, together with vectors for a range of DNA segment sizes (up to a million bp), allowed comprehensive gene/transcript cloning that isolated entire genomes (i.e., the human genome initiative).

56. The answer is e. *(Murray, pp 358–373. Scriver, pp 3–45. Lewis, pp 171–185.)* Despite some differences, protein synthesis in prokaryotes and eukaryotes is quite similar. The small ribosomal subunit is 30S in prokaryotes and 40S in eukaryotes. The large ribosomal subunit is 50S in prokaryotes and 60S in eukaryotes. The intact ribosome is consequently larger in eukaryotes (80S) and smaller in prokaryotes (70S). At the start of translation, initiation factors, mRNA, and initiation aminoacyl-tRNA bind to the dissociated small ribosomal subunit. The initiation tRNA in prokaryotes is N-formyl methionine in prokaryotes and simply methionine in eukaryotes. Only after the small ribosomal subunit is primed with mRNA and initiation aminoacyl-tRNA does the large ribosomal subunit bind to it. Once this happens, elongation factors bring the first aminoacyl-tRNA of the nascent protein to the A site. Then peptidyl transferase forges a peptide bond between the initiation amino acid and the first amino acid of the forming peptide. The now uncharged initiation tRNA leaves the P site and the peptidyl-tRNA from the A site moves to the now vacant P site with the two amino acids attached. The ribosome advances three bases to read the next codon and the process repeats. When the stop signal is reached after the complete polypeptide has been synthesized, releasing factors bind to the stop signal, causing peptidyl transferase to hydrolyze the bond that joins the polypeptide at the A site to the tRNA. Factors prevent the reassociation of ribosomal subunits in the absence of new initiation complex.

57. The answer is d. *(Murray, pp 358–373. Scriver, pp 3–45. Lewis, pp 185–204.)* Protein synthesis occurs in the cytoplasm, on groups of free ribosomes called polysomes, and on ribosomes associated with membranes, termed the rough endoplasmic reticulum. However, proteins destined for secretion are only synthesized on ribosomes of the endoplasmic reticulum and are synthesized in such a manner that they end up inside the lumen of the endoplasmic reticulum. From there the secretory proteins are packaged in vesicles. The Golgi apparatus is involved in the O-glycosylation and packaging of macromolecules into membranes for secretion.

58. The answer is b. *(Lewis, pp 358–373. Murray, pp 361–364. Scriver, pp 4571–4636.)* The insertion or deletion of nucleotides other than multiples of three will change the reading frame by which the linear nucleotides of RNA parsed three at a time (codons) into the linear amino acids of protein. Insertion or deletion of one or two nucleotides will disrupt this reading by threes, disrupt the reading frame, and produce frameshift mutations. A shift in the reading frame by one or two positions will completely change the sense of ensuing nucleotides, causing all subsequent codons to be read out of frame to produce different (nonsense) amino acid sequences. Furthermore, the shift in frame often introduces a stop codon very shortly after the frameshift and produces a truncated protein. Whether the amino acid sequence is garbled or truncated, a frameshift mutation will disrupt production of normal protein. In the case of frameshift mutations in the β-globin gene, production of β-globin protein will be reduced as with transcription or RNA processing mutations, causing another form of β-thalassemia when both β-globin gene copies are ineffective. Missense mutations are alterations in a single codon such that the three base triplet encodes for a different amino acid. Silent mutations are alterations in a single codon such that the new codon still encodes for the same amino acid. This is possible because of the degeneracy of the genetic code. Missense mutations may produce a protein with variant structure and function (e.g., as in a hemoglobinopathy) while silent mutations will have no effect on protein structure/function and may be called polymorphisms (harmless genetic variations).

59. The answer is e. *(Murray, pp 341–357. Scriver, pp 32219–3256.)* By using recombinant DNA techniques, mRNAs can be produced that yield chimeric proteins. When DNA encoding an amino terminal signal sequence is inserted upstream of the α-globin gene, the usual cytosolic α-globin becomes a secretory protein and is translocated into the lumen of endoplasmic reticulum. The signal sequence thus contains all the information needed to direct the translocation of protein across endoplasmic reticulum. For diseases with abnormal targeting to or abnormal storage of proteins in the endoplasmic reticulum, cleavage of the signal sequene can alter the targeting or lessen the accumulation. To be effective as therapy, the factors that modify protein structure in vitro must be introduced into the appropriate tissues in a sustaining manner. So far, such protein or enzyme therapy has only been effective when specific targeting mechanisms exist (like targeting of enzymes to lysosomes by adding mannose-6-phosphate signal residues) and when tissues are accessible (i.e., not protected by the blood-brain barrier).

60. The answer is c. *(Murray, pp 358–373. Scriver, pp 3–45. Lewis, pp 185–204.)* ATP is required for the esterification of amino acids to their corresponding tRNAs. This reaction is catalyzed by the class of enzymes known as aminoacyl-tRNA synthetases. Each one of these enzymes is specific for one tRNA and its corresponding amino acid:

$$\text{amino acid} + \text{tRNA} + \text{ATP} \rightarrow \text{aminoacyl-tRNA} + \text{AMP} + \text{PP}_i$$

As with most ATP hydrolysis reactions that release pyrophosphate, pyrophosphatase quickly hydrolyzes the product to P_i, which makes the reaction essentially irreversible. Since ATP is hydrolyzed to AMP and PP_i during the reaction, the equivalent of two high-energy phosphate bonds is utilized.

61. The answer is b. *(Murray, pp 358–373. Scriver, pp 3–45. Lewis, pp 185–204.)* During the course of protein synthesis on a ribosome, peptidyl transferase catalyzes the formation of peptide bonds. However, when a stop codon such as UAA, UGA, or UAG is reached, aminoacyl-tRNA does not bind to the A site of a ribosome. One of the proteins, known as a release factor, binds to the specific trinucleotide sequence present. This binding of the release factor activates peptidyl transferase to hydrolyze the bond between the polypeptide and the tRNA occupying the P site. Thus, instead of forming a peptide bond, peptidyl transferase catalyzes the hydrolytic step that leads to the release of newly synthesized proteins. Following release of the polypeptide, the ribosome dissociates into its major subunits.

62. The answer is e. *(Murray, pp 358–373. Scriver, pp 3–45. Lewis, pp 185–204.)* The template strand refers to the DNA strand that is transcribed into RNA. As for DNA, RNA is synthesized in the 5′ to 3′ direction. The template strand is always read in the 3′ to 5′ direction. The opposite DNA strand is known as the coding strand and has the same sequence as the RNA transcript, except that U replaces T in RNA. Choices b and d are DNAs, as they contain T instead of U.

63. The answer is d. *(Murray, pp 358–373. Scriver, pp 3–45. Lewis, pp 185–204.)* The two subunits of ribosomes are composed of proteins and rRNA. Ribosomes are found in the cytoplasm, in mitochondria, and bound to the endoplasmic reticulum. Transcription refers to the synthesis of RNA complementary to a DNA template and has nothing immediately to do with ribosomes.

64. The answer is c. *(Murray, pp 358–373. Scriver, pp 3–45.)* Two molecules of GTP are used in the formation of each peptide bond on the ribosome. In the elongation cycle, binding of aminoacyl-tRNA delivered by EF-2 to the A site requires hydrolysis of one GTP. Peptide bond formation then occurs. Translocation of the nascent peptide chain on tRNA to the P site requires hydrolysis of a second GTP. The activation of amino acids with aminoacyl-tRNA synthetase requires hydrolysis of ATP to AMP plus PP_i.

65. The answer is a. *(Murray, pp 358–373. Scriver, pp 3–45. Lewis, pp 185–204.)* Virulent strains of bacteria such as Mycoplasma pneumoniae, various Legionella species, and Bordetella pertussis that cause severe, life-threatening respiratory tract infections can often be successfully treated with erythromycin. The mechanism of action of erythromycin is to specifically bind the 50S subunit of bacterial ribosomes. Under normal conditions, after mRNA attaches to the initiation site of the 30S subunit, the 50S subunit binds to the 30S complex and forms the 70S complex that allows protein chain elongation to go forward. Elongation is prevented in the presence of erythromycin.

66. The answer is d. *(Murray, pp 358–373. Scriver, pp 3–45. Lewis, pp 185–204.)* The gene that produces the deadly toxin of Corynebacterium diphtheriae comes from a lysogenic phage that grows in the bacteria. Prior to immunization, diphtheria was the primary cause of death in children. The protein toxin produced by this bacterium inhibits protein synthesis by inactivating elongation factor 2 (EF-2, or translocase). Diphtheria toxin is a single protein composed of two portions (A and B). The B portion enables the A portion to translocate across a cell membrane into the cytoplasm. The A portion catalyzes the transfer of the adenosine diphosphate ribose unit of NAD_1 to a nitrogen atom of the diphthamide ring of EF-2, thereby blocking translocation. Diphthamide is an unusual amino acid residue of EF-2.

67. The answer is a. *(Murray, pp 358–373. Scriver, pp 3–45. Lewis, pp 185–204.)* Aminoacyl-tRNA synthetases are responsible for charging a tRNA with the appropriate amino acid for translation. Charging a tRNA is a two-step reaction. In the first step, the enzyme forms an aminoacyl-AMP enzyme complex in a reaction that requires one ATP. In the second step, the activated amino acid is attached to the appropriate tRNA and the enzyme and AMP are released.

68. The answer is d. *(Murray, pp 358–373. Scriver, pp 3–45. Lewis, pp 185–204.)* Prokaryotic ribosomes have a sedimentation coefficient of 70S and are composed of 50S and 30S subunits. Eukaryotic cytoplasmic ribosomes, either free or bound to the endoplasmic reticulum, are larger—60S and 40S subunits that associate to an 80S ribosome. Nuclear ribosomes are attached to the endoplasmic reticulum of the nuclear membrane. Ribosomes in chloroplasts and mitochondria of eukaryotic cells are more similar to prokaryotic ribosomes than to eukaryotic cytosolic ribosomes. Like bacterial ribosomes, chloroplast and mitochondrial ribosomes use a formylated tRNA. In addition, they are sensitive to many of the inhibitors of protein synthesis in bacteria.

69. The answer is b. *(Murray, pp 358–373. Lewis, 196–203. Scriver, pp1471–1488.)* The initiation of protein synthesis is a multistep process that includes several protein factors—eIF-4E and eIF-4G proteins that bind the mRNA cap, eIF-4A and eIF-4B proteins that bind to the 5′-end of mRNA and reduce its secondary structure. The eIF-3 proteins bind to the prior factors, linking them to the 40S ribosomal subunit and scanning for suitable AUG codons that will initiate peptide bond formation. This is usually the 5′-most AUG, but others may be selected by virtue of Kozak consensus sequences that surround it (GCC-AUG-UGG). Other protein factors regulate the rate of protein synthesis initiation by acting on eIF-4E, including those such as BP1 that bind and inactivate eIF-4E unless it is phosphorylated. Insulin and other growth factors act to phosphoryate BP-1 at several sites, releasing eIF-4E and stimlating initiation and protein synthesis. Though stimulation of protein synthesis by insulin is one plausible factor in increased fetal growth, other factors undoubtedly contribute to this complex process.

Once the EF factors, 40S subunit, and relaxed mRNA are associated (as a 43S preinitiation complex), it binds the 60S ribosomal subunit and its peptidyl transferase that is a component of the 28S rRNA—an example of a ribozyme. In translation, the P site of the ribosome is occupied by the peptidyl-tRNA, which has the growing peptide chain attached. The appropriate aminoacyl-tRNA enters the A site and the carboxyl group of the peptidyl tRNA undergoes nucleophilic attack by the α-amino group of the aminoacyl-tRNA, as catalyzed by peptidyl transferase. The peptide chain is transfered to the tRNA in the A site, which is subsequently displaced to the P site, freeing the A site to bind the next charged tRNA.

70. The answer is b. *(Murray, pp 344–357. Scriver, pp 3–45. Lewis, pp 190–196.)* Eukaryotic promoters are much more complex than bacterial promoters. The most common bacterial promoter elements are the −10 and −35 sequences, which are the recognition sites for RNA polymerase binding. In addition, bacterial promoters may have operators (repressor binding sites) and activator binding sites. Eukaryotic promoters have a core region that may contain a TATA box (which is bound by TBP, the TATA binding protein), an initiator sequence, and downstream promoter elements. Many promoters lack one or more of these elements. In addition, eukaryotic promoters have upstream elements such as GC boxes and CCAAT boxes that bind specific transcription factors (Sp1 and CTF, respectively). Enhancers are elements that increase or enhance the rate of transcription initiation from a promoter. Enhancers can be upstream or downstream of the transcription start site and can exert their effect from hundreds or thousands of bases away. In addition, enhancers are orientation-independent.

71. The answer is e. *(Murray, pp 358–373. Scriver, pp 3–45. Lewis, pp 185–204.)* Signal recognition particles (SRPs) recognize the signal sequence on the *N*-terminal end of proteins destined for the lumen of the endoplasmic reticulum (ER). SRP binding arrests translation and an SRP receptor facilitates import of the nascent protein into the ER lumen. A signal peptidase removes the signal sequence from the protein, which may remain in the membrane or be routed for secretion. Common to both eukaryotic and prokaryotic protein synthesis is the requirement for ATP to activate amino acids. The activated aminoacyl-tRNAs then interact with ribosomes carrying mRNA. Peptidyl transferase catalyzes the formation of peptide bonds between the free amino group of activated aminoacyl-tRNA on the A site of the ribosome and the esterified carboxyl group of the peptidyl-rRNA on the P site; the liberated rRNA remains on the P site.

72. The answer is a. *(Murray, pp 358–373, 498–513. Scriver, pp 5559–5628.)* The decreased amount of AAT protein, its abnormal mobility, and the engorgement of liver ER suggest a mutant AAT that is inefficiently transported from the ER to plasma. Since other plasma protein abnormalities were not mentioned, general deficiencies of protein synthesis arising from defective energy metabolism or defective signal recognition particles are unlikely. A mutation affecting the *N*-terminal methionine of AAT or its signal sequence should drastically decrease its synthesis and import to the ER lumen. This would not explain the engorgement of liver ER. The usual binding of the signal recognition particle to the signal sequence of AAT, followed by import into the ER lumen, seems intact. An altered amino acid necessary for signal peptidase cleavage of the signal sequence of AAT might be invoked, but a general deficiency of the signal peptidase should disrupt many secreted proteins and be an embryonic lethal mutation. AAT deficiency (107400) is a well-characterized autosomal dominant disease with common ZZ, SZ, and SS genotypes that can cause childhood liver disease and adult emphysema. The Z and S mutations alter AAT conformation and interfere with its secretion from ER to plasma. Lack of AAT protection from proteases in lung is thought to cause the thinning of alveolar walls and dysfunctional "air sacs" of emphysema.

73. The answer is e. *(Murray, pp 374–395. Scriver, pp 175–192. Lewis, pp 389–390.)* Gene therapy refers to a group of techniques by which gene structure or expression is altered to ameliorate a disease. Because of ethical and practical difficulties, germ-line therapy involving alterations of genes in primordial germ cells is not being explored in humans. Although germ-line genetic engineering is being performed in animals with the goals of improved breeding or agricultural yield, it alters the characteristics of offspring rather than the treated individuals. Somatic cell gene therapy is targeted to an affected tissue or group of tissues in the individual and is most effective if stem cells such as bone marrow can be treated. Somatic cell gene therapy offers the hope of replacing damaged tissue without the rejection problems of transplantation. For autosomal recessive disorders, only one of the two defective alleles must be replaced or supplemented.

74. The answer is a. *(Murray, pp 374–414. Scriver, pp 175–192. Lewis, pp 397–416.)* Challenges for gene therapy include the construction of recombinant viral genomes that can propagate the replacement gene (gene constructs or vectors), delivery of the altered gene to the appropriate tissues (gene targeting), and recombination at the appropriate locus so that replacement of the defective gene is achieved (site-specific recombination). The latter step positions DNA sequences in the vector so that the replacement gene pairs and recombines precisely with homologous DNA in the native gene. *Ex vivo* transfection (introduction of vector DNA into patient cells outside the body) is an ideal method for gene targeting if the engineered cells can repopulate the tissue/organ in question. Transfection of bone marrow stem cells with a functional adenosine deaminase gene, followed by bone marrow transplantation back to the patient, has been successful in restoring immunity to children with severe deficiency. Even when tissue targeting and precise gene replacement are feasible, mimicking the appropriate patterns of gene expression can be a substantial barrier to gene therapy. Injection of deficient enzymes into plasma (enzyme therapy) has been successful in disorders such as Gaucher disease (231000)—storage of lipids in the spleen and bone—and takes advantage of cellular pathways that target enzymes to lysosomes.

75. The answer is c. *(Murray, pp 374–395. Scriver, pp 175–192. Lewis, pp 377–396.)* After the locus responsible for a genetic disease is mapped to a particular chromosome region, "candidate" genes can be examined for molecular abnormalities in affected individuals. The connective tissue abnormalities in Stickler syndrome (108300) make the COL2A1 collagen locus an attractive candidate for disease mutations, prompting analysis of COL2A1 gene structure and expression. Western blotting detects gene alterations that interfere with protein expression, while use of the reverse transcriptase-polymerase chain reaction (RT-PCR) detects alterations in mRNA levels. Each analysis should detect one-half the respective amounts of COL2A1 protein or mRNA in the case of a promoter mutation that abolishes transcription of one COL2A1 allele. Southern blotting detects nucleotide changes that alter DNA restriction sites, but this is relatively insensitive unless large portions of the gene are deleted. Fluorescent *in situ* hybridization (FISH) analysis using DNA probes from the COL2A1 locus is a sensitive method for detecting deletions of the entire locus, and DNA sequencing of the entire gene provides the gold standard for detecting any alteration in the regulatory or coding sequences. Nucleotide sequence changes are still subject to interpretation, since they may represent polymorphisms that do not alter gene function. Population studies and/or in vitro studies of gene expression are often needed to discriminate DNA polymorphisms from mutations that disrupt gene function. For any autosomal locus, the interpretation of molecular analyses is complicated by the presence of two homologous copies of the gene.

76. The answer is e. *(Murray, pp 374–414. Scriver, pp 1857–1896. Lewis, pp 185–204.)* Missense mutations, which cause the substitution of one amino acid for another, may significantly alter the function of the resultant protein without altering the size of DNA restriction fragments detected by Southern blotting. In this case, Northern blot results would most likely also be normal. Single-base changes may also result in nonsense mutations. Large insertions or deletions in the exon or coding regions of the gene alter the Southern blot pattern and usually ablate the activity of one gene copy. In the case of an autosomal locus like that for ornithine aminotransferase, the homologous allele remains active and gives 50% enzyme activity (heterozygote or carrier range with a normal phenotype). Similar effects on enzyme activity would be predicted from complete gene deletions at one locus, while duplication might produce 150 or 50% of normal enzyme activity depending on the status of promoter sites.

77. The answer is b. *(Murray, pp 396–414. Scriver, pp 4517–4554. Lewis, pp 234, 296.)* Red cell hemolysis after drug exposure suggests a red cell enzyme defect, most easily confirmed by enzyme assay to demonstrate deficient activity. A likely diagnosis here is glucose-6-phosphate dehydrogenase (G6PD) deficiency (305900), probably the most common genetic disease (it affects 400 million people worldwide). Tropical African and Mediterranean peoples exhibit the highest prevalence because the disease, like sickle cell trait, confers resistance to malaria. DNA analysis is available to demonstrate particular alleles, but simple enzyme assay is sufficient for diagnosis. More than 400 types of abnormal G6PD alleles have been described, meaning that most affected individuals are compound heterozygotes. The phenotype of jaundice and red blood cell hemolysis with anemia is triggered by a variety of infections and drugs, including a dietary substance in fava beans. Sulfonamide and related antibiotics as well as antimalarial drugs are notorious for inducing hemolysis in G6PD-deficient individuals. G6PD deficiency exhibits X-linked recessive inheritance, explaining why male offspring but not the parents become ill when exposed to antimalarials.

78. The answer is b. *(Murray, pp 396–414. Scriver, pp 3421–3452. Lewis, pp 402–403.)* All of the modes of therapy are theoretically possible, and enzyme therapy (i.e., injection of purified enzyme) has been successful in several lysosomal deficiencies, particularly those in which the central nervous system is not affected [i.e., Gaucher disease (231000)]. Unfortunately, antibodies frequently develop to the injected enzyme and limit the term of successful enzyme delivery. Heterologous bone marrow transplant, preferably from a related donor, offers the most realistic and effective therapy since the graft provides a permanent source of enzyme. Bone marrow transplants do have a 10% mortality, however, and the enzyme diffuses poorly into the central nervous system. Somatic gene therapy (i.e., delivery of enzyme to somatic cells via viral vectors or transfected tissue) is now possible; however, targeting of the gene product to appropriate tissues and organelles is still a problem. Transfected autologous bone marrow transplant (i.e., marrow from the patient) has been used in a few cases of adenosine deaminase deficiency, an immune disorder affecting lymphocytes. Germ-line gene therapy requires the insertion of functional genes into gametes or blastomeres of early embryos prior to birth. The potential for embryonic damage, lack of knowledge regarding developmental gene control, and ethical controversies regarding selective breeding or embryo experimentation make germ-line therapy unrealistic at present.

79. The answer is e. *(Murray, pp 358–373. Scriver, pp 3–45. Lewis, pp 397–416.)* Because chromosomes are large chains of DNA comprising several thousand genes (links of chain), even small deletions will remove tens to hundreds of genes. Deletions involving the autosomes (chromosomes 1–22) will reduce genes within the deletion from diploid to haploid dosage, decreasing the amount of mRNA produced from these genes (answer e). The other answers concern changes in epigenesis—histone acetylation, DNA methylation, small RNA decoration—or a change in gene sequence that may not occur if the deletion cuts between genes. Changes in epigenesis undoubtedly occur with chromosome rearrangements (e.g., translocations, duplicated segments, interstitial deletions between chromosome ends) that make new links between noncontiguous chromosome segments. Epigenetic changes likely contribute to the diverse phenotypic effects of trisomies, where an extra dose of normal chromosomal DNA sequence is added to cells (e.g., trisomy 21 causing Down syndrome).

80. The answer is c. *(Murray, pp 358–373. Scriver, pp 3635–3643. Lewis, pp 185–204.)* The replacement of the codon UAC with UAA would be a nonsense mutation since UAC encodes tyrosine and UAA is a "stop" signal (see Fig. 8). Instead of proceeding through the mRNA segment, the ribosome would be signaled to stop glucocerebrosidase synthesis, resulting in a shortened peptide that would be unable to catalyze glucocerebride cleavage. Homozygous nonsense mutation affecting both glucocerebrosidase alleles would result in no enzyme produced and no ability for the cells to break down stored lipids. Most glucocerebrosidase mutations cause amino acid substitutions (missense mutations) with less impact on enzyme function; such mutations cause gradual lipid accumulation with adult onset of symptoms. Nonsense mutations will cause more severe enzyme deficiencies with resulting childhood onset and neurologic disability due to accumulation of lipids in brain (neuropathic forms of Gaucher disease). A suppressor mutation moderates the impact of nonsense mutations, usually through changes in the anticodon of transfer RNA. They are well-known in simpler organisms but not well characterized in mammals. The addition or deletion of nucleotides results in a frameshift mutation.

81. The answer is d. *(Murray, pp 358–373. Scriver, pp 3–45. Lewis, pp 205–216.)* The change in Gordon's DNA coding strand sequence from TAC to GAC, changing AUG to CUG in mRNA, is a missense mutation that substitutes the amino acid leucine for methionine. Not only will it affect the conformation of the translated protein, altering its mobility on electrophoresis, but it also ablates AUG codon for methionine that is used as an initiation signal for the ribosomal complex to begin translation of the mRNA. Reduced synthesis of the protein with diminished signal on Western blotting would also be expected. Transcription of mRNA should not be affected, so the answers indicating absent or unusual bands by Northern blotting can be eliminated. Note that the change from T (thymine, a pyrimidine) to G (guanine, a purine) is a transversion with change in base class rather than a transition that substitutes one purine or pyrimidine for another. Transversions will usually have more severe consequences than transitions, and both will be less severe than frameshift or nonsense mutations that garble or truncate the protein product.

82. The answer is e. *(Murray, pp 341–357. Lewis, pp 194–195; Scriver, pp 2717–2721.)* The apoB gene, which encodes apolipoprotein B, is transcribed in the liver normally and the mRNA is translated into a 100-kDa protein (apoB100). In the intestine, however, the apoB mRNA is edited by the enzyme cysteine deaminase, which alters a CAA codon (encoding a glutamine) to UAA (a stop codon). This change results in synthesis of a 48-kDa form of apolipoprotein B (apoB48) that lacks the carboxy-terminal end. The apoB100 and apoB48 proteins serve different functions in the liver and the intestine. A mutation that ablates apoB mRNA editing and its resulting apoB48 protein product in intestine could interfere with lipid absorption and production of VLDL and LDL in plasma. Other answers besides *e* indicate processes that would affect mRNA transcription, not protein size.

Although RNA editing is not widespread, there are a growing number of other examples. Alternative RNA splicing is a much more common means of generating alternative forms of a protein. In splicing, intron sequences are removed and exon (protein coding) sequences are joined together. Use of alternative splice sites can include or exclude certain exons, resulting in different primary sequence, conformation, and size of a protein. RNA splicing will usually preserve the carboxy-terminal exon since it is needed for mRNA polyadenylation and its transport from nucleus to cytoplasm.

83. The answer is b. *(Murray, pp 341–357. Scriver, pp 2717–2721. Lewis, pp 185–204.)* The structures of glycine and alanine are quite similar, with the -H side group of glycine being replaced with the $-CH_3$ side group of alanine. Consequently, a mutation causing such a change, particularly near the carboxy-terminus is unlikely to produce a dysfunctional protein. Similarly, the third position of mRNA codons is least crucial for amino acid coding due to "wobble"—similar or identical amino acids are often produced regardless of the third codon nucleotide (see Table 3). In contrast, a mutation inserting two bases into DNA and mRNA will change the reading frame of translation, producing a truncated (misread termination codon) or garbled amino acid sequence with apoB dysfunction. Introns are spliced out of RNA and do not encode segments of the protein product unless splicing is defective; intronic mutations should therefore not disrupt protein function unless they affect the splice sites near exon-intron junctions.

84. The answer is b. *(Murray, pp 358–373. Scriver, pp 525–537. Lewis, pp 185–204.)* The undermethylation of IGF2 alleles in sperm as compared to methylated and undermethylated alleles in diploid adult tissues suggests that the gene is imprinted. During germ cell formation, certain chromosome regions are patterned differently or "imprinted" in males versus females, producing different levels of maternal versus paternal allele expression in tissues of the resulting embryos and adults. These imprinting patterns are associated with DNA methylation at key CpG dinucleotide sites, up- or down-regulating allele transcription and expression. Biparental origin of alleles in diploid tissues is thus necessary for normal levels of gene expression, a balance disrupted by uniparental disomy (both copies of a chromosome and its alleles from one parent) or loss of imprinting (LOI) of one allele. Imprinted genes are often growth factors, perhaps arising to regulate embryofetal growth but persisting in diploid tissues as potential sources of cell proliferation and tumors. The specific increased IGF2 expression in WIlms tumor suggests it is a potential regulator of cell proliferation rather than rates of mutation. The fact that one allele can increase expression and cause a tumor suggests IGF2 is an oncogene rather than a tumor suppressor that must have both alleles inactivated to produce a tumor.

85. The answer is b. *(Murray, pp 358–373. Scriver, pp 3–45. Lewis, pp 185–204.)* The following mutations were shown in the DNA changes:

a. Missense (Cys to Leu)
b. Nonsense (Tyr to stop)
c. Missense (Ser to Phe)
d. Harmless (Tyr to Tyr)
e. Missense (Leu to Phe)

Most of the mutations shown result in a missense effect, with a different amino acid being incorporated into the same site in a protein. This may or may not have an effect depending on its location. Some single-base mutations are harmless because of the degeneracy of the genetic code, whereby more than one triplet code exists for all amino acids except tryptophan and methionine. Choice a contains two mutations, one degenerate and the other missense.

DNA coding: 3′-ACGACGACG-5′ to 3′-ACAAACACG-5′
mRNA: 5′-UGCUGCUGC-3′ to 5′-UGUUUGUGC-3′
Protein: Cys-Cys-Cys to Cys-Leu-Cys

Nonsense mutations occur when the reading of the normal termination signal is changed. This can occur by mutation to a stop signal as in choice b, by deletions near a stop codon, or by insertions.

86. The answer is c. *(Murray, pp 374–395. Scriver, pp 525–537. Lewis, pp 205–216.)* Southern analysis using methylation-sensitive or insensitive endonuclease restriction in the first two panels of the figure suggests both p57 alleles in the tumor are methylated. Only the larger fragment is detected in the patient sample when restricted with methylation-sensitive endonuclease (second panel). The accompanying Northern blot shows markedly decreased amounts of p57 mRNA, supporting a connection between p57 allele methylation and silencing of expression. The maternal allele of p57 is undermethylated and expressed in normal tissues, and its loss of imprinting (methylation) is one of the few situations where epigenetic silencing appears to be the sole carcinogenic event.

87. The answer is d. *(Murray, pp 374–395. Scriver, pp 3–45.)* Several operons in *Escherichia coli*, including the lac operon, are subject to catabolite repression. In the presence of glucose, there is decreased manufacture of cyclic AMP (cAMP) by adenylate cyclase. Low glucose levels increase production of cAMP, which binds to the catabolite activator protein (CAP). The cAMP-CAP complex binds to the promoters of several responsive operons at catabolite activator protein (CAP) binding sites, greatly enhancing transcription of operon RNA. This positive control stimulates use of more exotic metabolites when glucose is not available and conserves energy when glucose is plentiful. High levels of glucose lower cAMP levels and direct metabolism toward constitutive glucose pathways such as glycolysis.

88. The answer is c. *(Murray, pp 374–395. Scriver, pp 3–45. Lewis, pp 185–204.)* Certain regulatory elements act on genes on the same chromosome ("cis"), while others can regulate genes on the opposite chromosome ("trans"). The terminology makes analogy to carbon-carbon double bonds, where two modifying groups may both be above or below the bond (cis) or opposite it (trans). Cis regulatory elements like the lac operator and promoter or mammalian enhancers are usually DNA sequences (regulatory sequences) adjoining or within the regulated gene. Transregulatory elements like the lac repressor protein or mammalian transcription factors are usually diffusible proteins (regulatory factors) that can interact with adjoining target genes or with target genes on other chromosomes. Classification of bacterial elements as cis or trans requires mating experiments where portions of a second chromosome are introduced by transduction (with bacteriophage) or conjugation (with other bacteria). The distinction between cis and trans is fundamental for understanding how regulators work.

89. The answer is d. *(Murray, pp 374–395. Scriver, pp 3–45. Lewis, pp 64–65.)* Mammalian regulatory factors are much more diverse than those of bacteria, possessing several types of structural domains. Activators of transcription, such as steroid hormones, may enter the cell and bind to regulatory factors at specific sites called ligand-binding domains; these intracellular "receptors" are analogous to G protein-linked membrane receptors that extend into the extracellular space. Response elements are not regulatory factors but DNA sequences near the transcription site for certain types of genes (e.g., steroid-responsive and heat shock-responsive genes). Regulatory factors interact with specific DNA sequences through their DNA-binding domains and with other regulatory factors through transcription-activating domains. Some regulatory factors have antirepressor domains that counteract the inhibitory effects of chromatin proteins (histones and nonhistones).

90. The answer is d. *(Murray, pp 341–357, 374–395. Scriver, pp 3–45. Lewis, pp 205–216.)* The POMC gene provides a mammalian example in which several proteins are derived from the same RNA transcript. Unlike the polycistronic mRNA of the bacterial lactose operon, mammalian cells generate several mRNAs or proteins from the same gene by variable protein processing or by alternative splicing. Variable protein processing preserves the peptide products of some gene regions but degrades those from others. Alternative splicing would often produce proteins composed of different exon combinations with the same terminal exon and carboxy-terminal peptide, but could remove the terminal exon in some proteins and produce different C-terminal peptides. Different transcription factors or enhancers in different brain regions could regulate the total amounts of POMC gene transcript but not the types of protein produced. Elongation of protein synthesis involves GTP cleavage but is not differentially regulated in mammalian tissues.

91. The answer is a. *(Murray, pp 374–395. Scriver, pp 4571–4636. Lewis, pp 205–216.)* Imbalance of globin chain synthesis occurs in the thalassemias. Deficiency of α-globin chains (α-thalassemia—141900) is common in Asian populations and may be associated with abnormal hemoglobins composed of four β-globin chains (hemoglobin H) or (in fetuses and newborns) of four γ-globin chains (hemoglobin Bart's). Mutation in a transcription factor necessary for expression of α-globin could ablate α-globin expression, since the same factor could act in trans on all four copies of the α-globin genes (two α-globin loci). Mutation of a regulatory sequence element that acts in cis would inactivate only one α-globin gene, leaving others to produce α-globin in reduced amounts (mild α-thalassemia). Deletions of one α-globin would produce a similar mild phenotype, and deficiencies of transcription factors regulating α- and β-globin genes would not produce chain imbalance.

92. The answer is d. *(Murray, pp 374–395. Scriver, pp 4571–4636. Lewis, pp 220–225.)* Missense mutations are those in which a single base change (point mutation) results in a codon that encodes for a different amino acid residue. The effects of these types of mutations can range from very minor or even undetectable to major, depending on the importance of the altered residue to protein folding and function. Nonsense mutations are also point mutations in which the affected codon is altered to a stop (nonsense) codon, resulting in a truncated protein. Frameshift mutations are due to one or two base pair insertions or deletions such that the reading frame is altered. These mutations generally lead to truncated proteins as well, since in most protein coding regions the unused reading frames contain numerous stop codons.

93. The answer is b. *(Murray, pp 374–395. Scriver, pp 3–45. Lewis, pp 171–184.)* The boys have an X-linked recessive condition called α-thalassemia/mental retardation or ATR-X syndrome (301040). The X-encoded gene has an unknown function in the brain as well as being a factor that regulates α-globin gene transcription. In order to affect all four α-globin genes, the X-encoded gene must produce a transacting factor; second mutations altering enhancers or promoters would be cis-acting and affect only one α-globin gene. Pseudogenes are functionless gene copies, so altered expression would not influence α-globin chain synthesis.

94. The answer is c. *(Murray, pp 580–597. Scriver, pp 645–664. Lewis, pp 331–454.)* This case is an example of Burkitt lymphoma, which may affect the tonsils or other lymphoid tissues. The translocation places the myc oncogene on chromosome 8 downstream of the very active heavy-chain locus on chromosome 14, activating myc gene expression in B-cells and their derivatives. The translocation is likely an aberrant form of the normal DNA rearrangements that generate unique heavy-chain genes in each B-cell. The translocation joins one chromosome 8 to one chromosome 14, leaving their homologues unaffected. The cause for the phenotype must therefore be transacting, since cis-acting effects would pertain only to the translocated loci and not affect the homologous untranslocated loci. Activation of a tumor-promoting gene (oncogene) on chromosome 8 could produce an enlarged tonsil, while underactivity of immunoglobulin production due to one-half expression could decrease immune function but would not completely ablate the processes in choices a, b, d, and e. At the genetic level, transacting events are autosomal dominant in that one of the two homologous loci is abnormal and produces a phenotype. Mutations of cis-acting events must disrupt both homologous loci to produce phenotypes, making them autosomal recessive at the genetic level.

Acid-Base Equilibria, Amino Acids, and Protein Structure/Function

Acid-Base Equilibria, Amino Acids, and Protein Structure

Questions

DIRECTIONS: Each item below contains a question or incomplete statement followed by suggested responses. Select the **one best** response to each question.

95. A 2-day-old neonate becomes lethargic and uninterested in breast-feeding. Physical examination reveals hypotonia (low muscle tone), muscle twitching that suggests seizures, and tachypnea (rapid breathing). The child has a normal heartbeat and breath sounds with no indication of cardiorespiratory disease. Initial blood chemistry values include normal glucose, sodium, potassium, chloride, and bicarbonate (HCO_3^-) levels; initial blood gas values reveal a pH of 7.53, partial pressure of oxygen (Po_2) normal at 103 mmHg, and partial pressure of carbon dioxide (Pco_2) decreased at 27 mmHg. Which of the following treatment strategies is most appropriate?

a. Administer alkali to treat metabolic acidosis
b. Administer alkali to treat respiratory acidosis
c. Decrease the respiratory rate to treat metabolic acidosis
d. Decrease the respiratory rate to treat respiratory alkalosis
e. Administer acid to treat metabolic alkalosis

96. A newborn with tachypnea and cyanosis is found to have a blood pH of 7.1. A serum bicarbonate is measured as 12 mM, but the blood gas machine that would determine the partial pressures of oxygen (Po_2) and carbon dioxide (Pco_2) is broken. Recall the pK_a of 6.1 for carbonic acid (reflecting the HCO_3^-/CO_2 equilibrium in blood) and the fact that the blood CO_2 concentration is equal to the Pco_2 in mmHg (normal value = 40 mmHg) multiplied by 0.03. Which of the following treatment strategies is most appropriate?

a. Administer oxygen to improve tissue perfusion and decrease metabolic acidosis
b. Administer oxygen to decrease respiratory acidosis
c. Increase the respiratory rate to treat respiratory acidosis
d. Decrease the respiratory rate to treat respiratory acidosis
e. Administer medicines to decrease renal hydrogen ion excretion

97. A 72-year-old male with diabetes mellitus (222100) is evaluated in the emergency room because of lethargy, disorientation, and long, deep breaths (Kussmaul respirations). Initial chemistries on venous blood demonstrate high glucose at 380 mg/dL (normal up to 120) and a pH of 7.3. Recalling the normal bicarbonate (22–28 mM) and Pco_2 (33–45 mmHg) values, which of the following additional test results is consistent with the man's pH and breathing pattern?

a. A bicarbonate of 5 mM and Pco_2 of 10 mmHg
b. A bicarbonate of 15 mM and Pco_2 of 30 mmHg
c. A bicarbonate of 15 mM and Pco_2 of 40 mmHg
d. A bicarbonate of 20 mM and Pco_2 of 45 mmHg
e. A bicarbonate of 25 mM and Pco_2 of 50 mmHg

98. Several families are studied whose affected individuals have nephrogenic diabetes insipidus (125800). This disease causes childhood symptoms of polyuria (frequent urination), polydipsia (constant thirst and frequent drinking), poor growth, and hypernatremia (increased serum sodium concentration). Administration of antidiuretic hormone was not curative, focusing attention on a renal water loss due to a transport defect. A gene named aquaporin-2 was cloned from renal tubular epithelium, its amino acid sequence derived, and structural domains hypothesized to facilitate separation of mutations from benign variants (polymorphisms). The hypothesized structure contained several transmembrane domains demarcated by β-turns, and these potential water channels were found to be mutated in affected individuals. Which of the following amino acids is most suggestive of β-turns?

a. Arginine and lysine
b. Aspartic acid and glutamic acid
c. Leucine and valine
d. Glycine and proline
e. Tryptophan and tyrosine

99. A teenager presents with acute abdominal pain and is noted to have mildly yellow whites of the eyes (scleral icterus). Blood counts indicate a low hemoglobin concentration and the blood smear shows sphere-shaped instead of biconcave red blood cells. The teen's mother reports that she, her father, and several other relatives have anemia, and that they have been diagnosed with a form of spherocytosis (182900) that is caused by mutations in the ankyrin structural protein of erythrocytes. The student on the case is asked to prepare discussion of clinical-molecular correlation on morning rounds, and downloads a diagram of ankyrin structure and amino acid sequence. The structure has domains of antiparallel α-helices, which facilitate stacking of ankyrins into ordered arrays. As the student attempts correlation of ankyrin sequence and structure, α-helical domains could be best identified by the absence of which of the following amino acids?

a. Alanine
b. Cysteine
c. Histidine
d. Proline

100. A child presents to a pediatrician after being removed from his parents because of severe neglect. The pediatrician notes the child is undersized with sparse hair, boggy subcutaneous tissue, and a hopeless, depressed look. Marasmus is suspected, and supported with laboratory studies that include a low serum protein concentration. The pediatrician institutes a gradual regimen of increased calories and nutrition, gradual because rapid feeding will produce diarrhea and further protein loss. This is because long-term starvation leads to low protein concentrations, reduced osmotic pressure, and acidosis in the tissues, producing the extra tissue fluid (edema) and catabolic state of marasmus. Marasmus and related starvation conditions (like the swollen abdomen and reddish hair of kwashiorkor) demonstrate the importance of proteins in maintaining tissue hydration and pH. The greatest buffering capacity at physiologic pH would be provided by a protein rich in which of the following amino acids?

a. Lysine
b. Histidine
c. Aspartic acid
d. Valine
e. Leucine

101. A 1-year-old infant presents with several fractures, and a protective services investigation ensues. Laboratory evaluation shows mild anemia, a serum pH of 7.2, and a urine pH that is anomalously high at 8.5. Review of the radiographs shows some increased bone density of the skull and limbs, and the diagnosis is changed from battered child to a form of osteopetrosis (259730). This condition is caused by mutations in the gene for one form of carbonic anhydrase, the enzyme catalyzing reversible hydration of carbon dioxide ($CO_2 + H_2O \leftrightarrows H_2CO_2 \leftrightarrows H^+ + HCO_3^-$). The discrepant blood and urine pH values in the patient are best explained by which of the following?

a. Decreased renal carbonic anhydrase with reduced conversion and excretion of bicarbonate in urine
b. Increased renal carbonic anhydrase with reduced conversion and excretion of bicarbonate into urine
c. Decreased renal carbonic anhydrase with reduced formation and excretion of hydrogen ion into urine
d. Decreased renal carbonic anhydrase with increased formation and excretion of hydrogen ion into urine
e. Increased renal carbonic anhydrase with reduced formation and excretion of hydrogen ion into urine

102. A 2-year-old child has been healthy until she developed a severe gastroenteritis with progressive sleepiness and fatigue. On presentation to her pediatrician, she has obvious signs of dehydration with no tears on crying, dry mucous membranes, tenting of her skin (retention of a skin fold when pinched), and lack of urination. Her respiratory rate is normal and her lips pink, suggestive of good aeration. Initial laboratory values indicate a low glucose with normal electrolyte values (sodium of 140, potassium of 4.5, chloride of 110) except for bicarbonate (8) and pH (7.1). She does not have glucose (dextrostix negative) or ketones (ketostix negative) in her urine. These values are most consistent with which of the following?

a. A first episode of diabetes mellitus
b. Respiratory acidosis due to lethargy and poor breathing
c. Respiratory acidosis suggestive of a toxin ingestion
d. Metabolic acidosis with anion gap suggesting buildup of a negatively charged metabolite
e. Metabolic acidosis without anion gap suggestive of hidden ketones.

103. A severe form of osteogenesis imperfecta (166210) was noted where newborn infants have extremely deformed limbs and chest, causing them to die shortly after birth because their chest wall is not adequate for respiration. This "type II" severe form was initially thought to be autosomal recessive as opposed to autosomal dominant for the milder type I, but was later shown to involve mutations in type I collagen like other forms of osteogenesis imperfecta. Recall that collagen is a fibrous protein consisting of three peptide chains entwined in a triple helix, formed by a repeating amino acid motif (where X or Y can be any amino acid). Which of the following shows the repeating 3-amino acid motif most compatible with collagen triple helix formation and the mutation most likely to cause severe osteogenesis imperfecta?

a. Pro-X-Y mutated to Gly-X-Y in one repeat
b. Ala-X-Y mutated to Leu-X-Y in one repeat
c. Ala-X-Y mutated to Gly-X-Y in one repeat
d. Gly-X-Y mutated to Ala-X-Y in one repeat
e. Gly-X-Y mutated to Pro-X-Y in one repeat

104. A male infant does well in the nursery but seems to have a reaction to cereal introduced at age 6 weeks. The infant begins vomiting severely, often spewing vomitus across the crib (projectile vomiting). Concern about food allergy persists until an experienced surgeon sits with her hand over the infant's stomach for 20 minutes at the bedside, feeling a small oval shape that has been described as an olive. The surgeon obtains electrolytes and blood gases preparatory to anesthesia. Which of the combinations of laboratory results below and their interpretations are most likely for this infant?

a. Low P_{CO_2}, normal bicarbonate, normal chloride, high pH—pure respiratory alkalosis
b. Low P_{CO_2}, low bicarbonate, low pH, low chloride—compensated metabolic acidosis
c. Normal P_{CO_2}, low bicarbonate, low pH, normal chloride—pure metabolic acidosis
d. High P_{CO_2}, normal bicarbonate, low pH , normal chloride—pure respiratory acidosis
e. Normal P_{CO_2}, high bicarbonate, high pH, low chloride—pure metabolic alkalosis

105. A 1-year-old female presents with growth failure and mild elevation of blood urea nitrogen and creatinine (suggesting decreased kidney function). No hormonal or dietary causes of her growth failure are found, and her mother informs her pediatrician that the child seems to avoid light. Referral to an ophthalmologist reveals unusual crystals in her cornea. Measurement of her blood amino acids reveals an unusual peak, which on analysis breaks down into an amino acid with a sulfhydryl group. The derived amino acid furthermore seems to have an ionizable side group with a pK of about 8.3. Which of the following is the most likely amino acid?

a. Lysine
b. Methionine
c. Cysteine
d. Arginine
e. Glutamine

106. A 60-year-old man is brought to his physician from an institution for severe mental deficiency. The physician reviews his family history and finds he has an older sister in the same institution. Their parents are deceased but reportedly had normal intelligence and no chronic diseases. The man sits in an odd position as though he was sewing, prompting the physician to obtain a ferric chloride test on the man's urine. This test turns color with aromatic (ring) compounds, including certain amino acids, and a green color confirms the physician's diagnosis. Which of the following amino acids was most likely detected in the man's urine?

a. Glycine
b. Serine
c. Glutamine
d. Phenylalanine
e. Methionine

107. Water, which constitutes 70% of body weight, may be said to be the "cell solvent." Which of the following properties of water most contributes to its ability to dissolve compounds?

a. Strong covalent bond formed between water and salts
b. Hydrogen bond formed between water and biochemical molecules
c. Hydrophobic bond formed between water and long-chain fatty acids
d. Absence of interacting forces
e. Fact that the freezing point of water is much lower than body temperature

108. A 5-year-old girl displays decreased appetite, increased urinary frequency, and thirst. Her physician suspects new-onset diabetes mellitus (222100) and confirms that she has elevated urine glucose ketones. Which of the following blood values is most compatible with diabetic ketoacidosis?

	pH	Bicarbonate (mM)	Arterial P_{CO_2}
a.	7.05	16.0	52
b.	7.25	20.0	41
c.	7.40	24.5	39
d.	7.66	37.0	30
e.	7.33	12.0	21

109. A child presents with severe vomiting, dehydration, and fever. Initial blood studies show acidosis with a low bicarbonate and an anion gap (the sum of sodium plus potassium minus chloride plus bicarbonate is 40 and larger than the normal 12 ± 2). Preliminary results from the blood amino acid screen show two elevated amino acids, both with nonpolar side chains. A titration curve performed on one of the elevated species shows two ionizable groups with approximate pKs of 2 and 9.5. Which of the following pairs of elevated amino acids is most likely elevated?

a. Aspartic acid and glutamine
b. Glutamic acid and threonine
c. Histidine and valine
d. Leucine and isoleucine
e. Glutamine and isoleucine

110. Which of the hemoglobin designations below best describes the relationship of subunits in the quaternary structure of adult hemoglobin?

a. $(\alpha_1\text{-}\alpha_2)(\beta_1\text{-}\beta_2)$
b. $\alpha_1\text{-}\alpha_2\text{-}\alpha_3\text{-}\alpha_4$
c. $\beta\text{-}\beta\text{-}\beta\text{-}\alpha$
d. $(\beta_1\text{-}\beta_2\text{-}\beta_3\text{-}\alpha_1)$
e. $(\alpha_1\text{-}\beta_1)\text{-}(\alpha_2\text{-}\beta_2)$

111. A 2-year old boy presents with frequent sinus and ear infections, including one, which progressed to staphylococcal bacteria in the blood (bacteremia) and bone infection (osteomyelitis). Family history indicated that his mother had a brother who died young of sepsis and that her mother had two brothers who died young. Suspicion of an X-linked immunoglobulin deficiency led to assay for a phosphokinase that is known to be deficient in Bruton X-linked agammaglobulinemia (300300). Which of the following amino acids could be used as an acceptor for the phosphate group in the Bruton kinase assay?

a. Cysteine
b. Leucine
c. Methionine
d. Tyrosine
e. Tryptophan

112. Blood is drawn from a child with severe anemia and the hemoglobin protein is degraded for peptide and amino acid analysis. Of the results below, which change in hemoglobin primary structure is most likely to correlate with the clinical phenotype of anemia?

a. Ile-Leu-Val to Ile-Ile-Val
b. Leu-Glu-Ile to Leu-Val-Ile
c. Gly-Ile-Gly to Gly-Val-Gly
d. Gly-Asp-Gly to Gly-Glu-Gly
e. Val-Val-Val to Val-Leu-Val

113. An adult with mild, chronic anemia does not respond to iron supplementation. Blood is drawn and the red cell hemoglobin is analyzed. Which of the following results is most likely if the patient has an altered hemoglobin molecule (hemoglobinopathy)?

a. Several proteins but only one red protein detected by high-performance liquid chromatography (HPLC)
b. Two proteins detected in normal amounts by Western blotting
c. Several proteins and two red proteins separated by native gel electrophoresis
d. Two labeled bands a slight distance apart after SDS-gel electrophoresis and reaction with labeled antibody to α- and β-globin
e. A reddish mixture of proteins retained within a dialysis membrane

114. A teenage boy presents with chest pain on exertion. He is noted to be very tall and thin, with lax joints that enable him to do tricks for his friends. His chest is very concave (pectus excavatum), and he has flat feet. His physician suspects Marfan syndrome (154700) and orders DNA testing for fibrillin, the gene that causes Marfan syndrome. The physician explains that fibrillin gene testing is not very sensitive, because it is a large gene with many variations, and each Marfan family tends to have a different type of mutation. Which of the following amino acid changes (derived from the DNA sequence) would be most likely to represent a pathogenetic mutation rather than benign variation (polymorphism)?

a. gly-ser-ala to gly-ser-ser
b. gly-ser-ala to gly-ser-arg
c. gly-ser-ala to gly-ser-gly
d. gly-ser-ala to gly-ser-tyr
e. gly-ser-ala to gly-ser-ser

115. A child presents with multiple blisters over their extremities, first in response to scrapes or bruises, but then appearing regularly with illnesses or at contact sites for clothes, etc. The group of heritable diseases called epidermolysis bullosa (blistering skin—e.g., 131900) is suspected, and the diagnosis is confirmed by DNA testing with a mutation in the gene encoding type 5 keratin. The keratins are notable for their high content of which of the following?

a. Tyrosine
b. Proline
c. Cystine
d. Melanin
e. Serine

116. Parents bring in their 2-week-old child fearful that he has ingested a poison. They had delayed disposing one of the child's diapers, and noted a black discoloration where the urine had collected. Later, they realized that all of the child's diapers would turn black if stored as waste for a day or so. Knowing that phenol groups can complex to form colors, which of the following amino acid pathways are implicated in this phenomenon?

a. The phenylalanine, tyrosine, and homogentisate pathway
b. The histidine pathway
c. The leucine, isoleucine, and valine pathway
d. The methionine and homocystine pathway
e. The arginine and citrulline pathway (urea cycle)

117. Certain amino acids are not part of the primary structure of proteins but are modified after translation. In scurvy, which of the following amino acids that is normally part of collagen is not synthesized?

a. Hydroxytryptophan
b. Hydroxytyrosine
c. Hydroxyhistidine
d. Hydroxyalanine
e. Hydroxyproline

118. A newborn female has a large and distorted cranium, short and deformed limbs, and very blue scleras (whites of the eyes). Radiographs demonstrate multiple limb fractures and suggest a diagnosis of osteogenesis imperfecta (brittle bone disease-155210). Analysis of type I collagen protein, a triple helix formed from two α_1 and one α_2 collagen chains, shows a 50% reduction in the amount of type I collagen in the baby's skin. DNA analysis demonstrates the presence of two normal α_1 alleles and one normal α_2 allele. These results are best explained by which of the following?

a. Deficiency of α_1 collagen peptide synthesis
b. Inability of α_1 chains to incorporate into triple helix
c. Defective α_1 chains that interrupt triple helix formation
d. Incorporation of defective α_2 chains that cause instability and degradation of the triple helix
e. A missense mutation that alters the synthesis of α_1 chains

119. A child with tall stature, loose joints, and detached retinas is found to have a mutation in type II collagen. Recall that collagen consists of a repeating tripeptide motif where the first amino acid of each tripeptide is the same. Which of the following amino acids is the recurring amino acid most likely to be altered in mutations that distort collagen molecules?

a. Glycine
b. Hydroxyproline
c. Hydroxylysine
d. Tyrosine
e. Tryptophan

120. Children with urea cycle disorders present with elevated serum ammonia and consequent neurologic symptoms including altered respiration, lethargy, and coma. Several amino acids are intermediates of the urea cycle, having side ammonia groups that join with free carbon dioxide and ammonia to produce net excretion of ammonia as urea (NH_2CONH_2). Which of the following amino acids has an ammonia group in its side chain and is thus likely to be an intermediate of the urea cycle?

a. Arginine
b. Aspartate
c. Methionine
d. Glutamate
e. Phenylalanine

121. A child who was normal at birth shows developmental delay with coarsened facial features and enlarged liver and spleen by age 1 year. He is suspected of having I-cell disease (inclusion cell disease-252500), a lysosomal storage disease with progressive accumulation of complex carbohydrates and glycoproteins in organs. Affected individuals lack multiple enzymes in their lysosomes (with excess amounts in serum) because mannose-6-phosphate groups that target enzymes to lysosomes are not correctly synthesized. Which of the following techniques for purification of proteins could be used to isolate the putative lysosomal membrane protein that recognizes mannose-6-phosphate groups and transports enzymes into lysosomes?

a. Dialysis
b. Affinity chromatography
c. Gel filtration chromatography
d. Ion exchange chromatography
e. Electrophoresis

122. An adolescent presents with shortness of breath during exercise and is found to be anemic. A hemoglobin electrophoresis is performed that is depicted in the figure below. The adolescent's sample is run with controls including normal, sickle trait, and sickle cell anemia hemoglobin samples and serum. The adolescent is determined to have an unknown hemoglobinopathy. Which of the following lanes contains the adolescent's sample?

a. Lane A
b. Lane B
c. Lane C
d. Lane D
e. Lane E

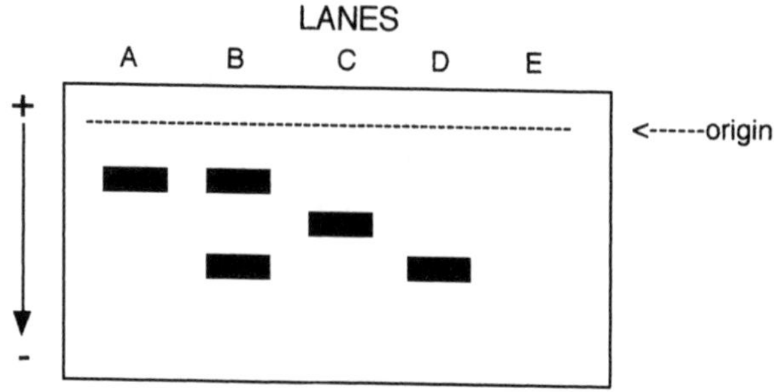

Electrophoretic Hemoglobin Patterns

123. An important enzyme for glycogen release is glycogen phosphorylase, deficiency of which can cause one form of glycogen storage disease (232700). The specific activity of glycogen phosphorylase increases from 2.5 U/mg homogenate protein to 325.5 U/mg protein after being bound to and eluted from a cation exchange column at pH 2.7. Which of the following is the correct conclusion based on this information?

a. The yield of enzyme is greater than 80%
b. The enzyme is negatively charged at pH 2.7
c. The enzyme is purified over 100-fold
d. The enzyme is globular in structure
e. The enzyme is in an activated state

124. A college student with a normal medical history collapses during an intramural basketball game. His friends think he is joking, then notice his blue color and call an ambulance. Resuscitation is unsuccessful and the autopsy reveals dilated cardiac chambers with increased thickness of the ventricular walls (hypertrophic, dilated cardiomyopathy). Electron microscopy of the heart muscle shows abnormal thick filaments, and the pathologist suspects a genetic disorder. Genes encoding which of the following proteins would be most likely to reveal the causative mutation?

a. α-Actinin
b. Actin
c. Myosin
d. Tropomyosin
e. Troponin

125. Which of the following proteolytic enzymes is activated by acid hydrolysis of the proenzyme form?

a. Carboxypeptidase
b. Chymotrypsin
c. Elastase
d. Pepsin
e. Trypsin

126. An infant is normal at birth but becomes lethargic after several feedings; the medical student describes an unusual smell to the urine but is ignored. Infection (sepsis) is suspected, and blood tests show normal white blood cell counts with a serum pH of 7.0. Electrolytes reveal an anion gap, and evaluation for an inborn error of metabolism shows an abnormal amino acid screen. The report states that branch-chain amino acids are strikingly elevated. Which of the following amino acids does the report refer to?

a. Arginine
b. Aspartic acid
c. Isoleucine
d. Lysine
e. Threonine

127. In comparing the secondary structure of proteins, which of the following descriptions applies to both the α helix and the β-pleated sheet?

a. All peptide bond components participate in hydrogen bonding
b. N-Terminals of chains are together and parallel
c. The structure is composed of two or more segments of polypeptide chain
d. N- and C-terminal ends of chains alternate in an antiparallel manner
e. The chains are almost fully extended

128. A child with speech delay is found to have a large, abnormal peak when blood amino acids are measured. The abnormal amino acid migrates towards the cathode, indicating a positively charged side group in addition to its carboxyl and amino groups. Which of the following amino acids is most probable?

a. Alanine
b. Glycine
c. Histidine
d. Leucine
e. Valine

129. The oxygen carrier of muscle is the globular protein myoglobin. Which of the following amino acids is highly likely to be localized within the interior of the molecule?

a. Arginine
b. Aspartic acid
c. Glutamic acid
d. Valine
e. Lysine

130. A child stops making developmental progress at age 2 years and develops coarse facial features with thick mucous drainage. Skeletal deformities including curved spine (kyphosis), thickened and short fingers, and curved limbs appear over the next year, and the child regresses to a vegetative state by age 10 years. The child's urine tests positive for glycosaminoglycans that include which of the following molecules?

a. Collagen
b. γ-Aminobutyric acid
c. Heparan sulfate
d. Glycogen
e. Fibrillin

131. Under normal conditions in blood, which of the following amino acid residues of albumin is neutral?

a. Arginine
b. Aspartate
c. Glutamine
d. Glutamate
e. Histidine

132. Several diseases (osteogenesis imperfecta, Ehlers-Danlos, sensorineural deafness) result from mutations in collagens, a large family of proteins that are important for connective tissue. Different types of collagens occur in bone, ligaments, joints, sclerae (whites of the eyes), and even the inner ear. Collagen peptides have repeating units of gly-X-Y, allowing them to form triple helices that lend structural support to tissues. Which of the following are characteristics of glycine that might account for its use as the initial amino acid in this repeat?

a. Acidic side groups to promote binding
b. Basic side groups to promote binding
c. Hydrophilic to facilitate water incorporation
d. Small molecular diameter compared to other amino acids
e. Optically active with asymmetry to direct the helix

133. Which of the following amino acids is aromatic (ring compound), and in a pathway leading to neurotransmitters and melanin?

a. Arginine
b. Cystine
c. Glutamine
d. Leucine
e. Proline
f. Serine
g. Tyrosine

134. Which of the following substances is primarily found in tendons?

a. Collagen
b. Fibrillin
c. Fibrin
d. Fibronectin
e. Troponin

135. Which of the following is primarily found in the extracellular matrix?

a. Collagen
b. Fibrin
c. Keratin
d. Proteoglycan
e. Troponin

136. The presence of which of the following structural arrangements in a protein strongly suggests that it is a DNA-binding, regulatory protein?

a. α helix
b. β bend
c. β sheet
d. Triple helix
e. Zinc finger

137. During synthesis of mature collagen fibers, which of the following steps occurs within the fibroblast?

a. Hydrolysis of procollagen to form collagen
b. Glycosylation of proline residues
c. Formation of a triple helix
d. Formation of covalent cross-links between molecules
e. Assembly of the collagen fiber

Acid-Base Equilibria, Amino Acids, and Protein Structure

Answers

95. The answer is d. *(Murray, pp 5–13. Scriver, pp 3–45. Lewis, pp 185–204.)* Brain injury or metabolic diseases that irritate the respiratory center may cause tachypnea in term infants, resulting in respiratory alkalosis. The increased respiratory rate removes ("blows off") carbon dioxide from the lung alveoli and lowers blood CO_2, forcing a shift in the indicated equilibrium toward the left:

$$CO_2 + H_2O \leftrightharpoons H_2CO_2 \leftrightharpoons H^+ + HCO_3^-$$

Carbonic acid (H_2CO_2) can be ignored because negligible amounts are present at physiologic pH, leaving the equilibrium:

$$CO_2 + H_2O \leftrightharpoons H^+ + HCO_3^-$$

The leftward shift to replenish the exhaled CO_2 of rapid breathing decreases the hydrogen ion concentration $[H^+]$ and increases the pH ($^-\log_{10}[H^+]$) to produce alkalosis (blood pH above the physiologic norm of 7.4).

Other answers are eliminated because the newborn does not have acidosis, defined as a blood pH below 7.4, either from excess blood acids (metabolic acidosis) or from slower or ineffective respiration with increased $[CO_2]$ (respiratory acidosis). The baby also does not have metabolic alkalosis, caused by loss of hydrogen ion from the kidney (e.g., with renal tubular disease) or stomach (e.g., with severe vomiting). Respiratory alkalosis is best treated by eliminating the underlying disease which will diminish the respiratory rate, elevate blood $[CO_2]$, force the above equilibrium to the right, elevate the $[H^+]$, and decrease the pH. The infant would prove to have a urea cycle disorder such as citrullinemia (215700) with neurologic effects (hypotonia, seizures) of high ammonia concentrations. Withdrawal of milk (protein) and other therapies decreased the ammonia, eliminated the seizures, and restored normal respiration.

96. The answer is a. *(Murray, pp 5–13. Scriver, pp 3–45. Lewis, pp 185–204.)* The equilibrium between an acid and its conjugate base is defined by the Henderson-Hasselbalch equation:

$$pH = pK_a + \log [\text{base}]/[\text{acid}] \text{ or } pH = 6.1 + \log [HCO_3^-]/[CO_2]$$

in the case of carbonic acid. Note that CO_2 is the effective acid and HCO_3^- the conjugate base for carbonic acid due to its complete dissociation in water. Given a pH of 7.1 in the cyanotic newborn, then $7.1 - 6.1 = 1 = \log (10) = \log [HCO_3^-]/[CO_2] = \log [HCO_3^-]/0.03 \times Pco_2$. Since the $[HCO_3^-]$ is 12 mM, the $Pco_2 \times 0.03$ must be 1.2 mM and the Pco_2 40 mmHg. This normal calculated value for Pco_2 means that the baby must have metabolic acidosis, a common accompaniment of hypoxia (low Po_2) that can be treated by providing oxygen or administering alkali to ameliorate the acidosis. A test administration of 100% oxygen is often given to see if an increase in Po_2 is obtained, because children with heart defects (like transposition of the great arteries) may have separate pulmonary and systemic circulations connected by a small shunt (patent ductus arteriosus) that allows minimal delivery of pulmonary oxygen to the tissues. Children who do not respond to oxygen will require extracorporeal membrane oxygen (ECMO) and immediate surgery to create a palliative shunt between circulations (e.g., widened foramen ovale).

Other answers are eliminated because a baby with respiratory acidosis, would have elevated Pco_2, treated by restoring ventilation to blow off CO_2. Renal treatment of acidosis by increasing acid excretion or alkali retention is not effective for severe hypoxia.

97. The answer is b. *(Murray, pp 5–13. Scriver, pp 1471–1488. Lewis, pp 185–204.)* The man is acidotic as defined by the pH lower than the normal 7.4. His hyperventilation with Kussmaul respirations can be interpreted as compensation by the lungs to blow off CO_2, lower Pco_2, increase $[HCO_3^-]/[CO_2]$ ratio, and raise pH. The correct answer therefore includes a low Pco_2, eliminating choices c through e. Using the Henderson-Hasselbalch equation indicates that the pH minus the pK for carbonic acid

(7.3 – 6.1 = 1.2) equals log [15]/[0.03 × 30 mmHg] or log [15/0.9]. These values correspond to those in choice b. The man has compensated his metabolic acidosis (caused by the accumulation of ketone bodies such as acetoacetic acid) by increasing his respiratory rate and volume. The treatment of diabetes is administration of insulin to restore glucose entry into cells, fluids to reverse dehydration, and potassium and/or phosphate administration to correct deficits caused by poor renal perfusion.

98. The answer is d. *(Murray, pp 5–13. Scriver, pp 3–45. Lewis, pp 185–204.)* A β-turn structure consists of four amino acids in which the first residue is hydrogen bonded to the fourth residue of the turn (see Fig. 7A). Glycine residues are small and flexible, while proline residues assume a cis or flattened conformation, making these residues amenable to tight turns. Transport proteins often have several membrane-spanning domains demarcated by β turns that allow them to exit and return back into the membrane. These transmembrane domains form channels that regulate transport of ions and water in organs like lung, gut, and kidney. Nephrogenic diabetes insipidus results when the kidney is less responsive to antidiuretic hormone excreted by the posterior pituitary, causing abnormal water excretion, dehydration, and electrolyte disturbances. Treatment is difficult and in part utilizes the paradoxical effect of some diuretics (e.g. chlorthiazide or Diuril) in restoring sodium balance.

99. The answer is d. *(Murray, pp 5–13. Scriver, pp 3–45. Lewis, pp 185–204.)* A stable α-helix requires hydrogen bonding between peptide bonds at four amino acid intervals (see Fig. 7B). Every peptide bond in the helix participates in this hydrogen bonding. Proline is uncommon in α-helices because it destabilizes the helix by introducing a kink and cannot hydrogen bond with other residues. Other residues with negative (glutamates, aspartates) or positive (lysine, arginine) charges will also destabilize the helix if present in large blocks. Ankyrin mutations that cause spherocytosis disrupt the α-helical domains and interfere with ankyrin stacking that contributes to red cell shape. The altered shape reduces red cell survival, increases hemolysis, and increases the amount of heme converted to bilirubin. Increased bilirubin may be seen in the whites of the eyes (sclerae) or skin as a yellow color (jaundice). Increased storage of bilirubin in the gall bladder may cause gall stones and inflammation (cholecystitis), leading to acute abdominal pain and sometimes requiring gall bladder removal (cholecystectomy).

100. The answer is b. *(Murray, pp 5–13. Scriver, pp 3–45. Lewis, pp 185–204.)* Proteins can be effective buffers of body and intracellular fluids. Buffering capacity is dependent on the presence of amino acids having ionizable side chains with pKas near physiologic pH. In the example given, only histidine has an ionizable imidazolium group that has a pK close to neutrality (pK = 6.0). Valine and leucine are amino acids with uncharged, branched side chains. Lysine has a very basic amino group (pK = 10.5) on its aliphatic side chain that is positively charged at physiologic pH, and aspartic acid has a side chain carboxyl (pK = 3.8) that is negative at pH 7.

101. The answer is c. *(Murray, pp 5–13. Scriver, pp 3–45. Lewis, pp 185–204.)* Several forms of carbonic anhydrase exist in human tissues, functioning to catalyze the reversible conversion of carbon dioxide and water to carbonic acid (which in turn dissociates into hydrogen ion and bicarbonate). The concentrations of carbon dioxide will be different among tissues, requiring carbonic anhydrases with different Kms and catalytic properties. The enzyme in renal tubular tissue is important for converting serum and tissue carbon dioxide into hydrogen ion and bicarbonate, allowing for excretion of hydrogen ion in diseases with acidosis. When the kidney cannot excrete hydrogen ion appropriately, a primary renal tubular acidosis ensues with paradoxically high urine pH (lower hydrogen ion concentration and higher pH) compared to serum pH. Renal tubular acidosis has secondary effects on calcification and bone resorption, causing the brittle and dense bones (literally, petrified bones) in the rare recessive osteopetrosis and renal tubular acidosis due to carbonic anhydrase deficiency (259730).

102. The answer is d. *(Murray, pp 5–13. Scriver, pp 3–45. Lewis, pp 185–204.)* Children with inborn errors of organic or fatty acid metabolism often present in the newborn period after separation from the maternal metabolism and ingestion of milk proteins. Those with milder mutations that yield some functional protein (partial enzyme activity) may maintain metabolic balance until an intercurrent illness exaggerates energy needs or causes anorexia/dehydration with need for fat reserves. Since separate enzyme pathways exist for breakdown of long, medium, or short chain fatty acids, deficiency in one (like medium chain fatty acylCoA dehydrogenase or MCAD) may not compromise the child until there are severe demands for fat breakdown and energy once carbohydrates and glycogen are depleted

(3–4 hours after feeds on average). Depletion of glycogen and inability to maintain glucose through gluconeogenesis may lead to low serum glucose (hypoglycemia), and ineffective fatty acid/organic acid breakdown will not yield the ketones seen in hypoglycemia from other causes or in diabetes mellitus where glucose cannot enter cells. Fatty or organic acids that build up due to the enzyme block manifest as hidden anions, causing the kidney to excrete bicarbonate in an effort to balance the major cations (Na^+, K^+) with anions (Cl^-, HCO_3^-). The sum of measured cations is thus greater than the sum of measured anions, producing an anion gap equal to the amount of organic anion. There are more unmeasured anions in normal serum (e.g., phosphates, sulfates) than unmeasured cations (e.g., magnesium, zinc cations) causing a usual anion gap of 8–12. Anion gaps over 20 (~26 in this case), particularly when a pH lower than 7.4 indicates the kidney can no longer compensate, are seen in organic acidemias/fatty acid oxidation disorders or toxic ingestions of anionic substances (e.g., aspirin to yield serum salicylates).

A first episode of diabetes can have transient low rather than high serum glucose, but the switch to normal fatty acid oxidation would produce abundant ketones. Respiratory acidosis should be associated with abnormal respiration and produce a higher bicarbonate to accompany elevated carbon dioxide. The negative ketostix test excludes significant ketone concentrations.

103. The answer is e. *(Lewis, pp 214–215. Murray, pp 30–39. Scriver, pp 5241–5286.)* Collagen is the most abundant fibrous protein and is found in connective tissue, bone, cartilage, skin, ligmants, and tendons as well as other tissues. Collagen consists of two strands of α_1 and one strand of α_2 collagen intertwined in a triple helix. The triple helix has 3.3 residues per turn. The triple helix is stabilized by hydrogen bonds between residues in different strands. The presence of glycine every third residue allows for very tight packing of each strand in the triple helix since glycines are small and confer flexibility. Mutations substituting a larger or differently configured amino acid for the glycine of one repeat would disrupt the tight packing at that position of the collagen strand and alter triple helix conformation; proline substitutions for glycine (answer e) would alter chain direction and be more disruptive than those with alanine (answer d). Substitutions of amino acids at the X-Y positions of a repeat would have less influence on packing, better preserving the triple helix structure. Mutations at positions in the α_1 chain would also be more severe, since two of these strands are incorporated with each triple helix. Milder mutations alter bone collagen to decrease bone thickness and cause susceptibility to fractures. More severe mutations interfere with bone formation during development, causing severe deformities of limbs and chest wall that are incompatible with life. More severe mutations also inhibit collagen synthesis in the sclerae (whites of the eyes), causing them to be thinner so the underlying blue choroid shows through.

104. The answer is e. (*Murray, pp 5–13. Scriver, pp 3–45. Lewis, pp 185–204.*) Pure metabolic acidosis (choice c) or pure metabolic alkalosis (choice e) exhibits abnormal bicarbonate and normal lung function. Pure respiratory acidosis (choice d) or alkalosis (choice a) is associated with normal renal function (and normal blood acids) with a normal bicarbonate and abnormal Pco_2. Choice b must involve compensation, since both the Pco_2 and bicarbonate are abnormal. The infant is affected with pyloric stenosis (179010), blocking the exit of stomach contents into the duodenum and causing vomiting. The blockage is caused by failure of pyloric tissue to regress by cell death during development, leaving a ball of muscular tissue surrounding the pyloric valve (gastro-duodenal junction). The preferred treatment is surgical, slicing the excess tissue (pyloromyotomy) to relieve the blockage. When diagnosis is delayed, infants can die because of severe metabolic alkalosis caused by expulsion of hydrochloric acid in stomach fluid.

105. The answer is c. (*Murray, pp 5–13. Scriver, pp 3–45. Lewis, pp 185–204.*) The amino acid cystine, essentially a dimer of cysteine, accumulates in the lysosomes of patients with cystinosis (219800). It has a sulfhydryl side group with a pKa of 8.3 that is different from the amino side groups of lysine, arginine, and glutamine (pKas 9–12). These patients exhibit progressive vision problems and renal failure, but these problems can be forestalled by cysteamine treatment, which complexes with cystine and allows egress from lysosomes.

106. The answer is d. (*Murray, pp 5–13. Scriver, pp 3–45. Lewis, pp 185–204.*) Before phenylketonuria (261600) was recognized in the 1930s, and before the advent of routine newborn metabolic screening, children with this autosomal recessive disorder developed severe mental retardation without other identifying symptoms. Although few children with developmental disability are placed in institutions today, the movement for release into home or halfway house care in the 1960s and 1970s was complicated by long-term residents who had not developed life skills. Thus, some older individuals in institutions have disorders that could have been detected by modern screening and would never have prompted institutionalization with modern care. Phenylalanine, with its benzene ring, is an essential amino acid that is converted to tyrosine by phenylhydroxylase, the enzyme (or its cofactor biopterin) that is deficient in phenylketonuria.

107. The answer is b. *(Murray, pp 5–13. Scriver, pp 3–45. Lewis, pp 185–204.)* Water molecules have a dipole nature and dissolve salts because of attractions between the water dipoles and the ions that exceed the force of attraction between the oppositely charged ions of the salt. In addition, the latter force is weakened by the high dielectric constant of water. Nonionic but polar compounds are dissolved in water because of hydrogen bonding between water molecules and groups such as alcohols, aldehydes, and ketones.

108. The answer is e. *(Murray, pp 180–189. Scriver, pp 1471–1488. Lewis, pp 185–204.)* In the presence of insulin deficiency, a shift to fatty acid oxidation produces the ketones such as acetoacetate that cause metabolic acidosis. The pH and bicarbonate are low, and there is frequently some respiratory compensation (hyperventilation with deep breaths) to lower the Pco_2, as in choice e. A low pH with high Pco_2 would represent respiratory acidosis (choices a and b—the low-normal bicarbonate values in these choices indicate partial compensation). Choice d represents respiratory alkalosis as would occur with anxious hyperventilation (high pH and low Pco_2, partial compensation with high bicarbonate). Choice c illustrates normal values.

109. The answer is d. *(Murray, pp 14–20. Scriver, pp 1971–2006. Lewis, pp 185–204.)* Leucine and isoleucine have nonpolar methyl groups as side chains. As for any amino acid, titration curves obtained by noting the change in pH over the range of 1–14 would show a pK of about 2 for the primary carboxyl group and about 9.5 for the primary amino group; there would be no additional pK for an ionizable side chain. Recall that the pK is the point of maximal buffering capacity when the amounts of charged and uncharged species are equal (see answer to question 104). Aspartic and glutamic acids (second carboxyl group), histidine (imino group), and glutamine (second amino group) all have ionizable side chains that would give an additional pK on the titration curve. The likely diagnosis here is maple syrup urine disease, which involves elevated isoleucine, leucine, and valine together with their ketoacid derivatives. The ketoacid derivatives cause the acidosis, and the fever suggests that the metabolic imbalance was worsened by an infection.

110. The answer is e. *(Murray, pp 14–20. Scriver, pp 3–45. Lewis, pp 185–204.)* Adult hemoglobin, or hemoglobin A, is composed of four polypeptide chains. Two of the chains are α chains and two are β chains. The chains are held together by noncovalent interactions. The hemoglobin tetramer can best be represented as being composed of two dimers, each containing the two different polypeptides. Thus the designation (α_1-β_1) (α_2-β_2), which refer to dimers 1 and 2, respectively, is the most correct way to refer to the quaternary structure of adult hemoglobin. Hydrophobic interactions are thought to be the main noncovalent interactions holding all four polypeptides together.

111. The answer is d. *(Murray, pp 14–20. Scriver, pp 3–45. Lewis, pp 185–204.)* Serine, threonine, and tyrosine can all be phosphorylated on their side-chain hydroxyl group. In addition, histidine, lysine, arginine, and aspartates are common targets for phosphorylation by protein kinases. Phosphorylation by protein kinases and dephosphorylation by protein phosphatases is a common method for regulating protein activity. In Bruton agammaglobulinemia (300300), deficiency of a tyrosine kinase prevents normal B-cell development. B-cells are the arm of the immune system responsible for making immunoglobulins, so children with B-cell deficiencies have frequent and overwhelming bacterial infections with normal T-cell function (resistance to viral infections).

112. The answer is b. *(Murray, pp 14–20. Scriver, pp 3–45. Lewis, pp 185–204.)* Primary protein structures denote the sequence of amino acids held together by peptide bonds (carboxyl groups joined to amino groups to form amide bonds). The types of amino acids then determine the secondary structure of peptide regions within the protein, sometimes forming spiral α_1-helices or flat pleated sheets. These regional peptide secondary structures then determine the overall three-dimensional tertiary structure of a protein, which is vital for its function. Amino acid substitutions that alter the charge of an amino acid side chain, like the change from glutamic acid (charged carboxyl group) to valine (nonpolar methyl groups) in choice b, are most likely to change the secondary and tertiary protein structure. A change in hemoglobin structure can cause instability, decreased mean cellular hemoglobin concentration (MCHC), and anemia. A change from glutamic acid to valine at position 6 in the β-hemoglobin chain is the mutation responsible for sickle cell anemia (602903).

113. The answer is c. *(Murray, pp 40–48. Scriver, pp 3-45. Lewis, pp 185–204.)* In the technique of polyacrylamide gel electrophoresis (PAGE), the distance that a protein is moved by an electrical current is proportional to its charge and inversely proportional to its size. Patients with normal hemoglobin A have two α-globin and two β_1-globin chains, each encoded by a pair of normal globin alleles. Mutation in one α- or β-globin allele alters the primary amino acid sequence of the encoded globin peptide. If the amino acid change alters the charge of the peptide, then the hemoglobin tetramer assembled with the mutant globin peptide has a different charge and electrophoretic migration than the normal hemoglobin tetramer. The electrophoresis of native (undenatured) hemoglobin therefore produces two species (two bands) rather than one, each retaining its heme molecule and red color. If the hemoglobins were first denatured into their α- and β-globin chains as with SDS-polyacrylamide gel electrophoresis, then the similar size of the α- or β-globin peptides would cause them to move closely together as two colorless bands. Identification of these peptides as globin would require use of labeled antibody specific for globin (Western blotting). Because the sodium dodecyl sulfate (SDS) detergent covers the protein surface and causes all proteins to be negatively charged, the distance migrated is solely dependent (inversely proportional) on protein size. High-performance liquid chromatography (HPLC) uses ionic resins to separate proteins by charge. The columns are run under high pressure, rapidly producing a series of proteins that are separated from most negative to most positive (or vice versa, depending on the charge of the ionic resin). A mutant hemoglobin with altered charge should produce a second red protein in the pattern. In dialysis, semipermeable membranes allow smaller proteins to diffuse into the outer fluid, but not larger proteins such as hemoglobin.

114. The answer is b. *(Murray, pp 14–20. Scriver, pp 5241–5286. Lewis, pp 185–204.)* The amino acids gly (glycine), ser (serine), and alanine (ala) have uncharged and small side groups (the serine hydroxyl group will not be ionized at near-neutral biological pHs of 7–7.4). Replacement of the alanine group with another small and uncharged amino acid would be less likely to alter fibrillin conformation and function than replacement with a charged amino acid like arginine (ammonium group with positive charge on side chain). Although Marfan syndrome (154700) is relatively common at 1 in 3000 births, fibrillin DNA testing remains difficult because the gene is large and susceptible to mutations throughout its length. DNA diagnosis thus requires complete sequencing of the gene in suspect patients, which is cost-prohibitive for commercial laboratories. Once a sequence variation is found, its pathogenicity can be assessed by testing for its presence in the normal parents.

115. The answer is c. *(Murray, pp 40–48. Scriver, pp 3–45. Lewis, pp 185–204.)* Keratins are a type of intermediate filament that comprises a large portion of many epithelial cells. The characteristics of skin, nails, and hair are all due to keratins. Keratins contain a large amount of the disulfide amino acid cystine. Approximately 14% of the protein composing human hair is cystine. This is the chemical basis of depilatory creams, which are reducing agents that render keratins soluble by breaking the disulfide bridges of these insoluble proteins. Mutations in keratins also alter the adherent properties of keratins and keratin-rich tissues, causing fragility (epidermolysis with blisters) or aggregation (hyperkeratosis) of skin cells.

116. The answer is a. *(Murray, pp 249–263. Scriver, pp 1971–2006.)* Lack of the enzyme homogentisate oxidase causes the accumulation of homogentisic acid, a metabolite in the pathway of degradation of phenylalanine and tyrosine. Homogentisate, like tyrosine, contains a phenol group. It is excreted in the urine, where it oxidizes and is polymerized to a dark substance upon standing. Under normal conditions, phenylalanine is degraded to tyrosine, which is broken down through a series of steps to fumarate and acetoacetate. The dark pigment melanin is another end product of this pathway. Deficiency of homogentisate oxidase is called alkaptonuria (black urine—203500), a mild disease discovered by Sir Archibald Garrod, the pioneer of biochemical genetics. Garrod's geneticist colleague, William Bateson, recognized that alkaptonuria, like nearly all enzyme deficiencies, exhibits autosomal recessive inheritance.

117. The answer is e. *(Murray, pp 481–497. Scriver, pp 5241–5286.)* Hydroxyproline and hydroxylysine are not present in newly synthesized collagen. Proline and lysine residues are modified by hydroxylation in a reaction requiring the reducing agent ascorbic acid (vitamin C). The enzymes catalyzing the reactions are prolyl hydroxylase and lysyl hydroxylase. In scurvy, which results from a deficiency of vitamin C, insufficient hydroxylation of collagen causes abnormal collagen fibrils. The weakened collagen in teeth, bone, and blood vessels causes tooth loss, brittle bones with fractures, and bleeding tendencies with bruising and bleeding gums.

118. The answer is d. *(Murray, pp 30–39. Scriver, pp 5241–5286.)* Collagen peptides assemble into helical tertiary structures that form quaternary triple helices. The triple helices in turn assemble end to end to form collagen fibrils that are essential for connective tissue strength. Over 15 types of collagen contribute to the connective tissue of various organs, including the contribution of type I collagen to eyes, bones, and skin. The fact that only one of two α_2 alleles is normal in this case implies that a mutant α_2 allele could be responsible for the disease (even if the α_2 locus is on the X chromosome, since the baby is female with two X chromosomes). The mutant α_2 collagen peptide would be incorporated into half of the type I collagen triple helices, causing a 50% reduction in normal type I collagen. (A mutant α_1 collagen peptide would distort 75% of the molecules because two α_1 peptides go into each triple helix.) The ability of one abnormal collagen peptide allele to alter triple helix structure with subsequent degradation is well-documented and colorfully named protein suicide or, more properly, a dominant-negative mutation.

119. The answer is a. *(Murray, pp 30–39. Scriver, pp 3–45. Lewis, pp 185–204.)* The primary structure of collagen peptides consists of repeating tripeptides with a gly-X-Y motif, where gly is glycine and X and Y are any amino acid. The small CH_2 group connecting the amino and carboxyl groups of glycine contrasts with the larger connecting groups and side chains of other amino acids. The small volume of glycine molecules is crucial for the α helix secondary structure of collagen peptides. This in turn is necessary for their tertiary helical structure and their assembly into quaternary tripeptide, triple-helix structures. The most severe clinical phenotypes caused by amino acid substitutions in collagen peptides are those affecting glycine that prevent a helix formation. The child has a disorder called Stickler's syndrome (108300) that exhibits autosomal dominant inheritance.

120. The answer is a. *(Murray, pp 30–39. Scriver, pp 3–45. Lewis, pp 185–204.)* Arginine is an amino acid used in proteins that is also part of the urea cycle. Citrulline and ornithine are amino acids not used in proteins but important as urea cycle intermediates. Aspartate is condensed with citrulline to form argininosuccinate in the urea cycle, and acetylglutamate is a cofactor in the joining of carbon dioxide with ammonia to form carbamoyl phosphate at the beginning of the urea cycle.

121. The answer is b. *(Murray, pp 30–39. Scriver, pp 3–45. Lewis, pp 185–204.)* Each of the techniques listed separates proteins from each other and from other biologic molecules based on characteristics such as size, solubility, and charge. However, only affinity chromatography can use the high affinity of proteins for specific chemical groups or the specificity of immobilized antibodies for unique proteins. In affinity chromatography, a specific compound that binds to the desired protein—such as an antibody, a polypeptide receptor, or a substrate—is covalently bound to the column material. A mixture of proteins is added to the column under conditions ideal for binding the protein desired, and the column is then washed with buffer to remove unbound proteins. The protein is eluted either by adding a high concentration of the original binding material or by making the conditions unfavorable for binding (e.g., changing the pH). The other techniques are less specific than affinity binding for isolating proteins. Dialysis separates large proteins from small molecules. Ion exchange chromatography separates proteins with an overall charge of one sort from proteins with an opposite charge (e.g., negative from positive). Gel filtration chromatography separates on the basis of size. Electrophoresis separates proteins on the principle that net charge influences the rate of migration in an electric field.

Inclusion-cell disease (mucolipidosis II—252500) can result from deficiency in either of two phosphotransferase enzymes that put mannose-6-phosphate groups on degradative enzymes, targeting them to lysosomes. Mucolipidosis II with multiple mistargeted enzymes is thus similar to but more severe than disorders like Hunter syndrome (iduronate sulfatase deficiency—309900) that result from deficiency of a single lysosomal enzyme.

122. The answer is c. *(Murray, pp 30–39. Scriver, pp 3–45. Lewis, pp 185–204.)* Protein electrophoresis is an important laboratory technique for investigating red cell proteins such as hemoglobin or plasma proteins such as the immunoglobulins. The proteins are dissolved in a buffer of low pH where the amino groups of amino acid side chains are positively charged, causing most proteins to migrate toward the negative electrode (anode). Red cell hemolysates are used for hemoglobin electrophoresis, plasma (blood supernatant with unhemolyzed red cells removed) for plasma proteins. Serum (blood supernatant after clotting) would not contain red cells but would contain many blood enzymes and proteins. In sickle cell anemia, the hemoglobin S contains a valine substitution for the glutamic acid at position 6 in hemoglobin A. Hemoglobin S thus loses two negative charges (loss of a glutamic acid carboxyl group on each of two β-globin chains) compared to hemoglobin A. Hemoglobin S is thus more positively charged and migrates more rapidly toward the anode than hemoglobin A (Fig. 17). Lane B must represent the heterozygote with sickle cell trait (hemoglobins S and A), establishing lane A as the normal and lane D as the sickle cell anemia sample. The hemoglobin in lane C migrates differently from normal and hemoglobin S, as would befit an abnormal hemoglobin that is different from S. Lane E must be serum, which does not contain red blood cells.

123. The answer is c. *(Murray, pp 30–39. Scriver, pp 3–45. Lewis, pp 185–204.)* Proteins can be separated on the basis of their overall charge at a given pH by ion exchange chromatography. At low pH, all proteins have an overall positive charge because carboxyl groups are protonated. Thus, proteins tend to bind to a cation exchange column that has immobilized the negative charges. Usually negatively charged sulfonic polystyrene resin is used, and Na charges are exchanged for the positively charged protein groups. Once binding has occurred, the pH and NaCl concentration of the eluting medium are increased, and proteins that have a low density of net negative charge emerge first, with those having a higher density of negative charge following. The only information that can be obtained from the information given in the question is that the enzyme has been purified over 100-fold. The turnover rate of the enzyme cannot be deduced. Likewise, the yield, which is the amount of original enzyme protein recovered, cannot be determined. The structure of the enzyme is not revealed by the information given.

124. The answer is c. *(Murray, pp 30–39, 556–579. Scriver, pp 5433–5432.)* Cardiac and skeletal muscle are similar in that both are striated and contain two kinds of interacting protein filaments. The thick filaments (15 nm in diameter) contain primarily myosin, while the thin filaments (7 nm in diameter) contain actin, troponin, and tropomyosin. The thick and thin filaments slide past one another during muscle contraction. Myosins are a family of proteins with heavy and light chains, and muscle myosins function as ATPases that bind to thin filaments during contraction. A particular cardiomyopathy (160760) is caused by mutations in the myosin 7 heavy chain gene, one of many causes of acute life-threatening events (ALTE) that can affect previously asymptomatic adults. ALTE are adult equivalents of sudden infant death syndrome (SIDS) or, more inclusively, sudden unexplained death syndrome (SUDS) that affect children. Congenital defects in muscle filaments, potassium channels, and the like, that affect cardiac contractility are substantial contributors to these tragic and unexpected disease categories—important reasons for annual and transitional (sports, precollege) physical examinations.

125. The answer is d. *(Murray, pp 30–39. Scriver, pp 3–45. Lewis, pp 185–204.)* Pepsin is secreted in a proenzyme form in the stomach. Unlike the majority of proenzymes, it is not activated by protease hydrolysis. Instead, spontaneous acid hydrolysis at pH 2 or lower converts pepsinogen to pepsin. Hydrochloric acid secreted by the stomach lining creates the acid environment. All the enzymes secreted by the pancreas are activated at the same time upon entrance into the duodenum. This is accomplished by trypsin hydrolysis of the inactive proenzymes trypsinogen, chymotrypsinogen, procarboxypeptidase, and proelastase. Primer amounts of trypsin are derived from trypsinogen by the action of enteropeptidase secreted by the cells of the duodenum.

126. The answer is c. *(Murray, pp 30–39. Scriver, pp 3–45. Lewis, pp 185–204.)* The carbon next to a carboxyl (C = O) group may be designated as the α carbon, with subsequent carbons as β, γ, δ, etc. α-Amino acids contain an amino group on their α-carbon, as distinguished from compounds like γ-aminobutyric acid, in which the amino group is two carbons down (γ-carbon). In α-amino acids the amino acid, carboxylic acid, and the side chain or R group are all bound to the central α-carbon, which is thus asymmetric (except when R is hydrogen, as for glycine). Amino acids are classified as acidic, neutral hydrophobic, neutral hydrophilic, or basic, depending on the charge or partial charge on the R group at pH 7. Hydrophobic (water-hating) groups are carbon-hydrogen chains like those of leucine, isoleucine, glycine, or valine. Basic R groups, such as those of lysine and arginine, carry a positive charge at physiologic pH owing to protonated amide groups, whereas acidic R groups, such as glutamic acid, carry a negative charge owing to ionized carboxyl groups. Threonine with its hydroxyl side chain is neutral at physiologic pH.

Leucine, isoleucine, and valine are amino acids with branched side groups, and they share a pathway for degradation that is deficient in children with maple syrup urine disease (248600). Their amino groups can be removed, but the resulting carboxy-acids accumulate with resulting acidosis, coma, and death unless a diet free of branch-chained amino acids is instituted.

127. The answer is a. *(Murray, pp 30–39. Scriver, pp 3–45. Lewis, pp 185–204.)* Regular arrangements of groups of amino acids located near each other in the linear sequence of a polypeptide are the secondary structure of a protein. The α helix, β sheet, and β bend are the secondary structures usually observed in proteins. In both the α helix and the β sheet, all the peptide bond components participate in hydrogen bonding. That is, the oxygen components of the peptide bond form hydrogen bonds with the amide hydrogens. In the case of the α helix, all hydrogen bonding is intrachain and stabilizes the helix. In the case of β sheets, the bonds are interchain when formed between the polypeptide backbones of separate polypeptide chains and intrachain when the β sheet is formed by a single polypeptide chain folding back on itself. While the spiral of the α helix prevents the chain from being fully extended, the chains of β sheets are almost fully extended and relatively flat. The chains of β sheets can be either parallel or antiparallel. When the N-terminals of chains run together, the chain or segment is considered parallel. In contrast, when N- and C-terminal ends of the chains alternate, the β-strand is considered antiparallel.

128. The answer is c. *(Murray, pp 14–30. Scriver, pp 3–45. Lewis, pp 185–204.)* Except for terminal amino acids, all α-amino groups and all α-carboxyl groups are utilized in peptide bonds. Thus only the side chains of amino acids may be ionizable in proteins. Seven of the twenty common amino acids have easily ionizable side chains. Lysine, arginine, and histidine have basic side chains (yielding a positive charge at neutral pH); aspartate and glutamate have acidic side chains (yielding a negative charge at neutral pH); and tyrosine and cysteine have hydroxyl/sulfydryl groups (ionizing only at basic pHs or within special environments of protein/enzyme active sites/channels).

Histidinemia (235800) is one of several abnormalities discovered when advances in ion exchange chromatography and paper electrophoresis made screening of blood and urine amino acids distributions feasible for patients. These diagnostic tests allowed confirmation of clinically defined disorders like phenylketonuria (261600), and revealed a host of new disorders like histidinemia or hyperprolinemia (239500). Although these disorders have been traced to specific enzyme deficiencies, their clinical significance is uncertain because many individuals with elevated screens do not have disease.

129. The answer is d. *(Murray, pp 30–39. Scriver, pp 3–45. Lewis, pp 185–204.)* The structure of myoglobin is illustrative of most water-soluble proteins. Globular proteins tend to fold into compact configurations with nonpolar cores. The interior of myoglobin is composed almost exclusively of nonpolar, hydrophobic amino acids like valine, leucine, phenylalanine, and methionine. In contrast, polar hydrophilic residues such as arginine, aspartic acid, glutamic acid, and lysine are found mostly on the surface of the water-soluble protein.

130. The answer is c. *(Murray, pp 30–39. Scriver, pp 3421–3452. Lewis, pp 185–204.)* Glycosaminoglycans (mucopolysaccharides) are polysaccharide chains that may be bound to proteins as proteoglycans. Each proteoglycan is a complex molecule with a core protein that is covalently bound to glycosaminoglycans—repeating units of disaccharides. The amino sugars forming the disaccharides contain negatively charged sulfate or carboxylate groups. The primary glycosaminoglycans found in mammals are hyaluronic acid, heparin, heparan sulfate, chondroitin sulfate, and keratan sulfate. Inborn errors of glycosaminoglycan degradation cause neurodegeneration and physical stigmata described by the outmoded term "gargoylism"—exemplified by Hurler syndrome (252800). Glycogen is a polysaccharide of glucose used for energy storage and has no sulfate groups. Collagen and fibrillin are important proteins in connective tissue. γ-aminobutyric acid is a γ-amino acid involved in neurotransmission.

131. The answer is c. *(Murray, pp 14–20. Scriver, pp 3–45. Lewis, pp 185–204.)* In blood and other solutions at physiologic pH (approximately 7), only terminal carboxyl groups, terminal amino groups, and ionizable side chains of amino acid residues in proteins have charges. The basic amino acids lysine, arginine, and histidine have positive charges (protonated amines). The acidic amino acids aspartate and glutamate have negative charges (ionized carboxyls). Glutamine possesses an uncharged but hydrophilic side chain.

132. The answer is d. *(Murray, pp 30–39. Scriver, pp 3–45. Lewis, pp 185–204.)* All α-amino acids have an asymmetric α-carbon atom to which an α-carboxyl group, an α-amino group, and an α-side chain are attached. Levorotary (L) isomers of amino acids compose proteins in nature. Because glycine has a hydrogen as its side chain, with two hydrogens, an amino group, and a carboxyl group on the α-carbon, it is the only optically inactive amino acid. Side chains contribute the distinctive properties at physiological pH to each amino acid (and hence proteins), which include: basic (positive); acidic (negative); neutral polar; neutral nonpolar; sulfur-containing (thiol); hydroxyl-containing; aromatic; hydrophobic; hydrophilic; branched; or straight-chained. Glycine is not a positively or negatively charged amino acid nor is it hydrophobic. Instead, glycine offers great flexibility to a peptide chain because of its small hydrogen side chain; thus, glycine is found in β-turns in proteins like the collagens.

133. The answer is g. *(Murray, pp 14–30. Scriver, pp 3–45. Lewis, pp 185–204.)* Amino acids are composed of an α-carbon atom bonded to carboxyl, amino, and side chain R groups. The α-carbon is so named because it is adjacent to the carboxyl group. The distinctive R side chains, with their variation in charge, shape, size, and reactivity, account for the diversity of protein conformations and functions. Aliphatic amino acids contain carbon chains as side groups (e.g., leucine, isoleucine, and valine). Aromatic amino acids have rings in their side groups, like phenylalanine and tyrosine. Those with carbon chains or rings are hydrophobic in nature, causing them to sequester together away from water in the interior of proteins. Polar amino acids have ionizable groups on their side chains, including basic amino acids (positively charged at neutral pH—lysine, arginine, histidine) and acidic amino acids (negatively charged at neutral pH—glutamate, aspartate). Polar amino acids are located on the outsides of proteins and moderate interactions of proteins with themselves and smaller molecules. Aromatic rings interact to produce colors, and the benzene ring of tyrosine is incorporated into melanin. Other branches of this pathway produce important neurotransmitters such as catecholamines and dopamine. External amino acids also provide substrates for enzymic modification of protein conformation and function, illustrated by the phosphorylation of tyrosine by kinases.

134. The answer is a. *(Murray, pp 30–39. Scriver, pp 3–45. Lewis, pp 185–204.)* Collagens are insoluble proteins that have great tensile strength. They are the main fibers composing the connective tissue elements of skin, bone, teeth, tendons, and cartilage. Collagen is composed of tropocollagen, a triple-stranded helical rod rich in glycine, proline, and hydroxyproline residues. Troponin is found in muscle, fibrillin in heart valves, blood vessels, and ligaments [it is defective in Marfan syndrome (154700)]. Fibrin is a component of blood clots and fibronectin is a component of extracellular matrix.

135. The answer is d. *(Murray, pp 30–39. Scriver, pp 3–45. Lewis, pp 185–204.)* The major macromolecular components of ground substance are proteoglycans, which are made up of polysaccharide chains attached to core proteins. The polysaccharide chains are made up of repeats of negatively charged disaccharide units. This polyanionic quality of proteoglycans allows them to bind water and cations and thus determines the viscoelastic properties of connective tissues. Collagen is the other major component of connective tissue besides ground substance. The cornified layer of epidermis derives its toughness and waterproof nature from keratin. Keratins are disulfide-rich proteins that compose the cytoskeletal elements known as intermediate filaments. Hair and animal horns are also composed of keratin. Troponin is a component of muscle, fibrin of blood clots.

136. The answer is e. *(Murray, pp 30–39. Scriver, pp 3–45. Lewis, pp 185–204.)* Regulatory proteins must bind with great specificity and high affinity to the correct portion of DNA. Several structural motifs have been discovered in DNA-regulatory proteins: the zinc finger, the leucine zipper, and the helix-turn-helix (found in homeotic proteins). Because of the uniqueness of these structural arrangements, their presence in a protein indicates that the protein might bind to DNA. The β sheet, β bend, and α helix are secondary structures found in polypeptide chains, and the triple helix is a tertiary structure composed of three polypeptides as in collagen.

137. The answer is c. *(Murray, pp 30–39. Scriver, pp 3–45. Lewis, pp 185–204.)* The connective tissue fiber collagen is synthesized by fibroblasts. However, because the length of the finished collagen fibers is many times greater than that of the cell of origin, a portion of assembly occurs extracellularly. The intracellular formation of the biosynthetic precursor of collagen, procollagen peptides pro-α_1(I) and pro-α_2, occurs in the following steps: (1) synthesis of polypeptides, (2) hydroxylation of proline and lysine residues, (3) glycosylation of lysine residues (proline residues are not glycosylated), (4) formation of the triple helix, and (5) secretion. Once outside the fibroblasts, procollagen molecules are activated by fibroblast-specific procollagen peptidases. Before specific proteolytic cleavage of procollagen, tropocollagen bundles do not assemble into collagen fibers. Once the collagen fibers are formed, aldo cross-links between lysine residues and histidine-aldo cross-links are formed. These cross-links covalently bind the collagen chains to one another. The extent and type of cross-linking determines the flexibility and strength of the collagen mass formed.

Protein Structure/Function

Questions

DIRECTIONS: Each item below contains a question or incomplete statement followed by suggested responses. Select the **one best** response to each question.

138. A 72-year-old woman with emphysema presents to the emergency room with fatigue and respiratory distress. Which of the following sets of arterial blood gas values would represent her condition and reflect a shift of the hemoglobin oxygen dissociation curve to the right?

a. pH 7.05, bicarbonate 15 mM, Pco_2 60, Po_2 88
b. pH 7.15, bicarbonate 10 mM, Pco_2 30, Po_2 88
c. pH 7.25, bicarbonate 15 mM, Pco_2 30, Po_2 88
d. pH 7.4, bicarbonate 24 mM, Pco_2 60, Po_2 88
e. pH 7.45, bicarbonate 15 mM, Pco_2 60, Po_2 88

139. The ability of hemoglobin to serve as an effective transporter of oxygen and carbon dioxide between lungs and tissues is explained by which of the following properties?

a. The isolated heme group with ferrous iron binds oxygen much more avidly than carbon dioxide
b. The α- and β-globin chains of hemoglobin have very different primary structures than myoglobin
c. Hemoglobin utilizes oxidized ferric iron to bind oxygen, in contrast to the ferrous ion of myoglobin
d. In contrast to myoglobin, hemoglobin exhibits greater changes in secondary and tertiary structure after oxygen binding
e. Hemoglobin binds proportionately more oxygen at low oxygen tension than does myoglobin

140. A 65-year-old obese male presents with pain radiating down the left arm and shortness of breath. A serum lactate dehydrogenase (LDH) level is obtained to evaluate possible myocardial infarction, and its activity is only slightly elevated. Shortly thereafter the laboratory calls, saying that a more detailed analysis of LDH does suggest myocardial damage. The managing physician knows that lactate dehydrogenase is composed of two different polypeptide chains arranged in the form of a tetramer. Which of the following is the likely correlation between LDH measures and the likelihood of myocardial infarction?

a. LDH is an enzyme specific to the endocardium
b. LDH is mainly localized in liver, and its elevation in cardiac disease occurs because of heart failure
c. LDH isozymes are composed of different subunit combinations, some released during inflammation following heart attacks
d. LDH isozymes are composed of different subunit combinations, some specific for heart and released with myocardial damage
e. LDH isozymes are composed of different subunit combinations, some specific for vascular endothelium and released with infarction

141. A 28-year-old woman presents to her obstetrician at week 23 of pregnancy, complaining of extreme fatigue. Evaluations of serum iron level and fetal well-being are normal, but the nurse notices a weak and irregular pulse. Chest x-ray reveals an enlarged heart and the electrocardiogram reveals a short PR interval and prolonged QRS, including a slurred-up stroke of the R wave called a delta wave. The ECG is read as showing Wolff-Parkinson-White syndrome, a condition with risks for paroxysmal supraventricular tachycardia. The physician considers treatment with calcium channel regulators, balancing their risks to mother and fetus. Contraction of cardiac and skeletal muscle is initiated by the binding of calcium to which of the following substances?

a. Actin
b. Actomyosin
c. Myosin
d. Tropomyosin
e. Troponin

142. A previously healthy 2-year-old becomes grey and dusky looking and is brought to his physician with suspicion of heart disease. Rather than doing a cardiac evaluation, the physician asks about the family's water supply and notes they are farmers using well water. The physician then provides some oxygen and vitamin C with rapid improvement of the child's color. The child's problem was most likely due to which of the following?

a. Nitrates in well water cause reduced hemoglobin (methemoglobin) and cyanosis in all families exposed
b. Cyanide in well water poisoning the respiratory chain
c. Nitrates in well water interacting with heterozygous methemoglobin reductase deficiency to produce methemoglobin
d. Nitrates in well water competing for hemoglobin oxygen binding, producing a sigmoidal binding curve
e. Carbon dioxide released by methane fuels causing decreased hemoglobin O_2 affinity

143. A child is evaluated for anemia and is found to have increased indirect bilirubin in serum and plasma free hemoglobin suggestive of hemolysis (lysis of red blood cells). Enzyme assays reveal deficiency of 2,3-diphosphoglycerate mutase, with low concentrations of 2,3-DPG in red cells. The child shows greater respiratory distress than expected for the degree of anemia. Which of the following best explains this?

a. Lower 2,3-bisphosphoglycerate (BPG) concentrations will shift the oxygen dissociation curve for hemoglobin to the right, with greater release of oxygen to tissues
b. Lower 2,3-bisphosphoglycerate (BPG) will shift the oxygen dissociation curve for hemoglobin to the right, with lesser release of oxygen to tissues
c. Lower 2,3-bisphosphoglycerate (BPG) will shift the oxygen dissociation curve for hemoglobin to the left, with greater release of oxygen to tissues
d. Lower 2,3-bisphosphoglycerate (BPG) will shift the oxygen dissociation curve for hemoglobin to the left, with lesser release of oxygen to tissues
e. Lower 2,3-bisphosphoglycerate (BPG) will destablize the red cell by allowing oxidation of hemoglobin

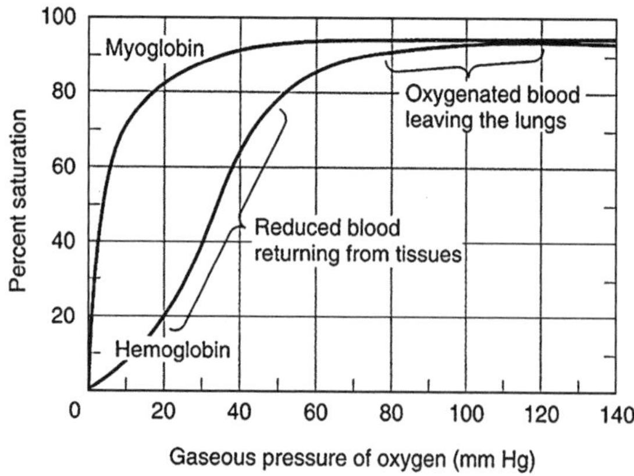

144. A young man with hypercholesterolemia is rushed to the hospital with crushing chest pain radiating to his left arm and a probable heart attack. Which of the following treatments should be considered?

a. A platelet transfusion
b. Heparin infusion
c. Thrombin infusion
d. Fibrinogen infusion
e. Tissue plasminogen activator infusion

145. A young college student presents to the health clinic with symptoms of increased urination (polyuria), avid thirst and water drinking (polydipsia), and weight loss without dieting. Significant in the family history is her father's death at age 42 of what was said to be "acute diabetes." Her father's sister and a paternal aunt also have diabetes, described as adult onset or type II. Laboratory evaluation reveals increased glucose in blood (hyperglycemia), urine (glucosuria), and urinary ketones. However, Western blotting of insulin species shows normal amounts of protein with a higher molecular size then usual. Which of the following is the most likely explanation?

a. Defective processing of proinsulin to insulin, causing decreased insulin action and diabetes mellitus
b. Defective insulin-like growth factors that must act in concert with insulin
c. Defective insulin receptors with reduced insulin action
d. Progressive fibrosis of pancreatic β-cells, leading to insulin deficiency
e. Defect in processing of a pituitary hormone that contains the insulin peptide

146. The substitution of valine for glutamate at position 6 on the two β chains in sickle cell hemoglobin causes which of the following?

a. Decreased polymerization of deoxyhemoglobin
b. Increased electrophoretic mobility at pH 7
c. Increased solubility of deoxyhemoglobin
d. More flexible red blood cells
e. Unchanged primary structure

147. An increased affinity of hemoglobin for O_2 may result from which of the following?

a. Acidosis
b. High 2,3-bisphosphoglycerate (BPG) levels within erythrocytes
c. High CO_2 levels
d. Low pH
e. Initial binding of O_2 to one of the four sites available in each deoxyhemoglobin molecule

148. A middle-aged man is brought to the emergency room in coma, well-known to the medical staff because of alcoholism and progressive liver disease. His current measure of serum glutamine-oxalate aminotransferase (SGOT), an enzyme used as a marker of liver cell damage, is reported as 1500 micromoles/min per mg protein, elevated but not as high as previous values in the 20,000 range. The lower SGOT activity contrasts with other measures of liver disease, including a serum ammonia in the 750 range (normal less than 30) and decreased amounts of coagulation factor proteins (these changes respectively account for the coma and bleeding tendencies of advanced liver disease). A call to the laboratory reveals an inexperienced technologist is on duty, who emphasizes he has performed the assay in the standard way. Which of the following is the most likely reason for the lower SGOT activity?

a. Measure of activity rather than specific activity
b. Inappropriate units for measure of specific activity
c. Substrate concentration similar to value of K_m
d. Lack of dilution with too much enzyme for substrate
e. Lack of dilution with too much substrate for enzyme

149. The functions of many enzymes, membrane transporters, and other proteins can be quickly activated or deactivated by phosphorylation of specific amino acid residues catalyzed by enzymes called what?

a. Cyclases
b. Kinases
c. Phosphatases
d. Proteases
e. Zymogens

150. The chemotherapy drug fluorouracil undergoes a series of chemical changes in vivo that result in a covalent complex such that it is bound to both thymidylate synthase and methylene-tetrahydrofolate. The inhibition of deoxythymidilate formation and subsequent blockage of cell division is due to which of the following?

a. Allosteric inhibition
b. Competitive inhibition
c. Irreversible inhibition
d. Noncovalent inhibition
e. Noncatalytic inhibition

151. The Lineweaver-Burk plot is used to graphically determine K_m and V_{max} for an enzyme that obeys classic Michaelis-Menten kinetics. When V is the reaction velocity at substrate concentration S, the y-axis experimental data in the Lineweaver-Burke plot are expressed as which of the following?

a. V
b. 1/V
c. S
d. 1/S
e. V/K_m

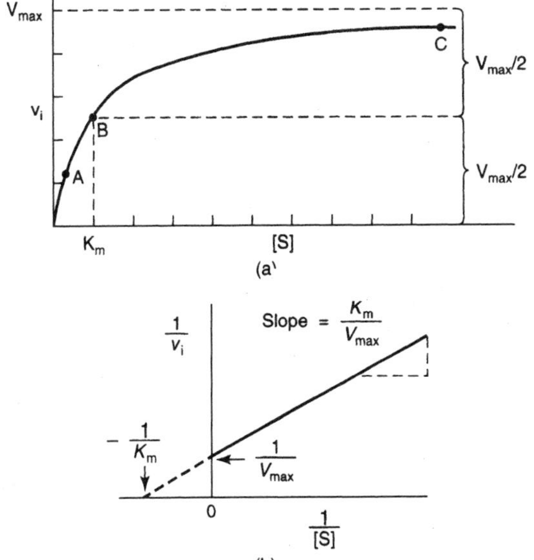

152. In the Lineweaver-Burk plot, which of the following is the V_{max} of an enzyme?

a. Reciprocal of the absolute value of the intercept of the curve with the x-axis
b. Reciprocal of the absolute value of the intercept of the curve with the y-axis
c. Absolute value of the intercept of the curve with the x-axis
d. Slope of the curve
e. Point of inflection of the curve

153. In the study of enzymes, a sigmoidal plot of substrate concentration ([S]) versus reaction velocity (V) may indicate which of the following?

a. Michaelis-Menten kinetics
b. Competitive inhibition
c. Noncompetitive inhibition
d. Cooperative binding

154. A noncompetitive inhibitor of an enzyme does which of the following?

a. Decreases V_{max}
b. Increases V_{max}
c. Decreases K_m and decreases V_{max}
d. Increases K_m and increases V_{max}
e. Increases K_m with no or little change in V_{max}

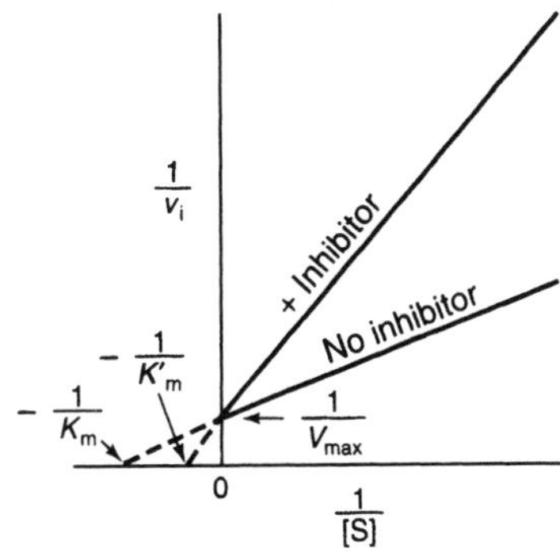

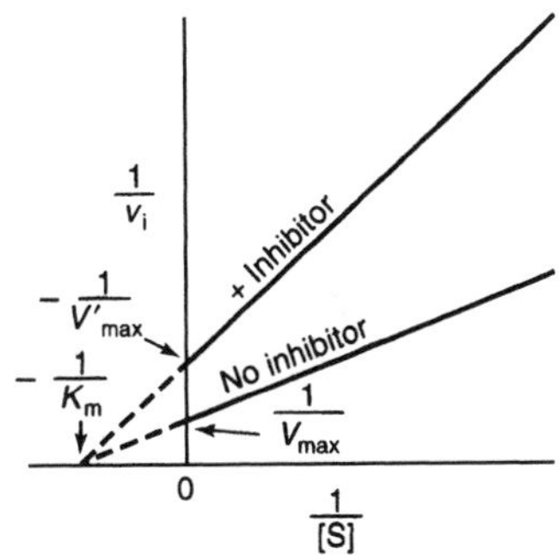

155. In the 1980s, biochemically oriented researchers focused on the enzyme superoxide dismutase (SOD) as a potential cause of Down syndrome. The trisomy (three doses) of chromosome 21 in that disorder would produce three copies of the SOD gene that is located on chromosome 21. SOD acts to remove superoxide anion free radical, catalyzing the reaction of two superoxide radicals with two hydrogen ions to form hydrogen peroxide and oxygen. Reasoning that the increased SOD activity and its excess peroxide products might cause embryonic birth defects, researchers constructed a mouse with three doses of the gene encoding SOD. Instead of simulating the multiple developmental changes of Down syndrome, mice with triplicated SOD loci had no abnormalities at all. Which of the following is the most likely fallacy in this research approach?

a. SOD enzyme assays with inadequate substrate concentration
b. Lack of attention to the concept of enzyme reserve, where most enzymes are present in excess of in vivo substrate concentrations
c. Lack of attention to colinked peroxidase loci that will also be increased in Down syndrome
d. Effects of human genetic mutations cannot be replicated in mice
e. Lack of attention to potential repressive mechanisms that negate extra doses of enzyme-encoding loci

156. A 2-year-old female presents with mildly enlarged liver, history of low blood sugar (hypoglycemia) on several occasions, and growth just below the third percentile for age (of concern because her parents are tall). Evaluation for glycogen storage disease includes glycogen phosphorylase enzyme assay, which is low-normal and does not increase with addition of cyclic AMP. Which of the following explanations is most likely?

a. Glycogen phosphorylase is activated by a cyclicAMP-regulated enzyme that is deficient in the patient
b. Glycogen phosphorylase is an allosteric enzyme regulated by a cyclic AMP binding site that is mutated in the patient
c. Glycogen phosphorylase gave a false normal value in the patient because it was not properly diluted to give excess substrate
d. Glycogen phosphorylase is subject to feedback inhibition by its product cyclic AMP
e. Glycogen is a complex substrate, so a linear relation of enzyme amount and activity cannot be expected.

157. Which of the following enzymes is regulated primarily through allosteric interaction?

a. Aspartate transcarbamoylase
b. Chymotrypsin
c. Glycogen phosphorylase
d. Glycogen synthase
e. Pyruvate dehydrogenase

158. Analysis of the fibroblast growth factor-3 (FGFR3) receptor gene demonstrated a common mutation in the receptor domain that causes achondroplasia (100800), while a lys650-to-glu change in the FGFR3 tyrosine kinase domain causes a much more severe phenotype called thanatophoric (death-loving) dwarfism (187600). Both phenotypes exhibit autosomal dominant inheritance, requiring one abnormal allele at the FGFR3 locus on chromosome 4. Which of the following is a likely molecular explanation for their difference in severity?

a. Binding of ligands to receptors is saturable like enzyme action, allowing defects to be compensated by increasing substrate concentrations
b. Signal transduction through tyrosine phosphorylation is an enzyme-mediated process requiring two abnormal alleles for phenotypic effects (recessive inheritance)
c. Fibroblast growth factor-3 is a large molecule that cannot achieve saturating concentrations
d. Binding of ligands to receptors is a linear process that is independent of ligand or receptor concentration
e. Binding of tyrosine phosphate to FGFR3 is an allosteric effect

159. Digestive enzymes such as pepsin, trypsin, and chymotrypsin are synthesized as inactive precursors. What are the preproteins of the active enzymes termed?

a. Kinases
b. Inducers
c. Isozymes
d. Phosphatases
e. Zymogens

160. Which of the following enzymes exhibits a hyberbolic curve when initial reaction velocity is plotted against substrate concentration?

a. Aspartate transcarbamoylase
b. Phosphofructokinase
c. Hexokinase
d. Pyruvate kinase
e. Lactate dehydrogenase

161. Children with cystinosis (219800) have growth delay, photosensitivity with crystals in the lens of their eyes, and progressive renal failure due to accumulation of cystine in cellular lysosomes. The defect involves a specific lysosomal membrane receptor that facilitates cystine egress, and an effective therapy has been found using oral cysteamine, a compound similar in structure to cystine. This therapy reflects the general principle that competitive inhibitors typically resemble the structure of which of the following?

a. Structure of enzyme or receptor protein
b. Structure of substrates or ligands that bind the enzyme/receptor
c. Structure of enzyme reaction products
d. Structure of the transition state in enzyme-catalyzed reactions
e. Structure of an allosteric regulator of enzyme/receptor activity

162. Which of the following is an explanation for rigor mortis?

a. Intracellular levels of ATP drop so ATP is not available to bind the S1 head of myosin; thus, actin does not dissociate from myosin
b. Intracellular levels of ATP drop so ATP is not available to bind the S1 head of myosin; thus, actin dissociates from myosin
c. Intracellular levels of ATP rise so ATP is available to bind the S1 head of myosin; thus, actin dissociates from myosin
d. Intracellular levels of ATP rise so ATP is available to bind the S1 head of myosin; thus, actin does not dissociate from myosin

163. Which of the following is the correct chronological order of the major biochemical events occurring during one cycle of skeletal muscle contraction and relaxation?

1. Actin is released from the complex
2. ATP binds S1 head of myosin
3. Power stroke
4. S1 head of myosin binds accessible actin
5. S1 head of myosin hydrolyzes ATP to ADP and P_i

a. 1, 2, 3, 4, 5
b. 5, 4, 3, 2, 1
c. 4, 2, 5, 3, 1
d. 2, 4, 5, 3, 1
e. 2, 5, 4, 3, 1

164. Inherited deficiency of the enzyme methylmalonyl CoA mutase (MMACoA mutase, 251000) causes serum and urine accumulation of methylmalonic acid with acidosis, neurologic degeneration and death. Recognition that pernicious anemia (due to deficiency of vitamin B12) can involve accumulation of methylmalonic acid led to successful treatment of some patients with MMACoA mutase deficiency using excess B12. Studies of purified MMACoA mutase enzyme from normal patients then showed enhanced mutase activity when B12 was added to the reaction mixture. These facts are best reconciled by which of the following explanations?

a. Vitamin B_{12} is a precursor for methylmalonic acid synthesis
b. Vitamin B_{12} is a prosthetic group for the enzyme methylmalonic acid Co A mutase
c. Vitamin B_{12} is a cofactor for the MMACoA mutase enzyme
d. Vitamin B_{12} is a competitive inhibitor of MMACoA mutase enzyme
e. Vitamin B_{12} is a feedback inhibitor of MMACoA mutase enzyme

Protein Structure/Function

Answers

138. The answer is a. *(Murray, pp 40–48. Scriver, pp 4571–4636.)* The woman would exhibit respiratory acidosis due to shortness of breath and decreased efficiency of gas exchange in the lungs. Emphysema involves dilated and dysfunctional alveoli from alveolar tissue damage, usually secondary to cigarette smoking. The hypoxia leads to tissue deoxygenation and acidosis, exacerbated by the hypercarbia (CO_2 accumulation) that distinguishes respiratory acidosis (higher bicarbonate than expected) from metabolic acidosis (very low bicarbonate, usually with low Pco_2 due to compensatory hyperventilation). Choice a shows the only set of values indicating acidosis (pH lower than 7.4), hypoxia (Po_2 lower than 95), and hypercarbia (Pco_2 greater than 44).

The tetrameric structure of hemoglobin allows cooperative binding of oxygen in that binding of oxygen to the heme molecule of the first subunit facilitates binding to the other three. This enhanced binding is due to allosteric changes of the hemoglobin molecule, accounting for its S-shaped oxygen saturation curve as compared with that of myoglobin (see the figure in question 143). At the lower oxygen saturations in peripheral tissues (Po_2 30–40), hemoglobin releases much more oxygen (up to 50% desaturated) than myoglobin with its single polypeptide structure. The amount of oxygen released (and CO_2 absorbed as carboxyhemoglobin) is further increased by the Bohr effect—increasing hydrogen ion (H^+) concentration (lowering pH) and increasing CO_2 partial pressure (Pco_2) shift the sigmoidal-shaped oxygen binding curve for hemoglobin further to the right.

139. The answer is d. *(Murray, pp 40–48. Scriver, pp 4571–4636.)* After binding of the first oxygen, hemoglobin shifts from a taut (T) state toward a relaxed (R) state with the ferrous iron in plane with the four planar pyrrole groups of heme. Binding of subsequent oxygen atoms requires less change of secondary, tertiary, and quaternary structure, producing the cooperative kinetics reflected in the sigmoidal oxygen binding curve (see the figure in question 143). Besides accounting for allosteric changes during oxygen binding, the tertiary folding of each hemoglobin chain and its quaternary (four-chain) structure produce preferred binding of oxygen due to steric restraint. Isolated heme binds carbon dioxide 25,000 times more strongly than oxygen, but in myoglobin and each hemoglobin chain, a histidine group interferes with the preferred mode of carbon dioxide binding such that oxygen is favored. The myoglobin molecule is virtually identical to the β-globin chain of hemoglobin, emphasizing again that the quaternary structure of four subunits in hemoglobin produces its sigmoidal oxygen binding curve, which provides for lung oxygen saturation and tissue desaturation with CO_2 loading. Because of this sigmoidal curve, hemoglobin binds proportionately less oxygen at low oxygen tension (low Po_2) than does myoglobin. Oxidation of the ferrous iron in myoglobin or hemoglobin to ferric ion abolishes oxygen binding, in contrast to the case with other proteins like cytochromes or catalase, where oxidation/reduction of iron modulates their function.

140. The answer is d. *(Murray, pp 49–59. Scriver, pp 4571–4636.)* Isozymes are multiple forms of a given enzyme that occur within a given species. Since isozymes are composed of different proteins, analysis by electrophoretic separation can be done. Lactate dehydrogenase is a tetramer composed of any combination of two different polypeptides, H and M. Thus the possible combinations are H4, H3M1, H2M2, H1M3, and M4. Although each combination is found in most tissues, M4 predominates in the liver and skeletal muscle, where as H4 is the predominant form in the heart. White and red blood cells as well as brain cells contain primarily intermediate forms. The M4 forms of the isozyme seem to have a higher affinity for pyruvate compared with the H4 form. Following a myocardial infarction, the H4 (LDH1) type of lactate dehydrogenase rises and reaches a peak approximately 36 hours later. Elevated LDH1 levels may signal myocardial disease even when the total lactate dehydrogenase level is normal.

141. The answer is e. *(Murray, pp 556–579. Scriver, pp 4571–4636.)* Calcium ions are the regulators of contraction of skeletal muscle. Calcium is actively sequestered in sarcoplasmic reticulum by an ATP pump during relaxation of muscle. Nervous stimulation leads to the release of calcium into the cytosol and raises the concentration from less than 1 mM to about 10 mM. The calcium binds to troponin C. The calcium-troponin complex undergoes a conformational change, which is transmitted to tropomyosin and causes tropomyosin to shift position. The shift of tropomyosin allows actin to interact with myosin and contraction to proceed.

Mutations affecting proteins involved in muscle contraction can present with low muscle tone and developmental delay in childhood, as chronic muscle cramps or fatigue, or with cardiomyopathies due to weakened heart muscle. Since cardiac muscle contraction is coordinated by electrical conduction from the sinus and atrioventricular nodes, muscle protein abnormalities can also interfere with cardiac rhythm. A specific mutation in troponin I can cause cardiomyopathy and the irregular cardiac rhythm known as Wolff-Parkinson-White syndrome (600858).

142. The answer is c. *(Murray, pp 40–59. Scriver, pp 4571–4636.)* Oxidizing agents can convert hemoglobin from its ferrous iron (Fe^{2+}) form to the ferric ion (Fe^{3+}) form (methemoglobinemia) that has poor oxygen-carrying capacity. Methemoglobin reductases in the red cell (with NADP or NADPH and cytochrome cofactors) keep the hemoglobin reduced. Autosomal dominant-acting mutations in the globin peptides, autosomal recessive deficiencies of methemoglobin reductase (e.g., 250800), or exogenous oxidizing agents (nitrates in well water) can produce significant amounts of methemoglobinemia with reduced blood oxygen and cyanosis. Vitamins C, E, and other antioxidants can oppose the action of oxidizing agents. Children who get severe methemoglobinemia from well water nitrates are heterozygotes (carriers) for methemoglobin reductase deficiency.

143. The answer is d. (Murray, pp 40–48. Scriver, pp 4571–4636.) In the oxygen dissociation curve, percent saturation of hemoglobin with oxygen on the y-axis is plotted against the amount of oxygen present in solution [the partial pressure of oxygen (Po_2)]—see the figure (Fig. A143 on page 186). Hemoglobin saturation varies from 0% to 100%. The O_2 pressure can vary from no oxygen in solution to high Po_2 levels. 2,3-bisphosphoglycerate (BPG) is present in concentrations similar to those of hemoglobin in red blood cells. BPG cross-links deoxyhemoglobin and lowers its affinity for oxygen, aiding the unloading of oxygen in capillaries. Thus, increased BPG shifts the oxygen dissociation curve to the right, while lower BPG will shift it to the left and reduce tissue oxygen delivery. Other factors include increased H^+ ions (lower pH in tissues) and increased CO_2 that enhance the release of O_2 from hemoglobin with shift of the curve to the right and better oxygen delivery. Conversely, the lower H^+ levels with increasing pH and decreasing CO_2 shift the curve leftward. Fetal hemoglobin has a greater affinity for O_2 under all conditions. Mixing of fetal with adult hemoglobin increases O_2 affinity and shifts the curve to the left.

144. The answer is e. *(Murray, pp 598–608. Scriver, pp 2863–2914.)* Many enzymes interact to regulate blood clotting. Plasmin is activated by proteolytic cleavage of its zymogen, plasminogen. The activating protease is called tissue plasminogen activator (tPA). Plasmin hydrolyzes fibrin clots to form soluble products and is used to dissolve clots in coronary arteries that cause myocardial infarction. Platelets, thrombin, and fibrinogen promote clotting through the intrinsic pathway and would be contraindicated in myocardial infarction. Platelets form a plug at the site of bleeding and bind prothrombin to facilitate its conversion to thrombin. Fibrinogen is the substrate acted on by thrombin to yield the fibrin mesh of blood clots. Heparin is a mucopolysaccharide that terminates clot formation by interfering with a number of steps in the coagulation cascade. Heparin inhibits the formation of clots, but cannot dissolve clots that have already formed.

145. The answer is a. *(Murray, pp 40–48. Scriver, pp 4571–4636.)* Insulin is secreted from the pancreatic β-cells as a propeptide called proinsulin with contiguous N-terminal A, internal C, and C-terminal B peptides. During processing, the C peptide is removed with joining of the A and B peptides (at sulfhydryl bonds) to form mature insulin. Rare families will exhibit autosomal dominant inheritance of mild, adult-onset diabetes due to decreased proinsulin processing and reduced amounts of insulin. They will have increased amounts of proinsulin in their blood, so the disease is called hyperproinsulinemia (176730). These individuals will be like juvenile diabetics who do not make insulin, but milder because they have one allele defective in the putative peptidase that processes proinsulin and another allele that is normal. They will respond normally to insulin, unlike many type II adult-onset diabetics who exhibit insulin resistance in their tissues.

146. The answer is b. *(Murray, pp 40–48. Scriver, pp 4571–4636.)* The carboxyl of glutamate at position 6 on the β-chain of normal hemoglobin is dissociated and negatively charged at pH 7. Substitution of uncharged valine for glutamate by mutation produces sickle cell hemoglobin, which is less negatively charged and has an increased electrophoretic mobility. Polymerization of the deoxygenated form of sickle hemoglobin occurs owing to the alteration of primary structure caused by the valine substitution. The insoluble, polymerized hemoglobin causes the erythrocyte to lose flexibility and to become rigid and sickle-shaped. The brittle cells produce anemia and block capillaries.

147. The answer is e. *(Murray, pp 40–48. Scriver, pp 4571–4636.)* In addition to its function as a carrier of O_2 and CO_2, hemoglobin buffers sudden additions of acid or base to the blood by virtue of the histidine 146 on each β chain. However, protonation of the imidazole of histidine causes deoxygenation of hemoglobin. Thus, decreased binding of O_2 occurs in the low-pH conditions of acidosis. 2,3-bisphosphoglycerate (BPG) binds specifically to deoxyhemoglobin; that is, BPG cross-links positively charged residues on the β-chain, thereby decreasing oxygen affinity and stabilizing the deoxygenated form of hemoglobin. The addition of each O_2 molecule to deoxyhemoglobin requires the breakage of salt links, such as those formed by 2,3-BPG. Each subsequent O_2 molecule requires the breakage of fewer salt links. Thus, initial O_2 binding actually results in an increased affinity for subsequent O_2 binding, which in turn results in a cooperative allosteric binding mechanism. CO_2 reacts reversibly with the amino acid terminals of hemoglobin to create carbaminohemoglobin, which is negatively charged and which forms salt bridges stabilizing deoxyhemoglobin. Hence, CO_2 binding lowers the affinity of hemoglobin for O_2.

148. The answer is d. *(Murray, pp 60–71. Scriver, pp 4571–4636.)* Enzyme assays require excess substrate such that the initial conversion of substrate to product will be maximal (V_{max}) and linear with time (substrate concentration [S] much above that concentration giving half-maximal reaction velocity = K_m). Substrate concentrations are usually expressed in terms of molarity, e.g., M = moles per liter, mM = millimoles per liter, μM = micromoles per liter. K_m, the Michaelis constant, is expressed in terms of substrate concentration. Under these reaction conditions, each unit of enzyme activity represents the amount of enzyme that converts a specific amount of substrate to a product within a given time. The standard units of activity are micromoles of substrate per minute. Specific activity relates the units of enzyme activity to the amount of protein present in the reaction, expressed as units of enzyme activity per milligram of protein. If the enzyme is pure (no proteins except the assayed enzyme are present), then the specific activity is maximal and constant for that particular enzyme (units of activity per milligram of enzyme).

Serum contains a complex mixture of enzymes and proteins, so the specific activity of enzymes like SGOT are related to milligrams of total serum protein. In severe liver disease with hepatocellular damage, large amounts of SGOT enzyme is released, causing excess enzyme in the amount of serum protein aliquoted into the standard assay. The hyperbolic relation of enzyme amount with reaction rate results in a plateau with excess enzyme, requiring that the serum be serially diluted until SGOT activity is linear with time. Without dilution, all enzyme amounts above the saturating value will measure as the same limiting activity, giving an underestimate of true SGOT activity. Other factors affecting SGOT activity will include small overestimates as the total serum protein decreases with liver disease (most proteins are synthesized in the liver) and eventual destruction of all liver cells (cirrhosis) so that there is no new enzyme to be released.

149. The answer is b. *(Murray, pp 72–79. Scriver, pp 4571–4636.)* A variety of highly regulated protein kinases can cause activation or deactivation of certain key regulatory proteins by covalent modification of specific serine, threonine, or tyrosine hydroxyl residues by phosphorylation. For example, skeletal muscle glycogen phosphorylase b is activated by phosphorylation of a single serine residue (serine 14) in each subunit of the dimers composing the enzyme. The phosphorylation reaction itself is catalyzed by phosphorylase kinase. Protein phosphatases can quickly reverse such effects. Activated muscle glycogen phosphorylase a is deactivated by a specific phosphatase that hydrolyzes the phosphoryl group off of serine 14. Whether the phosphorylated or dephosphorylated form of a protein predominates depends on the relative activities of the kinase versus the phosphatase.

150. The answer is c. *(Murray, pp 60–71. Scriver, pp 4571–4636.)* Since rapidly multiplying cancer cells are dependent on the synthesis of deoxythymidilate (dTMP) from deoxyuridylate (dUMP), a prime target in cancer therapy has been inhibition of dTMP synthesis. The anticancer drug fluorouracil is converted in vivo to fluorodeoxyuridylate (FdUMP), which is an analogue of dUMP. FdUMP irreversibly forms a covalent complex with the enzyme thymidylate synthase and its substrate N5,N10-methylene-tetrahydrofolate. This is a case of suicide inhibition, where an enzyme actually participates in the change of a substrate into a covalently linked inhibitor that irreversibly inhibits its catalytic activity.

151. The answer is b. *(Murray, pp 60–71. Scriver, pp 4571–4636.)* The Michaelis-Menten equation can be rearranged to its reciprocal as the Lineweaver-Burk equation:

$$V_i = \frac{V_{max}[S]}{K_m + [S]} \text{ and } \frac{1}{V_i} = \frac{K_m + [S]}{V_{max}[S]} \text{ or } \frac{1}{V_i} = \frac{K_m}{V_{max}} \times \frac{1}{[S]} + \frac{1}{V_{max}}$$

In the Lineweaver-Burk plot, the reciprocal of velocity 1/V is plotted on the y-axis against the reciprocal of substrate concentration 1/S on the x-axis (see figure below [Fig. A151]). Direct graphic determination of V_{max} is made by measuring the y intercept (= $1/V_{max}$ when $1/S = 0$). Direct graphic measurement of the K_m is made by measuring the x intercept ($= -1/K_m$ when $1/V = 0$). The slope is K_m/V_{max}.

152. The answer is b. *(Murray, pp 60–71. Scriver, pp 4571–4636.)* By plotting a reciprocal of the Michaelis-Menten equation, a straight-line Lineweaver-Burk plot is produced and the Michaelis constant (K_m) and the maximal rate (V_{max}) can be readily derived. The y intercept is $1/V_{max}$, while the x intercept is $-1/K_m$. Thus, a reciprocal of these absolute values yields V_{max} and K_m.

153. The answer is d. *(Murray, pp 60–71. Scriver, pp 4571–4636.)* Allosteric enzymes, unlike simpler enzymes, do not obey Michaelis-Menten kinetics. Often, one active site of an allosteric enzyme molecule can positively affect another active site in the same molecule. This leads to cooperativity and sigmoidal enzyme kinetics in a plot of [S] versus V. The terms competitive inhibition and noncompetitive inhibition apply to Michaelis-Menten kinetics and not to allosteric enzymes.

154. The answer is a. *(Murray, pp 60–71. Scriver, pp 4571–4636.)* In contrast to competitive inhibitors, noncompetitive inhibitors are not structural analogues of the substrate. Consequently, noncompetitive inhibitors bind to enzymes in locations remote from the active site. For this reason, the degree of inhibition is based solely upon the concentration of inhibitor and increasing the substrate concentrations do not compete with or change the inhibition. Therefore, unlike the increase in K_m seen with competitive inhibition, in noncompetitive inhibition V_{max} decreases while K_m usually remains the same. While competitive inhibitors can be overcome at sufficiently high concentration of substrate, noncompetitive inhibition is irreversible. (See figure [Fig. A154] below.)

155. The answer is b. *(Murray, pp 60–71. Scriver, pp 4571–4636.)* Nearly all enzymes in mammalian cells are present in excess of that needed for maximal reaction rates with in vivo substrate concentrations, a state called enzyme reserve. This is why nearly all metabolic disorders caused by enzyme deficiencies are inherited as autosomal recessive; mutation of one allele leaves another normal allele with 50% of enzyme amounts, still enough for maximal reaction. Diseases caused by single genes (Mendelian diseases), including those due to enzyme deficiencies (i.e., autosomal recessive metabolic disorders), can be modelled quite well in mice. These single locus diseases are quite different from those with multiple excess or deficient loci due to duplication or deletion of chromosome material.

156. The answer is a. *(Murray, pp 60–71. Scriver, pp 4571–4636.)* Many enzymes that catalyze initial or rate-limiting reactions in metabolic pathways are subject to allosteric effects, where cofactors or substrates (effectors) activate the enzyme and end-products of the pathway inhibit the enzyme (feedback inhibition). The binding of an effector to the regulatory subunit of an allosteric enzyme causes a conformational change that either increases or decreases the activity of the enzyme's separate catalytic site. There are also cascades of regulation illustrated by the glycogen phosphorylases of liver and muscle. Each are responsive to cAMP through inhibitor proteins, phosphorylation of phosphorylase kinase, and phosphorylation of phosphorylase kinase that then acts on phosphorylase. Several types of mutations that alter activity or allosteric regulation of glycogen phosphorylase or its kinase have been characterized (e.g., glycogen storage disease type IV, 232700).

157. The answer is a. *(Murray, pp 60–79. Scriver, pp 4571–4636.)* Aspartate transcarbamoylase, which controls the rate of pyrimidine synthesis in mammals, is negatively inhibited by the allosteric effector cytidine triphosphate, an end product of pyrimidine synthesis. The allosteric modulation occurs via the binding of effectors at the regulatory site of the enzyme. Noncovalent bonds are formed during the binding between effector and enzyme. In contrast, all the other enzymes are activated or deactivated by covalent modification. Chymotrypsinogen is secreted as an inactive proenzyme (zymogen) in pancreatic juice and is irreversibly activated by trypsin cleavage of a specific peptide bond. Glycogen phosphorylase is reversibly activated by phosphorylation of a specific serine residue. At the same time, glycogen synthase is reversibly deactivated by phosphorylation of a specific serine residue, thereby preventing a futile cycle of breakdown and resynthesis of glycogen. Pyruvate dehydrogenase also is reversibly inactivated by phosphorylation of a specific serine residue. In all four enzymes, a single, discrete, covalent modification leads to conformational changes that allow the switching on or off of enzyme activity.

158. The answer is a. *(Murray, pp 60–71. Scriver, pp 4571–4636.)* Many events of cell growth/metabolism, including those of differentiation and embryonic development, are controlled by signal transduction. A smaller signal molecule (ligand) interacts with membrane, intracellular, or nuclear receptors to initiate a cascade of protein changes. Ligand-receptor interaction is a saturable process much like enzyme-substrate interaction, and analogous reciprocal plots can reveal saturating ligand concentrations and the number of ligand molecules bound per receptor molecule. Ligand binding can initiate conformational changes in the receptor, activating processes like DNA binding (transcriptional activation/repression), membrane permeability (transport, conductivity), or cascades of protein phosphorylation (ATP, GTP, cAMP-mediated kinase reactions). Protein conformational changes are rapid, with cascades "channeled" within protein complexes so as to be obligate and unresponsive to surrounding metabolites. Mutations in the tyrosine kinase site of FGFR3 are less dependent on surrounding FGF3 concentrations, perhaps explaining why thanatophoric dwarfism (187600) has more severe limb and rib shortening (with asphyxia) than achondroplastic dwarfism (100800).

159. The answer is e. *(Murray, pp 76, 477.)* These digestive enzymes are proteases and are secreted as inactive zymogens; the active site of the enzyme is masked by a small region of its peptide chain, which is removed by hydrolysis of a specific peptide bond. Synthesis of proteases as zymogens is a mechanism that ensures that proteases will only be active when and where they are needed as inappropriate protease activity would be expected to have a very deleterious effect on the cell.

160. The answer is e. *(Murray, pp 49–79. Scriver, pp 4571–4636.)* Nonregulatory enzymes, such as lactate dehydrogenase, typically exhibit a hyperbolic saturation curve when initial velocity is plotted against substrate concentration (see the equation in answer 151). Enzymes at key points in metabolic pathways are typically allosteric—their velocities at a given substrate concentration may be altered due to effects of metabolites in the pathway. Allosteric enzymes typically exhibit sigmoidal kinetics. Examples of allosteric enzymes include aspartate transcarbamoylase, which is inhibited by cytidine triphosphate (CTP); phosphofructokinase, which is inhibited by adenosine triphosphate (ATP) and activated by fructose 2,6-bisphosphate; hexokinase, which is inhibited by glucose-6-phosphate; and pyruvate kinase, which is inhibited by ATP. Allosteric enzymes produce sigmoidal kinetics when substrate concentration is plotted against reaction velocity. In contrast, hyperbolic plots are observed with Michaelis-Menten enzymes. The binding of effector molecules, such as end products or second messengers, to regulatory subunits of allosteric enzymes can either positively or negatively regulate catalytic subunits.

161. The answer is b. *(Murray, pp 64–71.)* Ligand-receptor and substrate-enzyme reactions are both saturable processes with similar dependence of reaction rate on ligand/substrate and receptor/substrate concentrations. Competitive inhibitors function by binding to the substrate or ligand-binding portion of the active site and thereby block access to the substrate. Thus, the structures of competitive inhibitors tend to resemble the structures of the substrate and are often called substrate or ligand analogs. The effects of competitive inhibitors can be overcome by raising the concentration of the substrate. The amount the substrate must be increased is dependent on the concentration of the inhibitor, the affinity of the inhibitor for the enzyme, and the affinity of the substrate for the enzyme. For membrane receptors like that in the lysosome that is defective in cystinosis (219800), the reaction may be one of membrane transport such that internal substrate/ligand is in equilibrium with external substrate/ligand. Thus lysosome-internal cystine is substrate and lysosomal-external cystine a product, in a sense, such that lysosomal-external cysteamine will effectively decrease external cystine concentration and lead to egress of lysosomal cystine through its defective transporter.

162. The answer is a. *(Murray, pp 556–563.)* Rigor mortis is the stiffening of the body that occurs after death. Intracellular levels of ATP drop after death so that ATP is not available to bind the S1 head of myosin. Actin then cannot dissociate and remains bound to myosin. Therefore, the skeletal muscle remains contracted and relaxation, in which ATP bound to myosin complex is hydrolyzed to ADP and P_i, cannot occur.

163. The answer is b. *(Murray, pp 556–563.)* In the relaxation phase of skeletal muscle contraction, the S1 head of myosin hydrolyzes ATP to ADP and P_i, but the products remain bound. When contraction is stimulated (via the regulatory role of calcium in actin accesibility), actin becomes accessible and the actin-myosin-ADP-P_i complex is formed. Formation of the complex results in relase of P_i. This is followed by release of ADP, which is accompanied by a conformational change in the head of of myosin. This conformational change results in the power stroke in which actin filaments are being pulled past the myosin about 10 nm toward the center of the sarcomere. Another molecule of ATP is now able to bind the S1 head of myosin, forming an actin-myosin-ATP complex. The ATP-bound myosin has a low affinity for actin and thus actin dissociates from the complex.

164. The answer is c. *(Murray, pp 556–563.)* Small molecules may be integral parts of enzymes (prosthetic groups) or cofactors that participate in enzyme-substrate interaction or conversion. Prosthetic groups cannot be dissociated from the enzyme by dilution and thus will not be obvious components of the enzyme reaction when reconstitituted in the test tube. Cofactors, like vitamin B_{12} for methylmalonyl CoA mutase, associate reversibly with enzymes or substrates and can be added in vitro to obtain enhancement of the catalyzed reaction(s). Competitive or feedback inhibitors interact at substrate or allosteric binding sites of the enzyme, reducing effective substrate concentration and reaction rate or converting the enzyme to a less active conformation. Vitamin B_{12} (cyanocobalamin) is a cofactor for MMACoA mutase, accelerating the conversion of methylmalonic acid to succinyl CoA through activity of its cobalt group. Certain defects in MMACoA mutase can be ameliorated by intramuscular B_{12} injections so that effective B_{12} concentration and mutase activity are increased.

Intermediary Metabolism

Carbohydrate Metabolism

Questions

DIRECTIONS: Each item below contains a question or incomplete statement followed by suggested responses. Select the **one best** response to each question.

165. A previously normal 2-month-old female is evaluated because of jittery spells several hours after meals. A low blood glucose value is noted, and physical examination demonstrates a liver edge some two finger breadths below the right costal margin. Percussion of the right chest and abdomen confirms that the liver width is slightly enlarged. Hospital testing reveals that the infant can increase her blood glucose after breast feeding but that it is not maintained at normal levels 3–4 hours after feeding. Which of the following is the most likely diagnosis?

a. Intestinal malabsorption of lactose
b. Galactosemia with inability to convert lactose to glucose
c. Fructosemia with inability to liberate sucrose from glucose
d. Glycogen storage disease
e. Growth hormone deficiency with inability to maintain glucose

166. Diarrhea from infection or malnutrition is the world's most prevalent killer of children. A child develops chronic diarrhea and liver inflammation in early infancy when the mother begins using formula that includes corn syrup. Evaluation of the child demonstrates sensitivity to fructose in the diet. Which of the following glycosides contains fructose and therefore should be avoided when feeding or treating this infant?

a. Sucrose
b. Oaubain
c. Lactose
d. Maltose
e. Streptomycin

167. Which of the following carbohydrates would be most abundant in the diet of strict vegetarians?

a. Amylose
b. Lactose
c. Cellulose
d. Maltose
e. Glycogen

168. A teenager is brought in by his parents after his physical education teacher gives him a failing grade. The teacher has scolded him for malingering because he drops out of activities after a few minutes of exercise, complaining of leg cramps and fatigue. A stress test is arranged with sampling of blood metabolites and monitoring of exercise performance. Which of the following results after exercise would support a diagnosis of glycogen storage disease in this teenager?

a. Increased oxaloacetate, decreased glucose
b. Increased glycerol and glucose
c. Increased lactate and glucose
d. Increased pyruvate and stable glucose
e. Stable lactate and glucose

169. Recent statistics indicate alcohol abuse costs the United States $184 billion annually, more than cancer ($107 billion) or obesity ($100 billion). In 2001, 47% of those between ages 12 and 20 years admitted to drinking, 30% of these to binge drinking in the past month. Chronic alcoholics require more ethanol than do nondrinkers to become intoxicated because of a higher level of a specific enzyme. However, independent of specific enzyme levels, the availability of what other substance is rate-limiting in the clearance of ethanol?

a. NADH
b. NAD^+
c. FADH
d. FAD^+
e. NADPH

170. In lung diseases such as emphysema or chronic bronchitis, there is chronic hypoxia that is particularly obvious in vascular tissues such as the lips or nail beds (cyanosis). Certain genetic diseases like α1-antitrypsin deficiency (107400) predispose to emphysema, as do environmental exposures like cigarette smoking or asbestos. Poorly perfused areas exposed to chronic hypoxia have decreased metabolic energy for tissue maintenance and repair. Which of the following is an important reason for this?

a. Increased hexokinase activity owing to increased oxidative phosphorylation
b. Increased ethanol formation from pyruvate on changing from anaerobic to aerobic metabolism
c. Increased glucose utilization via the pentose phosphate pathway on changing from anaerobic to aerobic metabolism
d. Decreased ATP generation and increased glucose utilization on changing from aerobic to anaerobic metabolism
e. Decreased respiratory quotient on changing from carbohydrate to fat as the major metabolic fuel

171. Following a fad diet meal of skim milk and yogurt, an adult female patient experiences abdominal distention, nausea, cramping, and pain followed by a watery diarrhea. This set of symptoms is observed each time the meal is consumed. Which of the following is the most likely diagnosis?

a. Steatorrhea
b. Lactase deficiency
c. Maltose deficiency
d. Sialidase deficiency
e. Lipoprotein lipase deficiency

172. Asians and Native Americans may flush and feel ill after drinking small amounts of ethanol in alcoholic beverages. This reaction is due to genetic variation in an enzyme that metabolizes the liver metabolite of alcohol, which is which of the following?

a. Methanol
b. Acetone
c. Acetaldehyde
d. Hydrogen peroxide
e. Glycerol

173. Children with glycogen storage disease may exhibit symptoms due to altered liver (types I, III, IV, VI, VIII) or muscle (types V, VII) metabolism. Which of the following conversions explains the difference in these presentations?

a. Conversion of glycogen to lactate in liver
b. Conversion of glycogen and lactate to glucose in liver
c. Conversion of glycogen to glucose in muscle
d. Conversion of glycogen to alanine in muscle
e. Conversion of glycogen to glucose-6-phosphate in liver

174. A child is evaluated because of chronic anemia, slightly enlarged spleen, increased reticulocyte count, and mild elevation of indirect-reacting (unconjugated) bilirubin in serum. Incubation of the child's red cells with glucose yield decreased amounts of ATP as compared to controls, even in the presence of aeration (added oxygen). The child's anemia is explained by the fact that ATP is produced by which of the following pathways?

a. Glycogen breakdown
b. Glycolysis
c. Oxidative phosphorylation
d. Pentose phosphate cycle
e. Lactate conversion to glucose (Cori cycle)

175. A middle-Eastern family presents for evaluation because their infant son died in the nursery with severe hemolysis and jaundice. The couple had two prior female infants who are alive and well, and the wife relates that she lost a brother in infancy with severe hemolysis induced after a viral infection. The physician suspects glucose-6-phosphate dehydrogenase deficiency (305900), implying defective synthesis of which of the following compounds?

a. Deoxyribose and NADP
b. Glucose and lactate
c. Lactose and NADPH
d. Ribose and NADPH
e. Sucrose and NAD

176. A newborn begins vomiting after feeding, becomes severely jaundiced, has liver disease, and cloudy lenses of the eyes suggestive of cataracts. Treatment for possible sepsis is initiated, and the urine is found to have reducing substances. A blood screen for galactosemia is positive, and lactose-containing substances are removed from the diet. Lactose is toxic in this case because of which of the following?

a. Excess glucose accumulates in the blood
b. Galactose is converted to the toxic substance galactitol (dulcitol)
c. Galactose competes for glucose during hepatic glycogen synthesis
d. Galactose is itself toxic in even small amounts
e. Glucose metabolism is shut down by excess galactose

177. Which of the following best explains why fructose is often used as a carbohydrate substitute in special foods for patients with diabetes mellitus?

a. Fructose is a better substrate for hexokinase
b. Fructose stimulates residual insulin release
c. Fructose has a specific kinase in liver that allows bypass of phosphofructokinase
d. Fructose is phosphorylated and cleaved to triose phosphates, which cannot be used for gluconeogenesis
e. Hexokinase phosphorylates fructose in extrahepatic tissues, and its activity will not be affected by high glucose concentrations in diabetes

178. A normal female infant begins having jittery spells, vomiting, and falloff in growth when introduced to fruits and vegetables at age 6 months. Serum tests reveal low glucose and increased blood lactate, and her physician suspects hereditary fructose intolerance (229600), which is a deficiency of the enzyme aldolase B. The symptoms and serum abnormalities of this disease are due to which of the following?

a. Accumulation of hexose phosphates, phosphate and ATP depletion, defective electron transport, and glycogen phosphorylase inhibition
b. Accumulation of triose phosphates, phosphate and ATP excess, defective glycolysis, and glycogen synthase inhibition
c. Accumulation of triose phosphates, phosphate and ATP depletion, defective electron transport, and glycogen synthase inhibition
d. Accumulation of hexose phosphates, phosphate and ATP depletion, defective electron transport, and glycogen phosphorylase stimulation
e. Accumulation of hexose phosphates, phosphate and ATP excess, defective electron transport, and glycogen phosphorylase stimulation

179. A child is evaluated for hypoglycemia and lactic acidosis and noted to have an enlarged liver. Biopsy reveals stored glycogen, and a glycogen storage disease is suspected. Assay of usual glycogen enzyme deficiencies in the liver specimen is normal, so the metabolic consultant recommends assay of rarer enzyme deficiencies that influence glycogen metabolism. These enzymes would most likely include which of the following?

a. Hexokinase
b. cAMP-dependent protein kinase
c. Glucose-6-phosphate dehydrogenase
d. Phosphofructokinase
e. fructose-1,6-diphosphatase

180. An infant with hypoglycemia and a palpable liver is evaluated for possible glycogen storage disease. The parents have immigrated from Russia, and report that the child's older brother was diagnosed with a "debrancher" enzyme deficiency with similar glycogen storage. This diagnosis would imply accumulation of glycogen with which type of glucose linkages?

a. Linear $\alpha 1 \rightarrow 4$ linkages with branching $\alpha 1 \rightarrow 6$ linkages
b. Linear $\alpha 1 \rightarrow 6$ linkages with branching $\beta 1 \rightarrow 4$ linkages
c. Linear $\beta 1 \rightarrow 4$ linkages only
d. Linear $\beta 1 \rightarrow 6$ linkages only
e. Branching $\beta 1 \rightarrow 6$ linkages only

181. A 7-year-old female presents with dehydration after 3 days of vomiting and diarrhea. Her parents mention that a sibling was diagnosed with a type of diabetes that spilled sugar into the urine but did not need treatment. A urine Clinitest for reducing sugars is strongly positive, but the physician obtains a blood glucose level that is normal; a urine glucose oxidase test on the urine is also negative for glucose. Further analysis of the urine reveals a small amount of fructose and a large amount of an unidentified pentose that is most likely which of the following?

a. Galactose
b. Glucose
c. Lactose
d. Mannose
e. Xylulose

182. Certain carbohydrates can be recognized as reducing substances in urine by the Clinitest reaction, a tablet that combines with sugars to form a green color reaction. Among these is glucose with a C1 aldehyde group and four asymmetric carbons that generate 16 isomeric forms including galactose and mannose. Other hexose isomers have a ketone group at C2 (ketoses), which like the aldehyde can produce a reduction reaction. Which of the following is a ketose isomer of glucose?

a. Fructose
b. Galactose
c. Glucofuranose
d. Glucopyranose
e. Mannose

183. After a term uncomplicated gestation, normal delivery, and unremarkable nursery stay, a 10-day-old female is readmitted to the hospital because of poor feeding, weight loss, and rapid heart rate. Antibiotics are started as a precaution against sepsis, and initial testing indicates an unusual echocardiogram with a very short PR interval and a large heart on x-ray. Initial concern about a cardiac arrhythmia changes when a large tongue is noted, causing concern about glycogen storage disease type II (Pompe disease—232300—Table 3). Which of the following best explains why Pompe disease is more severe and lethal compared to other glycogen storage diseases?

a. The deficiency is a degradative rather than synthetic enzyme
b. The deficiency involves a liver enzyme
c. The deficiency involves a lysosomal enzyme
d. The deficiency causes associated neutropenia
e. The deficiency involves a serum enzyme

184. Which of the following explains why individuals with hyperlipidemia and/or gout should minimize their intake of sucrose and high-fructose syrups?

a. Fructose is initially phosphorylated by liver fructokinase
b. After initial modification, fructose is cleaved by a specific enolase
c. Fructose is converted to UDP-fructose
d. Fructose is ultimately converted to galactose
e. Fructose can be phosphorylated by hexokinase in adipose cells

185. Cellulose products are often used as solids (vehicles, binders) in pharmaceutical tablets and to provide texture in food products. They are inert ingredients because animals cannot metabolize cellulose, for which of the following reasons?

a. Cellulose is insoluble
b. They do not commonly consume cellulose
c. They do not have an enzyme to hydrolyze the β linkage
d. They do not have an enzyme to hydrolyze the branches

186. How many ATP molecules are generated by glycolysis of one glucose molecule?

a. One
b. Two
c. Four
d. Six
e. Twelve

187. A frequent presentation in the newborn period is transient hypoglycemia as the child adapts to separation from maternal glucose controls. Blood glucose is generally maintained at concentrations of 4.5–5.5 mmol/L but may rise to 6.5–7.2 mmol/L after feeding or decrease to 3.3–3.9 mmol/L in the fasting state. Which of the following enzymes plays an important role in regulating blood glucose levels after feeding?

a. Glucokinase
b. Glucose-6-phosphatase
c. Phosphofructokinase
d. Pyruvate kinase

188. A Nigerian medical student studying in the United States develops hemolytic anemia after taking the oxidizing antimalarial drug primaquine. Which of the following is the most likely cause of this severe reaction?

a. Glucose-6-phosphate dehydrogenase deficiency
b. Concomitant scurvy
c. Vitamin C deficiency
d. Diabetes
e. Glycogen phosphorylase deficiency

189. Which of the following events occurs during formation of phosphoenolpyruvate from pyruvate during gluconeogenesis?

a. CO_2 is consumed
b. Inorganic phosphate is consumed
c. Acetyl-CoA is utilized
d. ATP is generated
e. GTP is generated

190. Among the many molecules of high-energy phosphate compounds formed as a result of the functioning of the citric acid cycle, one molecule is synthesized at the substrate level. In which of the following reactions does this occur?

a. Citrate → α-ketoglutarate
b. α-Ketoglutarate → succinate
c. Succinate → fumarate
d. Fumarate → malate
e. Malate → oxaloacetate

191. Which of the following statements correctly describe human glucose metabolism?

a. Liver is impermeable to glucose in the absence of insulin
b. Pancreatic β-cells, liver and brain are freely permeable to glucose due to specific glucose transporters
c. Liver glucokinase phosphorylates glucose at high rates under all conditions
d. Extrahepatic tissues are permeable to glucose when glucagon is present
e. Liver takes up glucose when serum glucose is normal but releases it when serum glucose is high

192. Which of the following two compounds are the primary products of the pentose phosphate pathway?

a. NAD^+ and ribose
b. NADH and ribose
c. $NADP^+$ and ribose
d. NADPH and ribose
e. NAD^+ and glucose
f. NADH and glucose
g. $NADP^+$ and glucose
h. NADPH and glucose

193. Which of the following is an energy-requiring step of glycolysis?

a. Glucokinase
b. Lactate dehydrogenase
c. Phosphoglycerate kinase
d. Pyruvate kinase

194. Which of the following is a primary substrate for gluconeogenesis?

a. Galactose
b. Glycerol
c. Glycogen
d. Sucrose

195. A child has ingested cyanide from her parents' garage and is rushed to the emergency room. Which of the following components of the citric acid cycle will be depleted first in this child?

a. NAD^+ cofactor
b. Citrate synthase
c. Aconitase
d. Citrate production
e. Acetyl-CoA production

196. A 6-month-old male becomes ill after fruits and vegetables are added to his diet of breast milk. Mother feels that he used to become colicky when she ate fruit, although her pediatrician did not think this was significant. After 1 month of these new foods, the child has stopped gaining weight and the pediatrician feels an enlarged liver. Initial blood tests show a mild acidosis (pH 7.2) with increased lactic acid and low blood glucose. The Clinitest reaction is positive for reducing substances in the urine, but the glucose oxidase test is negative for glucosuria. A glycogen storage disease is suspected, and a liver biopsy dose shows mildly increased glycogen with marked cellular damage suggestive of early cirrhosis. Assays for type IV glycogen storage disease are negative (Table 3), and the initial frozen urine sample is reanalyzed and found to contain fructose. The most likely diagnosis and the reasons for hypoglycemia and glycogen accumulation is which of the following?

a. Hereditary fructose intolerance with inhibition of liver phosphorylase
b. Hereditary fructose intolerance with inhibition of glycogen synthase
c. Essential fructosuria with inhibition of glycogen synthase
d. Essential pentosuria with inhibition of liver phosphorylase
e. Essential fructosuria with allosteric stimulation of glycogen synthase

197. Disorders with abnormalities of the respiratory chain present with central nervous system and muscle symptoms (seizures, low tone) due energy deficiency. A preliminary test to decide if a patient may have a mitochondrial electron transport disorders examines the ratio of pyruvate to that of its product under resting conditions. What is the ratio and how would it be affected by abnormal electron transport?

a. Pyruvate/Acetyl-CoA—increased
b. Pyruvate/Acetyl-CoA—decreased
c. Pyruvate/Glucose—decreased
d. Pyruvate/Lactate—increased
e. Pyruvate/Lactate—decreased

198. Which enzyme reaction of the citric acid cycle leads to production of ATP (or GTP) by substrate-level phosphorylation?

a. Aconitase
b. Citrate synthase
c. Fumarase
d. Isocitrate dehydrogenase
e. α-ketoglutarate dehydrogenase
f. Malate dehydrogenase
g. Succinate dehydrogenase
h. Succinate thiokinase

199. Which of the following compounds is recycled in the citric acid cycle and thus serves a catalytic role?

a. Acetyl-CoA
b. Citrate
c. Oxaloacetate
d. Succinate

200. A child presents with low blood glucose (hypoglycemia), enlarged liver (hepatomegaly), and excess fat deposition in the cheeks (cherubic facies). A liver biopsy reveals excess glycogen in hepatocytes. Deficiency of which of the following enzymes best explains this phenotype?

a. α-1,1-glucosidase
b. α-1,1-galactosidase
c. α-1,4-glucosidase
d. α-1,4-galactosidase
e. α-1,6-galactosidase

201. What is the role of glucagon?

a. To stimulate the citric acid cycle
b. To stimulate gluconeogenesis
c. To stimulate glycolysis
d. To stimulate the pentose phosphate pathway

202. Fasting is observed in many religions and occurs with food shortages or fad diets. A man goes on a hunger strike and confines himself to a liquid diet with minimal calories. Which of the following would occur after 4–5 hours?

a. Decreased cyclic AMP and increased liver glycogen synthesis
b. Increased cyclic AMP and increased liver glycogenolysis
c. Decreased epinephrine levels and increased liver glycogenolysis
d. Increased Ca^{2+} in muscle and decreased glycogenolysis
e. Decreased Ca^{2+} in muscle and decreased glycogenolysis

203. After a meal, blood glucose enters cells and is stored as glycogen, particularly in the liver. Which of the following is the donor of new glucose molecules in glycogen?

a. UDP-glucose-1-phosphate
b. UDP-glucose
c. UDP-glucose-6-phosphate
d. Glucose-6-phosphate
e. Glucose-1-phosphate

204. Which of the following statements about the structure of glycogen is true?

a. Glycogen is a copolymer of glucose and galactose
b. There are more branch residues than residues in straight chains
c. Branch points contain α1ϕ4 glycosidic linkages
d. New glucose molecules are added to the C1 aldehyde group of chain termini, forming a hemiacetal
e. The monosaccharide residues alternate between D- and L-glucose

205. The citric acid cycle occurs in which subcellular compartment?

a. Cytosol
b. Endoplasmic reticulum
c. Golgi
d. Mitochondria
e. Nucleus

206. McArdle's disease (type V glycogen storage disease, 232600, Table 3) causes muscle cramps and muscle fatigue with increased muscle glycogen. Which of the following enzymes is deficient?

a. Hepatic hexokinase
b. Muscle glycogen synthetase
c. Muscle phosphorylase
d. Muscle hexokinase
e. Muscle debranching enzyme

207. Which of the following is an example of a ketose sugar?

a. Fructose
b. Galactose
c. Glucose
d. Ribose
e. Xylose

Carbohydrate Metabolism

Answers

165. The answer is d. *(Murray, pp 102–110, 145–152. Scriver, pp 1521–1551.)* Important carbohydrates include the disaccharides maltose (glucose-glucose), sucrose (glucose-fructose) and lactose (galactose-glucose), and the glucose polymers starch (cereals, potatoes, vegetables) and glycogen (animal tissues). Humans must convert dietary carbohydrates to simple sugars (mainly glucose) for fuel, employing intestinal enzymes and transport systems for enzymatic digestion and absorption. Simple sugars (galactose, fructose) are converted to glucose by liver enzymes, and the glucose is reversibly stored as glycogen. Enzymatic deficiencies in intestinal digestion (e.g., lactase deficiency in those with lactose intolerance), in sugar to glucose conversion (e.g., galactose to glucose conversion in galactosemia), or in glycogenesis/glycogenolysis (e.g., in those glycogen storage diseases) result in glucose deficiencies (low blood glucose or hypoglycemia) with potential accumulation and toxicity to hepatic tissues. The infant had been normal, excluding low glucose due to growth hormone deficiency, and could readily digest breast milk lactose with absorption and conversion to glucose. Low glucose during fasting and liver enlargement implies altered regulation of glycogen synthesis/release due to one of the enzyme deficiencies within the category of glycogen storage disease.

166. The answer is a. *(Murray, pp 163–172. Scriver, pp 1489–1520.)* Glycosides are formed by condensation of the aldehyde or ketone group of a carbohydrate with a hydroxyl group of another compound. Other linked groups (aglycones) include steroids with hydroxyl groups (e.g., cardiac glycosides such as digitalis or ouabain) or other chemicals (e.g., antibiotics such as streptomycin). Sucrose (α-D-glucose-β-1 $\rightarrow$ 2-D-fructose), maltose (α-D-glucose-α-1 $\rightarrow$ 4-D-glucose), and lactose (α-D-galactose-β-1 $\rightarrow$ 4-D-glucose) are important disaccharides. Fructose is among several carbohydrate groups known as ketoses because it possesses a ketone group. The ketone group is at carbon 2 in fructose, and its alcohol group at carbon 1 (also at carbon 6) allows ketal formation to produce pyranose and furanose rings as with glucose. Most of the fructose found in the diet of North Americans is derived from the disaccharide sucrose (common table sugar). Sucrose is cleaved into equimolar amounts of glucose and fructose in the small intestine by the action of the pancreatic enzyme sucrase. Deficiency of sucrase can also cause chronic diarrhea. Hereditary fructose intolerance (229600) is caused by deficiency of the liver enzyme aldolase B, which hydrolyzes fructose-1-phosphate.

167. The answer is c. *(Murray, pp 102–110. Scriver, pp 1521–1552.)* Cellulose, the most abundant compound known, is the structural fiber of plants and bacterial walls. It is a polysaccharide consisting of chains of glucose residues linked by β 1→ 4 bonds. Since humans do not have intestinal hydrolases that attack β 1→ 4 linkages, cellulose cannot be digested but forms an important source of "bulk" in the diet. Lactose is a disaccharide of glucose and galactose found in milk. Amylose is an unbranched polymer of glucose residues in $\alpha 1 \rightarrow 4$ linkages. Glycogen is a branched polymer of glucose with both $\alpha 1 \rightarrow 4$ and $\alpha 1 \rightarrow 6$ linkages. Maltose is a disaccharide of glucose, which is usually the breakdown product of amylose.

168. The answer is e. *(Scriver, pp 1521–1551. Murray, pp 145–152.)* Under circumstances of intense muscular contraction, the rate of formation of NADH by glycolysis exceeds the capacity of mitochondria to reoxidize it. Consequently, pyruvate produced by glycolysis is reduced to lactate, thereby regenerating NAD^+. Since erythrocytes have no mitochondria, accumulation of lactate occurs normally. Lactate goes to the liver via the blood, is formed into glucose by gluconeogenesis, and then reenters the bloodstream to be reutilized by erythrocytes or muscle. This recycling of lactate to glucose is called the Cori cycle. A somewhat similar phenomenon using alanine generated by muscles during starvation is called the glucose-alanine cycle. All of the other substances listed—oxaloacetate, glycerol, and pyruvate—can be made into glucose by the liver. In muscle, glycogenolysis is synchronized with contraction by epinephrine (through cyclicAMP) and calcium activation of phosphorylase. In those with muscle-specific phosphorylase defects (glycogen storage diseases V and VII), glucose is not mobilized as efficiently from glycogen, causing decreased contractile efficiency (cramping, fatigue), decreased yield of lactate from glycolysis, and maintenance of serum glucose by compensating liver metabolism.

169. The answer is b. *(Murray, pp 136–144. Scriver, pp 1521–1552.)* In humans, ethanol is cleared from the body by oxidation catalyzed by two NAD^+-linked enzymes: alcohol dehydrogenase and acetaldehyde dehydrogenase. These enzymes act mainly in the liver to convert alcohol to acetaldehyde and acetate, respectively. In chronic alcoholics, alcohol dehydrogenase may be elevated somewhat. The NADH level is significantly increased in the liver during oxidation of alcohol, owing to the consumption of NAD^+. This leads to a swamping of the normal means of regenerating NAD^+. Thus, NAD^+ becomes the rate-limiting factor in oxidation of excess alcohol.

170. The answer is d. *(Murray, pp 580–597. Scriver, pp 5559–5586.)* The exposure of tissues to chronic hypoxia makes them rely more on anaerobic metabolism for the generation of energy as ATP and other high-energy phosphates. Most tissues except for red blood cells can metabolize glucose under anaerobic or aerobic conditions (red blood cells do not have mitochondria for electron transport and must rely on other tissues to generate glucose back from lactate). In most tissues, a switch from aerobic to anaerobic metabolism greatly increases glucose utilization and decreases energy production. (A reduction of glucose utilization under anaerobic conditions in bacteria is known as the Pasteur effect after its discoverer). Under aerobic conditions, the cell can produce a net gain in moles of ATP formed per mole of glucose utilized that can be as high as 18 times that produced under anaerobic conditions. Thus the cell generates more energy and requires less glucose under aerobic conditions. Such increased ATP concentrations, together with the release of citrate from the citric acid cycle under aerobic conditions, allosterically inhibit the key regulatory enzyme of the glycolytic pathway, phosphofructokinase. Decreased phosphofructokinase activity decreases metabolism of glucose by glycolysis.

171. The answer is b. *(Murray, pp 474–480. Scriver, pp 1521–1552.)* In many populations, a majority of adults are deficient in lactase and hence intolerant to the lactose in milk. In all populations, at least some adults have lactase deficiency (223000). Since virtually all children are able to digest lactose, this deficiency obviously develops in adulthood. In lactase-deficient adults, lactose accumulates in the small intestine because no transports exist for the disaccharide. An outflow of water into the gut owing to the osmotic effect of the milk sugar causes the clinical symptoms. Steatorrhea, or fatty stools, is caused by unabsorbed fat, which can occur following a fatty meal in persons with a deficiency of lipoprotein lipase (238600). Sialidase deficiency (256550) causes accumulation of sialic acid–containing proteoglycans and neurodegeneration.

172. The answer is c. *(Murray, pp 212–218. Scriver, pp 1521–1552.)* The principal pathway for hepatic metabolism of ethanol is thought to be oxidation to acetaldehyde in the cytoplasm by alcohol dehydrogenase. Acetaldehyde is then oxidized, chiefly by acetaldehyde dehydrogenase within the mitochondrion, to yield acetate. Acetone, methanol, hydrogen peroxide, and glycerol do not appear in this biodegradation pathway. The genetic variations of acetaldehyde dehydrogenase have few phenotypic effects aside from sensitivity to alcoholic beverages and are extremely common in the affected populations. These characteristics qualify acetaldehyde dehydrogenase variation as an example of enzyme polymorphism.

173. The answer is b. *(Murray, pp 145–152. Scriver, pp 1521–1551.)* Glucose-1-phosphate is the first intermediate in the conversion of glycogen to glucose. The enzyme glycogen phosphorylase catalyzes this first step. The second intermediate, glucose-6-phosphate is subsequently converted to glucose by the enzyme glucose-6-phosphatase. This enzyme is found only in the liver and kidney; thus, these are the only tissues able to break down glycogen for use by other tissues. In tissues such as muscle, glycogen can be broken down to glucose-6-phosphate but can only be used in the cell in which it was produced. Glycolysis in muscle produces lactate, which must be converted to glucose by liver or kidney via the Cori cycle. Defects in liver glycogen metabolism therefore impair glucose-6-phosphate production or gluconeogenesis with resulting hypoglycemia and liver glycogen storage with or without toxicity (cirrhosis). Defects in muscle glycogen metabolism impair contraction (cramps, fatigue) with decreased serum lactate production during exercise and muscle glycogen accumulation (progressive weakness and atrophy).

174. The answer is b. *(Murray, pp 136–144. Scriver, pp 4637–4664.)* Glycolysis is the major source of ATP in cells lacking mitochondria, but is a minor source of ATP in tissues undergoing active oxidative phosphorylation. Anaerobic tissues (like muscle during exercise) or those without mitochondria (like erythrocytes) are dependent on glucose metabolism by glycolysis to lactate (through pyruvate) for production of ATP and energy. Defects in glycolytic enzymes (like hexokinase deficiency—235700) reduce ATP production in erythrocytes, shortening red cell lifespan with increased cell death (hemolysis). The increased hemolysis decreases red cell counts (anemia) with increased heme conversion to bilirubin, increased jaundice, and splenomegaly due to red cell storage. The increased heme load prior to liver metabolism increases indirect-reacting (unconjugated) bilirubin rather than increased conjugated or direct-reacting bilirubin from defective liver/gall bladder metabolism. Lactate produced by red cells and exercising muscle is converted to glucose by the liver, while pyruvate produced during glycolysis can be used for the synthesis of certain amino acids.

175. The answer is d. *(Scriver, pp 4517–4554; Murray, pp 163–167.)* Glucose-6-phosphate dehydrogenase (G6PD) is the first enzyme of the pentose phosphate pathway, a side pathway for glucose metabolism whose primary purpose is to produce ribose and NADPH. Its deficiency (305900) is the most common enzymopathy, affecting 400 million people worldwide. It contrasts with glycolysis in its use of NADP rather than NAD for oxidation, its production of carbon dioxide, its production of pentoses (ribose, ribulose, xylulose), and its production of the high-energy compound PRPP (5-phosphoribosyl-1-pyrophosphate) rather than ATP. Production of NADPH by the pentose phosphate pathway is crucial for reduction of glutathione, which in turn removes hydrogen peroxide via glutathione peroxidase. Erythrocytes are particularly susceptible to hydrogen peroxide accumulation, which oxidizes red cell membranes and produces hemolysis. Stresses like newborn adjustment, infection, or certain drugs can increase red cell hemolysis in G6PD-deficient individuals, leading to severe anemia, jaundice, plugging of renal tubules with released hemoglobin, renal failure, heart failure, and death. Since the locus encoding G6PD is on the X chromosome, the deficiency exhibits X-linked recessive inheritance with severe affliction in males and transmission through asymptomatic female carriers. Ribose-5-phosphate produced by the pentose phosphate pathway is an important precursor for ribonucleotide synthesis, but alternative routes from fructose-6-phosphate allow ribose synthesis in tissues without the complete cohort of pentose phosphate enzymes or with G6PD deficiency. The complete pentose phosphate pathway is active in liver, adipose tissue, adrenal cortex, thyroid, erythrocytes, testis, and lactating mammary gland. Skeletal muscle has only low levels of some of the enzymes of the pathway but is still able to synthesize ribose through fructose-6-phosphate.

176. The answer is b. *(Murray, pp 163–172. Scriver, pp 1553–1588.)* Lactose in breast milk and infant formula is converted by intestinal lactase to glucose and galactose that are efficiently absorbed. In galactosemia (230400), deficiency of galactose-1-phosphate uridyl transferase prevents the conversion of galactose into glucose-6-phosphate by the liver or erythrocytes. Most other organs do not metabolize galactose. The severe symptoms of galactosemia are caused by the reduction of galactose to galactitol (dulcitol) in the presence of the enzyme aldose reductase. High levels of galactitol cause cataracts, the accumulation of galactose-1-phosphate contributes to liver disease, and the accumulation of galactose metabolites in urine can be measured as reducing substances by the Clinitest method. Any carbohydrate, including glucose, with a C1 aldehyde registers as a reducing substance by Clinitest, so a Dextrostix (glucose only) test is often performed as a control. In normal children, galactose is first phosphorylated by ATP to produce galactose-1-phosphate in the presence of galactokinase. Next, galactose-1-phosphate uridyl transferase transfers UDP from UDP-glucose to form UDP-galactose and glucose-1-phosphate. Under the action of UDP-galactose-4-epimerase, UDP-galactose is epimerized to UDP-glucose. Finally, glucose-1-phosphate is isomerized to glucose-6-phosphate by phosphoglucomutase. Infants with suspected galactosemia must be withdrawn from breast-feeding or lactose formulas and placed on nonlactose formulas such as Isomil.

177. The answer is c. *(Murray, pp 163–172. Scriver, pp 1489–1520.)* Three enzymes for fructose metabolism, a specific fructokinase plus aldolase B and triokinase, are present at high levels in liver (also in kidney and small intestine). Fructokinase catalyzes the phosphorylation of fructose to fructose-1-phosphate, which is then split to D-glyceraldehyde and dihydroxyacetone by aldolase B. Triokinase converts D-glyceraldehyde to glyceraldehyde-3-phosphate, which can be metabolized further by glycolysis or be condensed with dihydroxyacetone phosphate by adolase to form fructose 1, 6-diphosphate, glucose-6-phosphate, and glucose as gluconeogenesis. Foods high in sucrose (glucose-fructose) such as syrups, beverages, or diabetic substitutes yield high concentrations of fructose in the portal vein. Fructose is catabolized more rapidly than glucose by its specific fructokinase, bypassing hexokinase that is regulated by fasting and insulin. It provides a fuel for glycolysis, but also increases fatty acid, VLDL, and cholesterol-LDL production that is not desirable in diabetes mellitus.

178. The answer is a. *(Murray, pp 163–172. Scriver, pp 1489–1520.)* Hereditary fructose intolerance (229600) is a defect in aldolase B, causing accumulation of fructose-1-phosphate and other hexose phosphates. The accumulated hexose phosphates deplete cellular phosphate pools, inhibiting generation of ATP through glycolysis or oxidative-phosphorylation (with increased lactate). Altered AMP/ATP ratios cause increased uric acid formation, and inhibition of glycogen phosphorylase by fructose phosphates produces hypoglycemia. Once recognized, hereditary fructose intolerance can be treated by elimination of fructose and sucrose from the diet.

179. The answer is b. *(Murray, pp 145–152. Scriver, pp 1521–1552.)* Glycogen storage diseases are a group of inherited enzyme deficiencies that cause accumulation of glycogen in liver, heart, or muscle. Glucose is the primary source of energy for most cells and excess glucose is stored as glycogen. Glycogen provides for short-term high-energy consumption in muscle and is an emergency energy supply for the brain. Glycogen stored in the liver can be converted back to glucose for release into the blood stream for use by other tissues. Glycogen synthesis and breakdown (glycogenolysis) are accomplished by separate pathways rather than reversible reactions. Glycogen synthase is active when dephosphorylated, glycogen phosphorylase when phosphorylated. Cyclic AMP-dependent protein kinases regulate these enzyme phosphorylations, integrating glycogen synthesis/breakdown with food and glucose availability (refer to Fig. 14 in the High-Yield Facts section). Besides deficiencies of phosphorylase (types V, VI) or phosphorylase kinase (VIII), deficiency of adenylyl kinase or cAMP-dependent protein kinase can alter glycogenesis/glycogenolysis regulation and produce glycogen storage (refer to High-Yield Fact Table 4). Deficiency of phosphofructokinase is compensated in liver but can lead to glycogen storage and exercise intolerance in muscle.

180. The answer is a. *(Murray, pp 145–152. Scriver, pp 1521–1552.)* Normal glycogen is composed of glucose residues joined in straight chains by $\alpha 1 \rightarrow 4$ linkages. At 4- to 10-residue intervals, a branch of $\alpha 1 \rightarrow 4$ linkages is initiated at an $\alpha 1 \rightarrow 6$ linkage. Glycogen particles can contain up to 60,000 glucose residues. In the absence of the debrancher enzyme, glycogen can be degraded only to the branch points, inhibiting release of glucose into the serum and causing glycogen storage. As noted in High-Yield Facts Table 4, Forbes/Cori or type 3 glycogen storage disease (232400) involves deficiency of debranching enzyme.

181. The answer is e. *(Murray, pp 163–172. Scriver, pp 1489–1520.)* Before urine test strips were designed with specific enzyme reagents like glucose oxidase, any sugar with a reducing aldehyde or ketone group would reduce the dye and produce a green color reaction. It was therefore important to differentiate glucosuria due to diabetes mellitus or renal tubular problems from other sugars in the urine, like galactose in galactosemia or fructose in essential fructosuria. The uronic acid pathway, like the pentose phosphate pathway, provides an alternate fate for glucose without generating ATP. Glucose-6-phosphate is converted to glucose-1-phosphate and reacted with UTP to form the higher energy compound UDP-glucose. UDP-glucose is converted to UDP-glucuronic acid that is a precursor for glucuronide units in proteoglycan polymers. Unused glucuronic acid is converted to xylulose and then to xylitol by a xylulose reductase, the enzyme deficiency in essential pentosuria (260800). In this "disease," which is better called a trait, excess xylulose is excreted into urine but causes no pathology. Pentoses (5-carbon sugars) are important in the pentose phosphate and uronic acid pathways, providing ribose for nucleic acid metabolism. The other sugars listed as options are all 6-carbon hexoses.

182. The answer is a. *(Murray, pp 102–110.)* Glucofuranose and glucopyranose are ring structures of glucose, with the majority of glucose in solution in the glucopyranose form. Galactose and mannose are epimers of glucose (an aldose), and fructose is the ketose isomer of glucose.

183. The answer is c. *(Murray, pp 145–152. Scriver, pp 1521–1552.)* Pompe disease has an early and severe onset compared to the other glycogen storage diseases listed in High-Yield Facts Table 4 because the defective α-glucosidase is a lysosomal enzyme. Accumulation of substances in the lysosome often leads to a more severe and progressive course, illustrated by the mucopolysaccharidoses like Hurler syndrome (607014) or the neurolipidoses like Tay-Sachs disease (272800). Patients with Pompe disease exhibit lysosomal glycogen accumulation in muscle (muscle weakness or hypotonia), brain (with developmental retardation), and heart (with a short PR interval and heart failure). The other glycogen storage diseases lead to glycogen accumulation in liver or muscle with correspondingly milder symptoms.

184. The answer is a. *(Murray, pp 163–172. Scriver, pp 1521–1552.)* Fructose is taken in by humans as sucrose, sucrose-containing syrups, and the free sugar. Fructose is mainly phosphorylated to fructose-1-phosphate by liver fructokinase. Aldol cleavage by fructose-1-phosphate-specific aldolase, not enolase, yields glyceraldehyde and dihydroxyacetone phosphate. The glyceraldehyde is phosphorylated to glyceraldehyde-3-phosphate by triose kinase, and both triose phosphates can enter glycolysis. Excess fructose from commercial foods can exercise adverse effects by raising blood lipids and uric acid. Fructose phosphorylation bypasses phosphofructokinase, a regulatory enzyme of glycolysis and provides excess glycerol metabolites and excess triglyceride/lipid biosynthesis. Fructose phosphorylation can also deplete liver cell ATP, lessening its inhibition of adenine nucleotide degradation and increasing production of uric acid. In adipocytes, fructose can be alternatively phosphorylated by hexokinase to fructose-6-phosphate. However, this reaction is competitively inhibited by appreciable amounts of glucose, as it is in other tissues.

185. The answer is c. *(Murray, pp 102–110.)* Glucose (glucopyranose) residues in cellulose are linked by $\beta 1 \rightarrow 4$ bonds in straight chains that humans cannot hydrolyze because they do not possess an enzyme to carry out this function. Cellulose is a structural constituent of plants and is strengthened by hydrogen bonds that cross-link the strands. Cellulose is insoluble and is a source of fiber in the diet.

186. The answer is b. *(Murray, pp 136–144. Scriver, pp 1471–1488.)* In the first steps of glycolysis, two ATPs are hydrolyzed, one in the phosphorylation of glucose to glucose-6-phosphate by glucokinase (hexokinase), and one in phosphorylation of fructose-6-phosphate to fructose 1,6-bisphosphate by phosphofructokinase. ATP is generated during conversion of 1, 3-bisphosphoglycerate to 3-phosphoglycerate by phosphoglycerate kinase and in the conversion of phosphoenolpyruvate to pyruvate by pyruvate kinase. Since two molecules of 1,3-bisphosphoglycerate are generated from one glucose molecule (and subsequently two molecules of phosphoenolpyruvate are generated), each of these steps results in generation of two ATPs. Thus, two ATPs are expended in the first step of glycolysis and four ATPs are subsequently generated in later stages, for a net total of two ATPs generated from glycolysis of one molecule of glucose.

187. The answer is a. *(Murray, pp 153–162. Scriver, pp 14171–1488.)* Glucokinase promotes uptake of large amounts of glucose by the liver. At normal glucose levels, the liver produces glucose from glycogen, but as glucose levels rise after feeding, the liver stops converting glycogen and instead takes up glucose. Insulin also plays a role in regulating blood glucose levels. Pancreatic β-cells produce insulin in response to hyperglycemia. Glucose uptake by the β-cells and phosphorylation by glucokinase stimulates secretion of insulin, which enhances glucose transport into adipose tissues and muscle and thus lowers blood glucose levels.

188. The answer is a. *(Murray, pp 163–170, 613–619. Scriver, pp 4517–4554.)* One of the world's most common enzyme deficiencies is glucose-6-phosphate-dehydrogenase deficiency (305900). This deficiency in erythrocytes is particularly prevalent among African and Mediterranean males. A deficiency in glucose-6-phosphate dehydrogenase blocks the pentose phosphate pathway and NADPH production. Without NADPH to maintain glutathione in its reduced form, erythrocytes have no protection from oxidizing agents. This X-linked recessive deficiency is often diagnosed when patients develop hemolytic anemia after receiving oxidizing drugs such as primaquine or after eating oxidizing substances such as fava beans.

189. The answer is a. *(Murray, pp 153–162. Scriver, pp 1521–1552.)* In the formation of phosphoenolpyruvate during gluconeogenesis, oxaloacetate is an intermediate. In the first step, catalyzed by pyruvate carboxylase, pyruvate is carboxylated with the utilization of one high-energy ATP phosphate bond:

$$\text{pyruvate} + \text{ATP} + \text{CO}_2 \rightarrow \text{oxaloacetate} + \text{ADP} + \text{P}_i$$

In the second step, catalyzed by phosphoenolpyruvate carboxykinase, a high-energy phosphate bond of GTP drives the decarboxylation of oxaloacetate:

$$\text{oxaloacetate} + \text{GTP} \rightarrow \text{phosphoenolpyruvate} + \text{GDP} + \text{CO}_2$$

In contrast to gluconeogenesis, the formation of pyruvate from phosphoenolpyruvate during glycolysis requires only pyruvate kinase, and ATP is produced.

190. The answer is b. *(Murray, pp 130–135. Scriver, pp 1521–1552.)* A molecule of guanosine triphosphate is synthesized from guanosine diphosphate and phosphate at the cost of hydrolyzing succinyl-CoA to succinate and CoA. This constitutes substrate-level phosphorylation, and, in contrast to oxidative phosphorylation, this is the only reaction in the citric acid cycle that directly yields a high-energy phosphate bond. The sequence of reactions from α-ketoglutarate to succinate is catalyzed by the α-ketoglutarate dehydrogenase complex and succinyl-CoA synthetase, respectively.

$$\alpha\text{-ketoglutarate} + NAD^+ + \text{acetyl-CoA} \rightarrow \text{succinyl-CoA} + CO_2 + NADH$$

$$\text{succinyl-CoA} + P_i + GDP \rightarrow \text{succinate} + GTP + \text{acetyl-CoA}$$

191. The answer is b. *(Murray, pp 157–160; Scriver, pp 1521–1552.)* Liver cells are permeable to glucose while extrahepatic tissues require insulin for glucose entry, reflecting different glucose transporters (GLUT) in different tissues. Liver hexokinase has a low K_m for glucose and acts at a constant rate, while glucokinase has a higher K_m for glucose and promotes glucose uptake at high concentrations as found in the portal vein after meals. The liver releases glucose at normal serum glucose concentrations but takes up glucose at high serum glucose concentrations. Insulin and glucagon act in opposing fashion to regulate serum glucose concentration. Insulin, secreted by the pancreatic β-cell in response to internal increases in glucose, ATP, and calcium influx, increases glucose uptake by muscle and adipose cells by recruiting glucose transporters to their plasma membranes. Glucagon, secreted by the pancreatic α-cells, stimulates cyclic AMP synthesis with increased gluconeogenesis and glycogenolysis to increase serum glucose concentrations.

192. The answer is d. *(Murray, pp 163–172. Scriver, pp 1434–1436.)* The pentose phosphate cycle does not produce ATP, but instead produces ribose and NADPH. $NADP^+$ is the hydrogen acceptor instead of NAD^+, as in glycolysis. In the oxidative phase of the pentose phosphate pathway,

NADPH is generated by glucose-6-phosphate dehydrogenase. NADPH is also generated by 6-phosphogluconate dehydrogenase. Ribose is generated in the nonoxidative phase.

193. The answer is a. *(Murray, pp 136–144. Scriver, pp 1433–1436.)* Glucokinase catalyzes the conversion of glucose to glucose-6-phosphate in the energy-requiring first step of glycolysis. ATP is also required in the conversion of fructose-6-phosphate to fructose 1,6-bisphosphate by phosphofructokinase. ATP is generated in the conversion of 1,3-bisphosphoglycerate to 3-phosphoglycerate by phosphoglycerate kinase and in the conversion of phophoenolpyruvate to pyruvate by pyruvate kinase.

194. The answer is b. *(Murray, pp 153–162. Scriver, pp 1471–1478.)* Gluconeogenesis refers to the pathway for converting noncarbohydrate precursors to glucose. Glycerol, lactate, propionate, and certain amino acids such as alanine are all substrates for gluconeogenesis. Glycogen is a glucose storage molecule that can readily be converted in the liver back to glucose for maintenance of blood glucose levels between meals.

195. The answer is a. *(Murray, pp 92–101, 130–135. Scriver, pp 2261–2274.)* Cyanide blocks respiration by displacing oxygen from hemoglobin. Oxidative phosphorylation in the mitochondria cannot proceed because cyanide cannot oxidize (remove electrons) from reduced cofactors like NADH. The citric acid cycle is the major pathway for generating ATP and reducing equivalents (NADH, H^+) from catabolism of carbohydrates, amino acids, and lipids. Inability to regenerate NAD^+ from NADH through mitochondrial oxidative phosphorylation depletes the cell of NAD^+ and inhibits the citric acid cycle. Failure to generate ATP by oxidative phosphorylation using NADH from the citric acid cycle depletes the cell of energy and leads to cell and tissue death (organ failure). Enzymes (citrate synthase, aconitase) and intermediates of the citric acid cycle (citrate, acetyl coenzyme A) need only be present in trace amounts because they are not consumed.

196. The answer is a. *(Murray, pp 136–144. Scriver, pp 1489–1520.)* Hereditary fructose intolerance (229600) is caused by deficiency of aldolase B that converts fructose-1-phosphate to dihydroxyacetone phosphate and glyceraldehydes. Fructose can be converted to fructose-1-phosphate (by fructokinase, the block in essential fructosuria, 229800) but accumulates with its phosphate and is diverted to fructose-1,6-bisphosphate. These compounds allosterically inhibit glycogen phosphorylase and cause hypoglycemia in the presence of abundant glycogen stores. The abnormal sequestration of phosphate interferes with ATP generation from AMP, depleting cellular energy sources with severe effects on liver or kidney. Affected individuals become nauseated when eating fructose and exhibit a natural aversion to fruits. If diagnosis is postponed and fructose is not minimized in the diet, they can undergo progressive liver and kidney failure with malnutrition and death. Countries like Belgium that use fructose in hyperalimentation solutions may observe patients with milder fructose intolerance who decompensate in the face of high serum concentrations.

197. The answer is e. *(Murray, pp 92–101. Scriver, pp 2261–2274.)* Under aerobic conditions, pyruvate is oxidized by pyruvate dehydrogenase to acetyl-CoA, which enters the citric acid cycle. The citric acid cycle generates reducing equivalents in the form of FADH and NADH that are converted to oxygen by the electron transport chain to yield abundant ATP. Under anaerobic conditions such as heavy exercise, pyruvate must be converted to lactate to recycle NADH to NAD^+ to allow glycolysis to continue. In mitochondrial disorders resulting from mutations in cytochromes or pyruvate dehydrogenase, there is deficient NADH oxidation and ATP production. Lactate will accumulate as it does normally in tissues without mitochondria (erythrocytes) or in tissues with exercise stress (like muscle). The lactate can accumulate in serum, causing a decreased pyruvate to lactate ratio and lactic acidosis that are typical signs of mitochondrial disease. These abnormalities also occur with circulatory failure (shock) or hypoxemia, so they are suspect for inborn errors only when cardiorespiratory function is normal. Glycolysis produces only 2 ATP compared to the coupling of citric acid intermediates with electron transport that produces 12 ATP per cycle; tissues highly dependent on the respiratory chain (nerves, muscle, retina) are predominantly affected in mitochondrial disorders—for example, Leigh disease. Suggestive signs like the decreased pyruvate/lactate ratio must be followed by more specific tests like muscle biopsy (ragged red fibers), eye examination (retinal pigmentation), or mitochondrial DNA analysis (deletions, point mutations) to diagnose highly variable mitochondrial diseases.

198. The answer is h. *(Murray, pp 130–135. Scriver, pp 2327–2356.)* The citric acid cycle produces 12 ATP per turn. Most of these ATP are generated by reoxidation of the NADH and $FADH_2$ molecules produced by the dehydrogenases. Isocitrate dehydrogenase, α-ketoglutarate dehydrogenase, and malate dehydrogenase each produce one NADH. Succinate dehydrogenase produces one molecule of $FADH_2$ per turn of the cycle. Reoxidation of each NADH results in formation of 3 ATP, and reoxidation of $FADH_2$ results in production of 2 ATP. Succinate thiokinase is the only enzyme that generates ATP directly by substrate-level phosphorylation.

199. The answer is c. *(Murray, pp 130–135. Scriver, pp 2327–2356.)* Acetyl-CoA is the entrance substrate to the citric acid cycle. Reaction between acetyl-CoA and oxaloacetate results in production of citrate. Citrate is subsequently metabolized to succinate and then back to oxaloacetate with production of two molecules of CO_2. Oxaloacetate is thus regenerated during the cycle and only acts as a catalyst.

200. The answer is c. *(Murray, pp 145–152. Scriver, pp 1521–1552.)* The child has symptoms of glycogen storage disease. Glycogen is a glucose polymer with linear regions linked through the C1 aldehyde of one glucose to the C4 alcohol of the next (α-1,4-glucoside linkage). There are also branches from the linear glycogen polymer that have α-1,6-glucoside linkages. Glycogen is synthesized during times of carbohydrate and energy surplus, but must be degraded during fasting to provide energy. Separate enzymes for breakdown include phosphorylases (α-1,4-glucosidases) that cleave linear regions of glycogen and debranching enzymes (α-1,6-glucosidases) that cleave branch points. Glucose-6-phosphatase is needed in the liver to liberate free glucose from glucose-6-phosphate, providing fuel for other organs. There is no glucose-6-phosphatase in muscle, and muscle glycogenolysis provides energy just for muscle with production of lactate. Deficiencies of more than eight enzymes involved in glycogenolysis, including those mentioned, can produce glycogen storage disease.

201. The answer is b. *(Murray, pp 145–152. Scriver, pp 1471–1488.)* Glucagon is a hormone in response to decreases in blood glucose. This hormone stimulates gluconeogenesis in the liver by increasing the level of cAMP, which in turn activates the cAMP-dependent protein kinase. This enzyme inactivates pyruvate kinase by phosphorylation and thus inhibits glycolysis.

202. The answer is b. *(Murray, pp 153–162. Scriver, pp 1521–1552.)* In the presence of low blood glucose, epinephrine or norepinephrine interacts with specific receptors to stimulate adenylate cyclase production of cyclic AMP. Cyclic AMP activates protein kinase, which catalyzes phosphorylation and activation of phosphorylase kinase. Activated phosphorylase kinase activates glycogen phosphorylase, which catalyzes the breakdown of glycogen. Phosphorylase kinase can be activated in two ways. Phosphorylation leads to complete activation of phosphorylase kinase. Alternatively, in muscle, the transient increases in levels of Ca^{2+} associated with contraction lead to a partial activation of phosphorylase kinase. Ca^{2+} binds to calmodulin, which is a subunit of phosphorylase kinase. Calmodulin regulates many enzymes in mammalian cells through Ca^{2+} binding.

203. The answer is b. *(Murray, pp 145–162. Scriver, pp 1521–1552.)* Upon entering cells, blood glucose is rapidly converted to glucose-6-phosphate by hexokinase or, in the case of the liver, by glucokinase. Glucose-6-phosphate is in equilibrium with glucose-1-phosphate via the action of phosphoglucomutase. Glucose-1-phosphate is activated by UTP to form UDP-glucose, which is added to glycogen by an $\alpha 1 \rightarrow 4$ linkage in the presence of glycogen synthase. To increase the solubility of glycogen and to increase the number of terminal residues, glycogen-branching enzyme transfers a block of about 7 residues from a chain at least 11 residues long to a branch point at least 4 residues from the last branch point. The branch is attached by an $\alpha 1 \rightarrow 6$ linkage.

204. The answer is d. *(Murray, pp 102–110. Scriver, pp 1521–1552.)* Glycogen is a highly branched polymer of α-D-glucose residues joined by $\alpha 1 \rightarrow 4$-glycosidic linkage. Under the influence of glycogen synthase, the C4 alcohol of a new glucose is added to the C1 aldehyde group of the chain terminus. The branched chains occur about every 10 residues and are joined in $\alpha 1 \rightarrow 6$-glycosidic linkages. Large amounts of glycogen are stored as 100- to 400-Å granules in the cytoplasm of liver and muscle cells. The enzymes responsible for making or breaking the $\alpha 1 \rightarrow 4$-glycosidic bonds are contained within the granules. Thus glycogen is a readily mobilized form of glucose.

205. The answer is d. *(Murray, pp 122–135, 2327–2356.)* In addition to the citric acid cycle, mitochondria also house the enzymes for β oxidation of fatty acids and oxidative phosphorylation. The cytosol is the site for glycolysis, glycogenesis, the pentose phosphate pathway, and fatty acid biosynthesis.

206. The answer is c. *(Murray, pp 145–152. Scriver, pp 1521–1552.)* Muscle phosphorylase deficiency leads to a glycogen storage disease—McArdle disease (232600)—that in young adults causes inability to do strenuous physical work because of muscular cramps resulting from ischemia. The compromised phosphorylation of muscle glycogen characteristic of McArdle disease compels the muscles to rely on auxiliary energy sources such as free fatty acids and ambient glucose.

207. The answer is a. *(Murray, pp 102–110.)* Glucose can form 16 different isomers. The orientation of the H and OH groups on the carbon atom adjacent to the CH_2OH group determines whether the sugar is the D- or L-isomer. Most of the monosaccharides in mammals are in the D form. Glucose can also form a ring structure with either a six-membered ring (glucopyranose) or a five-membered ring (glucofuranose). Epimers of glucose are isomers that differ in their configuration of the H and OH groups at the 2, 3, and 4 carbons. Mannose and galactose are the most biologically important epimers of glucose. Fructose is an isomer of glucose in which there is a keto group at the anomeric 2 carbon. Glucose is an aldose sugar with an aldehyde group at the anomeric carbon in position 1.

Bioenergetics and Energy Metabolism

Questions

DIRECTIONS: Each item below contains a question or incomplete statement followed by suggested responses. Select the **one best** response to each question.

208. A teenage boy presents to clinic complaining of muscle cramps on exercise. Past history indicates he had some coordination problems in childhood and received occupational therapy. Blood tests show an increased amount of lactic acid at rest, with dramatic increases on exercise testing. Simultaneous measures of capillary oxygenation by a surface probe were normal. The abnormality most likely involves which of the following?

a. Glycolysis in the lysosomes
b. Glycolysis in the cytosol
c. Respiratory chain in the mitochondria
d. Glycogen breakdown in the mitochondria

209. Children with respiratory chain disorders frequently have elevations of citric acid cycle intermediates like succinate or fumarate in their blood. Transfer of H^+/e^- pairs to electron transport carriers, decarboxylation, and substrate-level phosphorylation occur at some of the steps shown in the following diagram of the citric acid cycle. All three of these events occur at which of the following steps?

a. Step A
b. Step B
c. Step C
d. Step D
e. Step E

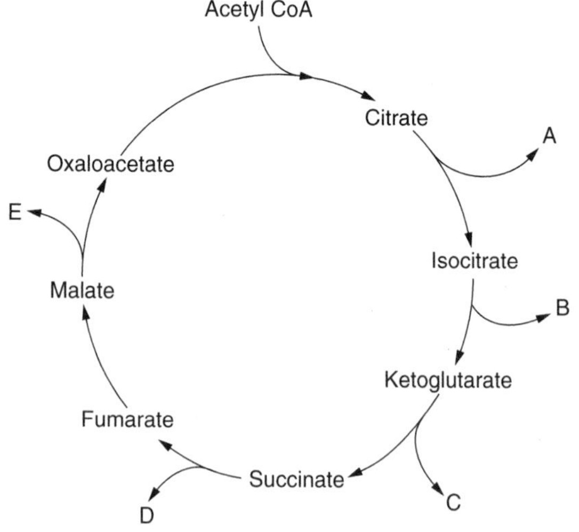

210. A comatose laboratory technician is rushed into the emergency room. She dies while you are examining her. Her most dramatic symptom is that her body is literally hot to your touch, indicating an extremely high fever. You learn that her laboratory has been working on metabolic inhibitors and that there is a high likelihood that she accidentally ingested one. Which of the following is the most likely culprit?

a. Barbiturates
b. Piericidin A
c. Dimercaprol
d. Dinitrophenol
e. Cyanide

211. Patients with deficiency of enzymes in the pentose phosphate cycle, such as those with glucose-6-phosphate dehydrogenase deficiency (305900), have increased red cell hemolysis and anemia. The hemolysis is related to membrane damage from accumulation of hydrogen peroxide, which in turn reflects inability to reduce oxidized glutathione. Which of the following redox pairs, due to its high redox potential, is crucial for glutathione reduction?

a. Fumarate/succinate
b. $NADP^+$/NADPH or NAD/NADH
c. Oxaloacetate/malate
d. Pyruvate/lactate
e. 6-Phosphogluconate/ribulose-5-phosphate

212. As electrons are received and passed down the transport chain shown below, the various carriers are first reduced with acceptance of the electron and then oxidized with loss of the electron. The drive for oxidation-reduction is ultimately provided by redox potential of oxygen to water. A patient poisoned by which of the following compounds has the most highly reduced state of most of the respiratory chain carriers?

a. Antimycin A
b. Rotenone
c. Carbon monoxide
d. Puromycin
e. Chloramphenicol

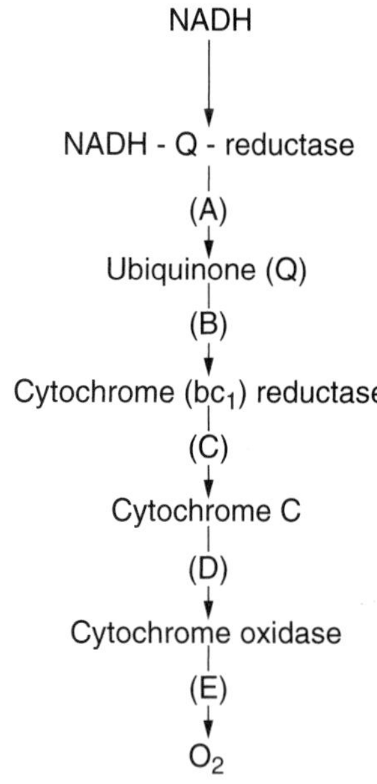

213. Dehydrogenases such as glucose-6-phosphate dehydrogenase serve to transfer H^+ from one substrate to another in coupled oxidation-reduction reactions, ultimately (in the respiratory chain) generating energy by oxygen/water reduction. Dehydrogenases can use which of the following compounds as an electron acceptor?

a. H_2O
b. NAD^+
c. O_2
d. Peroxide

214. Nicotine addiction from cigarette smoking is related to rates of conversion of nicotine to cotinine, carried out by a member of the cytochrome P450 enzyme family called P450PB (formerly CYP2A3 (122720). Individuals with variant alleles of the enzyme are predisposed towards nicotine addiction and the development of lung cancer. The P450 cytochromes are members of which family of oxidoreductases?

a. Catalase
b. Hydroperoxidase
c. Oxidase
d. Oxygenase

215. Which of the following compounds is a high-energy phosphate donor to ATP during glycolysis?

a. Glucose-6-phosphate
b. Glucose-1-phosphate
c. Phosphoenolpyruvate
d. Phosphoglyceric acid
e. Fructose-6-phosphate

216. A newborn is noted to maintain a frog-leg position with a weak cry and minimal spontaneous movement. A muscular dystrophy is suspected, and a serum enzyme is measured that reflects the abundance of a high energy storage molecule in muscle. Which of the following enzymes was measured?

a. Adenosine triphosphatase
b. Creatine phosphokinase
c. Glucose-1-phosphate dehydrogenase
d. Pyrophosphatase

217. The conversion of glucose to glucose-6-phosphate cannot take place in the cell unless the reaction is coupled to the hydrolysis of ATP. Which of the following correctly explains the reason why?

a. The reaction has a positive free energy
b. The reaction has a negative free energy
c. Glucose-6-phosphate is unstable
d. There is no enzyme capable of catalyzing this reaction

218. Which of the following enzymes allows the high-energy phosphate of ADP to be used in the synthesis of ATP?

a. Adenylyl kinase
b. ATPase
c. Inorganic pyrophosphatase
d. Nucleoside diphosphate kinase

219. In the figure below, which letter designates a reaction that may be catalyzed by different enzymes in different tissues, playing an important role in regulation of serum glucose levels?

a. Letter A
b. Letter B
c. Letter C
d. Letter D
e. Letter E

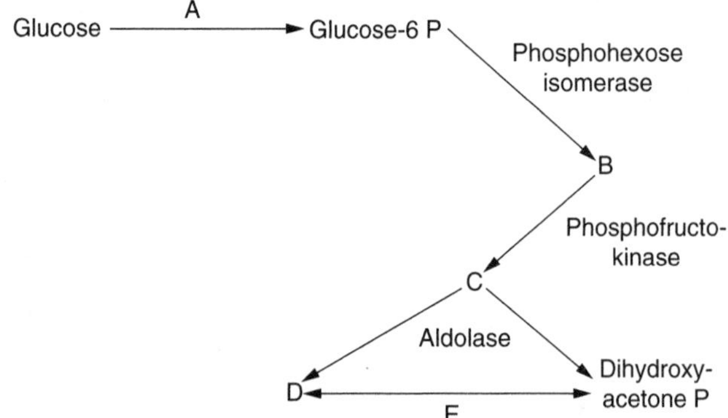

220. Which of the following reactions generates ATP during glycolysis?

a. Glucose-6-phosphate to fructose-6-phosphate
b. Glucose to glucose-6-phosphate
c. Fructose-6-phosphate to fructose-1,6-diphosphate
d. Phosphoenolpyruvate to pyruvate
e. Pyruvate to lactate

221. Which of the following enzymes catalyzes high-energy phosphorylation of substrates during glycolysis?

a. Pyruvate kinase
b. Phosphoglycerate kinase
c. Triose phosphate isomerase
d. Aldolase
e. Glyceraldehyde-3-phosphate dehydrogenase

222. Which of the following products of triacylglycerol breakdown and subsequent β oxidation may undergo gluconeogenesis?

a. Propionyl-CoA
b. Acetyl-CoA
c. All ketone bodies
d. Some amino acids
e. β-hydroxybutyrate

223. Which of the following regulates lipolysis in adipocytes?

a. Activation of fatty acid synthesis mediated by cyclic AMP
b. Activation of triglyceride lipase as a result of hormone-stimulated increases in cyclic AMP levels
c. Glycerol phosphorylation to prevent futile esterification of fatty acids
d. Activation of cyclic AMP production by insulin
e. Hormone-sensitive lipoprotein lipase

224. Oligomycin is one of several respiratory poisons with direct effects on the respiratory chain. These poisons inhibit synthesis of ATP during oxidative phosphorylation. Which of the following enzymes is directly inhibited by oligomycin?

a. Pyruvate kinase
b. Glucose-6-phosphate dehydrogenase
c. Enolase
d. ATPase (ATP synthase)
e. Phosphoenolpyruvate carboxykinase

225. Patients with fatty acid oxidation disorders are particularly susceptible to periods of fasting with disproportionate impact on muscular tissues. This is because, relative to energy from oxidation of glycogen (4 kcal/g or, when hydrated, 1.5 kcal/g), the yield from oxidation of triacylglyceride stores is which of the following?

a. 1 kcal/g
b. 2 kcal/g
c. 4 kcal/g
d. 9 kcal/g
e. 24 kcal/g

226. Which reaction in the figure below occurs in both muscle and liver but has substantially different qualities in the two?

a. Reaction A
b. Reaction B
c. Reaction C
d. Reaction D
e. Reaction E

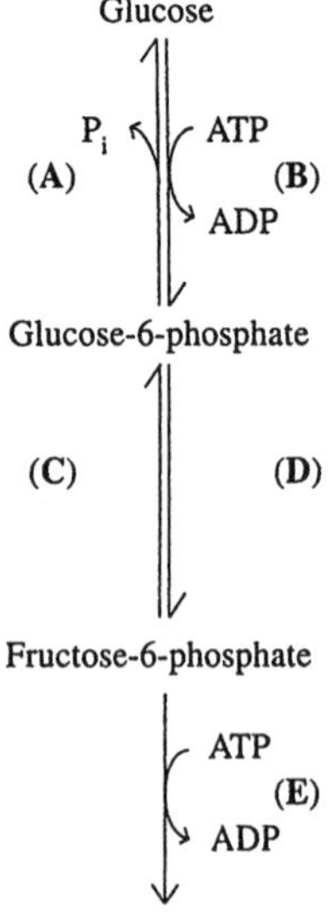

227. Nerve stimulation of skeletal muscle causes the release of calcium from sarcoplasmic reticulum and leads to muscle contraction. Simultaneously, the increased calcium concentration causes which of the following responses?

a. A dramatic rise in cyclic AMP levels
b. Inactivation of glycogen phosphorylase
c. Activation of phosphorylase kinase
d. Activation of cyclic AMP phosphodiesterase
e. Activation of protein phosphatase

228. A teenage girl is brought to the medical center complaining of fatigue that prevents participation in gym class. A consulting neurologist finds muscle weakness in the girl's arms and legs. Laboratory testing demonstrates elevated serum triacylglycerides esterified with long-chain fatty acids and borderline low glucose. Muscle biopsy shows increased numbers of lipid vacuoles. Which of the following is the most likely diagnosis?

a. Fatty acid synthase deficiency
b. Tay-Sachs disease
c. Carnitine deficiency
d. Biotin deficiency
e. Lipoprotein lipase deficiency

229. A newborn infant has a rapid respiratory rate, often due to retained fluid from delivery (transient tachypnea of the newborn). The child then has feeding problems due to low muscle tone (hypotonia), and this seems to have central (nervous system) rather than peripheral origin, implying an encephalopathy. A liver biopsy reveals a very low level of acetyl-CoA carboxylase, but normal levels of the enzymes of glycolysis, gluconeogenesis, the citric acid cycle, and the pentose phosphate pathway. Which of the following is the most likely cause of the infant's respiratory problems?

a. Low levels of phosphatidyl choline
b. Biotin deficiency
c. Ketoacidosis
d. High levels of citrate
e. Glycogen depletion

230. Patients with riboflavin deficiency will have lower FAD levels, while those with niacin deficiency will have lower NAD levels. How do oxidations involving NAD compare with those involving FAD?

a. NAD-linked oxidations generate 3 mol ATP per half mole of O_2 consumed, whereas FAD-linked oxidations only generate 2 mol ATP per half mole of O_2 consumed
b. FAD-linked oxidations generate 3 mol ATP per half mole of O_2 consumed, whereas NAD-linked oxidations only generate 2 mol ATP per half mole of O_2 consumed
c. Both oxidations generate 2 mol ATP per half mole of O_2 consumed
d. Both oxidations generate 3 mol ATP per half mole of O_2 consumed

231. Individuals with disorders of the respiratory chain are often placed on supplements containing riboflavin and coenzyme Q. Which of the following is the role of coenzyme Q (ubiquinone) in the respiratory chain?

a. It links flavoproteins to cytochrome b, the cytochrome of lowest redox potential
b. It links NAD-dependent dehydrogenases to cytochrome b
c. It links each of the cytochromes in the respiratory chain to one another
d. It is the first step in the respiratory chain

232. In the resting state, what is the primary condition that limits the rate of respiration?

a. Availability of ADP
b. Availability of oxygen
c. Availability of substrate
d. Availability of both ADP and substrate

233. Oxidative phosphorylation couples generation of ATP with which of the following?

a. Proton translocation
b. Substrate level phosphorylation
c. Electron flow through cytochromes
d. Reduction of NADH
e. Reduction of water

234. In the past, the uncoupler 2,4-dinitrophenol was used as a weight-reducing drug until side effects like fatigue and breathlessness precluded its use. How could the use of this drug result in weight loss?

a. 2,4-Dinitrophenol is an allosteric activator of ATP synthase and thus increases the rate of H^+ translocation and oxidation of fats and other fuels
b. 2,4-Dinitrophenol inhibits transport of pyruvate into the mitochondria. Fats are therefore metabolized to glycerol and subsequently to pyruvate, depleting fat stores
c. 2,4-Dinitrophenol allows oxidation of fats in adipose tissue without production of ATP. Fat oxidation can thus proceed continuously and fat stores will be used up
d. 2,4-Dinitrophenol causes ATP to be produced at a higher rate than normal, thus causing weight loss

235. Many compounds poison the respiratory chain by inhibiting various steps of oxidation or phosphorylation. Which of the following steps is inhibited by carbon monoxide and cyanide?

a. Oxidation step between cytochrome and coenzyme Q
b. Oxidation step involving direct reduction of oxygen
c. Uncoupling of oxidation from phosphorylation
d. Oxidation step between cytochromes c and b Allow oxidative phosphorylation in the presence of oligomycin

236. An important difference between respiratory chain inhibitors and uncouplers is which of the following?

a. The effect of respiratory chain inhibitors cannot be characterized spectroscopically, whereas that of uncouplers can
b. Uncouplers do not inhibit electron transport, but respiratory chain inhibitors do
c. Uncouplers are toxic substances, but respiratory chain inhibitors are not
d. Respiratory chain inhibitors allow leakage of protons across the membrane but uncouplers do not

237. Cholera toxin causes massive and often fatal diarrhea by which of the following mechanisms?

a. Inactivating G_i protein
b. Irreversibly activating adenylate cyclase
c. Locking G_s protein into an inactive form
d. Rapidly hydrolyzing G protein GTP to GDP
e. Preventing GTP from interacting with G protein

238. Why is the yield of ATP from the complete oxidation of glucose lower in muscle and brain than in kidney, liver, and heart?

a. Different shuttle mechanisms operate to transfer electrons from the cytosol to the mitochondria in the two sets of tissues
b. Muscle and brain cells have a lower requirement for ATP
c. There are fewer mitochondria in muscle and brain cells
d. There are fewer ATP synthases in muscle and brain cells

239. Children with a variety of organic acidemias will complex excess intermediates with carnitine as abnormal acylcarnitines and deplete free carnitine. The unavailability of carnitine to translocate fatty acids into mitochondria will cause which of the following?

a. Inhibition of ATP synthase
b. Depletion of NADH needed for oxidation
c. Inhibition of cytochrome oxidase
d. Inhibition of electron transfer from cytochromes to coenzyme Q
e. Uncoupling of oxidation from phosphorylation

240. The problem of regenerating NAD^+ from NADH for cytoplasmic processes by using mitochondria is solved in the most energy-efficient manner by which of the following?

a. Reversing the direction of enzyme reactions like pyruvate dehydrogenase
b. Locating certain cytochromes in the cytoplasm
c. Shuttling of coupled reaction substrates like malate to aspartate
d. Reversing the direction of glycolysis
e. Direct oxidation of NADH by cytochromes P450

241. A certain class of disease is produced because of the tissue's lack of certain metabolic pathways. Which one of the following tissues can metabolize glucose, fatty acids, and ketone bodies for ATP production?

a. Liver
b. Muscle
c. Hepatocytes
d. Brain
e. Red blood cells

Bioenergetics and Energy Metabolism

Answers

208. The answer is c. *(Murray, pp 80–101. Scriver, pp 2261–2296.)* Under conditions of plentiful oxygen (aerobic metabolism), pyruvate formed from glycolysis in the cytosol is metabolized to acetylCoA. Acetyl CoA enters the mitochondria and the citric acid cycle in the conversion of oxaloacetate to citrate, generating NADH and $FADH_2$ reducing equivalents that generate ATP through oxidation in the mitochondrial respiratory chain. In respiratory chain disorders, the disrupted electron transport chain does not function as well, causing more pyruvate to be converted to lactate in muscle with muscle weakness and cramping. Lactate from exercising muscle is normally converted to glucose by the liver, but excess lactate produced in severe respiratory chain disorders accumulates in serum to lower the pH (acidosis). Mitochondria are called the powerhouses of the cell since they contain the citric acid cycle and the respiratory chain that generates abundant ATP through oxidative phosphorylation.

209. The answer is c. *(Murray, pp 123–135. Scriver, pp 2367–2424.)* In the citric acid cycle, the conversion of α-ketoglutarate to succinate results in decarboxylation, transfer of an H^+/e^- pair to $NADH^+$, H^+, and the substrate-level phosphorylation of GDP to GTP. The series of reactions involved is quite complex. First, α-ketoglutarate reacts with NAD^+ + CoA to yield succinyl-CoA + CO_2 + NADH + H^+. These reactions occur by the catalysis of the α-ketoglutarate dehydrogenase complex, which contains lipoamide, FAD^+, and thiamine pyrophosphate as prosthetic groups. Under the action of succinyl CoA synthetase, succinyl CoA catalyzes the phosphorylation of GDP with inorganic phosphate coupled to the cleavage of the thioester bond of succinyl CoA. Thus, the production of succinate from α-ketoglutarate yields one substrate-level phosphorylation and the production of three ATP equivalents from NADH via oxidative phosphorylation.

210. The answer is d. *(Murray, pp 86–101. Scriver, pp 2361–2374.)* All of the poisons shown affect either electron transport or oxidative phosphorylation.

Dinitrophenol is unique in that it disconnects the ordinarily tight coupling of electron transport and phosphorylation. In its presence, electron transport continues normally with no oxidative phosphorylation occurring. Instead, heat energy is generated. The same principle is utilized in a well-controlled way by brown fat to generate heat in newborn humans and cold-adapted mammals. The biological uncoupler in brown fat is a protein called thermogenin. Barbiturates, the antibiotic piericidin A, the fish poison rotenone, dimercaprol, and cyanide all act by inhibiting the electron transport chain at some point.

211. The answer is b. *(Murray, pp 163–172. Scriver, pp 4517–4554.)* NAD^+/NADH is a favored redox couple used in pathways such as the citric acid cycle, glycolysis, and (with NADP/NADPH), the pentose phosphate pathway. Pyruvate/lactate is found as a redox couple in glycolysis, fumarate/succinate and oxaloacetate/malate in the citric acid cycle, and 6-phosphogluconate/ribulose-5-phosphate in the pentose phosphate pathway. The latter redox pair follows the glucose-6-phosphate to 6-phosphogluconate pair, both steps generating NADPH that is essential for reducing oxidized glutathione. Since reduction involves the gain of electrons (loss of hydrogen protons) and oxidation the loss of electrons (gain of hydrogen protons), oxygen to water has the highest drive for oxidation in biological systems and thus the highest positive reduction (Redox) potential of +0.82. The NAD^+/$NADP^+$ to NADH/NADPH couple has the highest redox potential with a negative value of –.32, and other coupled reactions like those in the answer options will have intermediate redox potentials, allowing the oxygen to water potential to drive all metabolic reactions through the process of respiration.

212. The answer is c. *(Murray, pp 163–172. Scriver, pp 4517–4554.)* The electron transport chain shown contains three proton pumps linked by two mobile electron carriers. At each of these three sites (NADH–Q reductase, cytochrome reductase, and cytochrome oxidase), the transfer of electrons down the chain powers the pumping of protons across the inner mitochondrial membrane. The blockage of electron transfers by specific point inhibitors leads to a buildup of highly reduced carriers behind the block because of the inability to transfer electrons across the block. In the scheme shown, rotenone blocks step A, antimycin A blocks step B, and carbon monoxide (as well as cyanide and azide) blocks step E. Therefore a carbon monoxide inhibition leads to a highly reduced state of all of the carriers of the chain. Puromycin and chloramphenicol are inhibitors of protein synthesis and have no direct effect on the electron transport chain.

213. The answer is b. *(Murray, pp 86–91, 163-172. Scriver, pp 4517–4554.)* Dehydrogenases are specific for their substrates but most use either NAD^+ or $NADP^+$as the coenzyme. Some dehydrogenases use flavin coenzymes similar to FMN and FAD used by the oxidases. The final steps in the conversion of oxygen to water in the respiratory chain is carried out by cytochrome oxidase (cytochrome a3) as part of complex IV. This final enzyme is an oxidase, defined by its use of oxygen to oxidize metabolites and form water or hydrogen peroxide. The prior cytochromes of the respiratory chain (b, c1, c, a) can be described as dehydrogenases, transferring electrons (or H^+ protons in reverse) by oscillation between ferric (Fe^{+++}) and ferrous (Fe^{++}) ions.

214. The answer is d. *(Murray, pp 86–91.)* Cytochrome P450 is a monooxygenase that can be reduced by NADH or NADPH and can in turn oxidize substrates by the hydroxylase cycle. In the liver, cytochrome P450 is found with cytochrome b_5 and plays an important role in detoxification.

215. The answer is c. *(Murray, pp 80–85. Scriver, pp 2367–2424.)* In order to serve as a high-energy phosphate donor to ATP, the compound must have a more negative standard free energy of hydrolysis than ATP. ATP has a free energy of hydrolysis of −30.5 kJ/mol (−7.3 kcal/mol). Phosphoenolpyruvate has a standard free energy of hydrolysis of −61.9 kJ/mol (−14.8 kcal/mol). Thus, this compound can donate a high-energy phosphate to ATP. The other listed compounds have less negative standard free energies and thus cannot serve as phosphate donors to ATP but may serve as phosphate acceptors.

216. The answer is b. *(Murray, pp 80–85. Scriver, pp 2367–2424.)* Creatine phosphate has a more negative standard free energy of hydrolysis than ATP, whereas ADP, glucose-1-phosphate, and pyrophosphate all have lower energy phosphate groups than ATP. When ATP is being utilized rapidly in skeletal muscle, creatine phosphate can be hydrolyzed and act as a phosphate donor to ADP to regenerate ATP. During resting periods when the ATP/ADP ratio is high, creatine can be phosphorylated to creatine phosphate to serve as storage for high-energy phosphate. The enzyme creatine phosphokinase (CPK) catalyzes this reaction, and its high concentration in muscle is transferred to serum in certain dystrophies where muscle breaks down. Elevated serum CPK levels can provide a hint that muscle weakness is due to inherent muscle problems rather than innervation from the brain or peripheral nerves.

217. The answer is a. *(Murray, pp 80–85. Scriver, pp 2367–2424.)* The reaction is endergonic and must be coupled to a more exergonic reaction such that the overall Gibbs free energy yield (ΔG) for the coupled reactions is negative. Coupling of ATP hydrolysis with energetically unfavorable reactions can not only allow the reaction to proceed in the forward direction, but can in some cases make the reaction irreversible if the free energy value is negative enough.

218. The answer is a. *(Murray, pp 80–85. Scriver, pp 2367–2424.)* Adenylyl kinase (myokinase) catalyzes the reaction: 2 ADP → ATP + AMP. Nucleoside diphosphate kinase allows the high-energy phosphate of nucleotide triphosphates other than ATP to serve as phosphate donors for ATP synthesis. Inorganic pyrophosphatase catalyzes the hydrolysis of PP_i. This reaction has a large ΔG of −27.6 kJ/mol and can drive reactions such as the activation of long-chain fatty acids by acyl-CoA synthetase in the forward direction.

219. The answer is a. *(Murray, pp 153–162. Scriver, pp 2367–2424.)* Glucose is immediately phosphorylated to form glucose-6-phosphate (G6P) after being transported into all extrahepatic cells by the enzyme hexokinase. Hexokinase has a very low K_m and thus extremely high affinity for glucose, virtually trapping glucose into entering the metabolic pathways of most tissues. G6P is the starting point for glycolysis, glycogenesis, and the pentose phosphate pathway. In contrast, the liver's hexokinase is called glucokinase and it is only active following a meal, when blood glucose levels are above about 5 mM. It has a relatively low affinity and high K_m. In this manner, the liver sequesters and stores glucose as glycogen for later distribution to tissues only when it is in excess.

220. The answer is d. *(Murray, pp 136–144. Scriver, pp 1471–1488.)* ATP is synthesized by two reactions in glycolysis. The first molecule of ATP is generated by phosphoglycerate kinase, converting 1,3-diphosphoglycerate to 3-phosphoglycerate. The second molecule of ATP is generated by pyruvate kinase, converting phosphoenolpyruvate to pyruvate.

221. The answer is e. *(Murray, pp 136–144. Scriver, pp 1471–1488.)* High-energy phosphate bonds are added to the substrates of glycolysis at three steps in the pathway. Hexokinase—or, in the case of the liver, glucokinase—adds phosphate from ATP to glucose to form glucose-6-phosphate. Strictly speaking, this is not always considered a step of the glycolytic pathway. Phosphofructokinase uses ATP to convert fructose-6-phosphate to fructose-1, 6-phosphate. Using NAD^+ in an oxidation-reduction reaction, inorganic phosphate is added to glyceraldehyde-3-phosphate by the enzyme glyceraldehyde-3-phosphate dehydrogenase to form 1,3-diphosphoglycerate. The enzymes phosphoglycerate kinase and pyruvate kinase transfer substrate high-energy phosphate groups to ADP to form ATP.

222. The answer is a. *(Murray, pp 180–189. Scriver, pp 2327–2356.)* Lipolysis of triacylglycerols yields fatty acids and glycerol. The free glycerol is transported to the liver, where it can be phosphorylated to glycerol phosphate and enter the glycolysis or the gluconeogenesis pathways at the level of dihydroxyacetone phosphate. Acetyl-CoA and propionyl-CoA are produced in the final round of degradation of an odd-chain fatty acid. Acetyl-CoA cannot be converted to glucose, but propionyl-CoA can. The three carbons of propionyl-CoA enter the citric acid cycle after being converted into succinyl-CoA. Succinyl-CoA can then be converted to oxaloacetate and enter the glycolytic scheme. Ketone bodies, including β-hydroxybutyrate, are produced from acetyl-CoA units derived from fatty acid β-oxidation. They may not be converted to glucose. Amino acids are not a product of triacylglycerol breakdown.

223. The answer is b. *(Murray, pp 180–189. Scriver, pp 2327–2356.)* Lipolysis is directly regulated by hormones in adipocytes. Epinephrine stimulates adenylate cyclase to produce cyclic AMP, which in turn stimulates a protein kinase. The kinase activates triglyceride lipase by phosphorylating it. Lipolysis then proceeds and results in the release of free fatty acids and glycerol. A futile reesterification of free fatty acids is prevented, since adipocytes contain little glycerol kinase to phosphorylate the liberated glycerol, which must be processed in the liver. Inhibition of lipolysis occurs in the presence of insulin, which lowers cyclic AMP levels. Lipoprotein lipase is not an adipocyte enzyme.

224. The answer is d. *(Murray, pp 92–101. Scriver, pp 2367–2424.)* Oligomycin inhibits mitochondrial ATPase and thus prevents phosphorylation of ADP to ATP. It prevents utilization of energy derived from electron transport for the synthesis of ATP. Oligomycin has no effect on coupling but blocks mitochondrial phosphorylation so that both oxidation and phosphorylation cease in its presence. The other enzymes catalyze coupling reactions that use or generate ATP; although tissues like erythrocytes (without mitochondria) and muscle (during exercise) may use glycolysis to generate ATP energy, they will fail in the long term if oxygen is not provided for respiration and ATP production by the mitochondria.

225. The answer is d. *(Murray, pp 180–189. Scriver, pp 2327–2356.)* Fats (triacylglycerols) are the most highly concentrated and efficient stores of metabolic energy in the body. This is because they are anhydrous and reduced. On a dry-weight basis, the yield from the complete oxidation of the fatty acids produced from triacylglycerols is approximately 9 kcal/g, compared with 4 kcal/g for glycogen and proteins. However, under physiologic conditions, glycogen and proteins become highly hydrated, whereas triacylglyceride stores remain relatively free of water. Therefore, although the energy yield from fat stores remains at approximately 9 kcal/g, the actual yields from the oxidation of glycogen and proteins are diluted considerably. Under physiologic conditions, fats yield three to four times the energy of glycogen stores. Patients with fatty acid oxidation disorders cannot switch to fat oxidation as efficiently when their glycogen is depleted by fasting, causing deficits in high energy requiring tissues like heart and skeletal muscle.

226. The answer is b. *(Murray, pp 136–144. Scriver, pp 2367–2424.)* The conversion of glucose to glucose-6-phosphate is different in liver and muscle. In muscle and most other tissues, hexokinase regulates the conversion of glucose to glucose-6-phosphate. When the major regulatory enzyme of glycolysis, phosphofructose kinase, is turned off, the level of fructose-6-phosphate increases and in turn the level of glucose-6-phosphate rises because it is in equilibrium with fructose-6-phosphate. Hexokinase is inhibited by glucose-6-phosphate. However, in the liver, glucose is phosphorylated even when glucose-6-phosphate levels are high because the enzyme regulating transformation of glucose into glucose-6-phosphate is glucokinase. Glucokinase is not inhibited by glucose-6-phosphate in the liver. Although hexokinase has a low K_m for glucose and is capable of acting on low levels of blood glucose, glucokinase has a high K_m for glucose and is effective only when glucose is abundant. Therefore, when blood glucose levels are low, muscle, brain, and other tissues are capable of taking up and phosphorylating glucose, whereas the liver is not. When blood glucose is abundant, glucokinase in the liver phosphorylates glucose and provides glucose-6-phosphate for the synthesis and storage of glucose as glycogen.

227. The answer is c. *(Murray, pp 180–189. Scriver, pp 2367–2424.)* Muscle contraction is caused by the release of calcium from the sarcoplasmic reticulum following nerve stimulation. In addition to stimulating contraction, the calcium released from the sarcoplasmic reticulum binds to a calmodulin subunit on phosphorylase kinase. This activates phosphorylase kinase, converting it from the D form to the A form. The activated phosphorylase then breaks down glycogen and provides glucose for energy metabolism during exercise. In this way, muscle contraction and glucose production from glycogen are coordinated by the transient increase of cytoplasmic calcium levels during muscle contraction.

228. The answer is c. *(Murray, pp 180–189. Scriver, pp 2297–2326.)* The most likely cause of the symptoms observed is carnitine deficiency. Under normal circumstances, long-chain fatty acids coming into muscle cells are activated as acyl-coenzyme A and transported as acyl-carnitine across the inner mitochondrial membrane into the matrix. A deficiency in carnitine, which is normally synthesized in the liver, can be genetic, but it is also observed in preterm babies with liver problems and dialysis patients. Blockage of the transport of long-chain fatty acids into mitochondria not only deprives the patient of energy production, but also disrupts the structure of the muscle cell with the accumulation of lipid droplets. Oral dietary supplementation usually can effect a cure. Deficiencies in the carnitine acyltransferase enzymes I and II can cause similar symptoms.

229. The answer is a. *(Murray, pp 180–189. Scriver, pp 2297–2326.)* Acetyl-CoA carboxylase deficiency drastically alters the ability of the patient to synthesize fatty acids. The fact that the infant was born at all is due to the body's ability to utilize fatty acids provided to it. However, all processes dependent on de novo fatty acid biosynthesis are affected. The lungs, in particular, require surfactant, a lipoprotein substance secreted by alveolar type II cells, to function properly. Surfactant lowers alveolar surface tension, facilitating gas exchange. It contains significant amounts of dipalmitoyl phosphatidylcholine. Palmitate is the major end product of de novo fatty acid synthesis. Acetyl-CoA carboxylase formation of malonyl-CoA is the first step of fatty acid synthesis. Biotin deficiency cannot be the problem because pyruvate carboxylase in gluconeogenesis is not affected. None of the other answers listed would result in all of the symptoms given.

230. The answer is a. *(Murray, pp 180–189. Scriver, pp 2297–2326.)* NAD-linked dehydrogenases generate one additional mole of ATP than flavoprotein-linked dehydrogenases. In the citric acid cycle, for example, three molecules of NADH and one molecule of $FADH_2$ are produced for each molecule of acetyl-CoA metabolized in one turn of the cycle. This leads to a total of 11 ATP produced by the respiratory chain for each turn of the citric acid cycle. An additional ATP is produced directly by substrate-level phosporylation.

231. The answer is a. *(Murray, pp 92–101.)* Coenzyme Q collects reducing equivalents from flavoprotein complexes and passes them along the chain to the cytochromes. Reducing equivalents from a number of substrates are passed through coenzyme Q in the respiratory chain, including flavin adenine dinucleotide ($FADH_2$) that is produced from metabolic reactions. Supplements of riboflavin (to boost flavin levels), coenzyme Q (available from health food stores), and carnitine (to facilitate entry of metabolites into mitochondria) have produced mild improvements in patients with respiratory chain disorders.

232. The answer is a. *(Murray, pp 92–101.)* An increase in ADP indicates the cell is in the working state and respiration will increase. In the resting state, the level of ADP should be low and thus respiration will be slow. During heavy workloads, such as during exercise, respiration may be regulated by the availability of oxygen or the limit of the capacity of the respiratory chain itself.

233. The answer is a. *(Murray, pp 92–101. Scriver, pp 2261–2274.)* Proton translocation across the mitochondrial membrane generates an electrochemical potential difference composed of a pH gradient and an electrical potential. This electrochemical potential difference is used to drive ATP synthase to form ATP. During this process NADH and water are oxidized, not reduced, by coupling with oxygen as the ultimate electron donor.

234. The answer is c. *(Murray, pp 92–101. Scriver, pp 2261–2274.)* Uncouplers such as 2,4-dinitrophenol dissociate oxidation from phosphorylation. Thus, ADP is not phosphorylated to produce ATP and respiration becomes uncontrolled as it tries to replenish ATP supplies. This leads to increased metabolic turnover (as in fat oxidation) in the attempt to generate ATP. Prolonged energy deficits will lead to fatigue in energy-dependent tissues like muscle or heart (cardiomyopathy), the latter being potentially lethal.

235. The answer is b. *(Murray, pp 92–101. Scriver, pp 2261–2274.)* Carbon monoxide and cyanide inhibit cytochrome oxidase, the terminal step of the respiratory chain that is driven by oxygen reduction to water. Barbiturates block transfer from cytochrome to coenzyme Q, antimycin A, and dimercaprol the step between cytochromes c and b, and dinitrophenol is an uncoupler that releases the respiratory chain from regulation by energy (phosphorylation) needs. Oligomycin blocks phosphorylation by inhibiting ATP synthase, thus shutting down its coupled oxidation.

236. The answer is b. *(Murray, pp 92–101. Scriver, pp 2261–2274.)* Uncouplers increase the permeability of the inner mitochondrial membrane to protons and reduce the electrochemical potential and inhibit ATP synthase. Respiratory chain inhibitors can include barbiturates, antibiotics such as antimycin A, and classic poisons such as cyanide and carbon monoxide. Barbiturates inhibit NAD-linked dehydrogenases by blocking the transfer of electrons from an iron-sulfur center to ubiquinone. Antimycin A inhibits the chain between cytochrome b and cytochrome c. Carbon monoxide and cyanide inhibit cytochrome oxidase and therefore totally arrest respiration.

237. The answer is b. *(Murray, pp 456–473. Scriver, pp 2367–2424.)* Cholera toxin is an 87-kDa protein produced by Vibrio cholerae, a gram-negative bacterium. The toxin enters intestinal mucosal cells by binding to G_{M1} ganglioside. It interacts with G_s protein, which stimulates adenylate cyclase. By ADP-ribosylation of G_s, the toxin blocks its capacity to hydrolyze bound GTP to GDP. Thus, the G protein is locked in an active form and adenylate cyclase stays irreversibly activated. Under normal conditions, inactivated G protein contains GDP, which is produced by a phosphatase catalyzing the hydrolysis of GTP to GDP. When GDP is so bound to the G protein, the adenylate cyclase is inactive. Upon hormone binding to the receptor, GTP is exchanged for GDP and the G protein is in an active state, allowing adenylate cyclase to produce cyclic AMP. Because cholera toxin prevents the hydrolysis of GTP to GDP, the adenylate cyclase remains in an irreversibly active state, continuously producing cyclic AMP in the intestinal mucosal cells. This leads to a massive loss of body fluid into the intestine within a few hours.

238. The answer is a. *(Murray, pp 92–101. Scriver, pp 2261–2274.)* Muscle and brain use the glycerophosphate shuttle to transfer reducing equivalents through the mitochondrial membrane. The glycerophosphate dehydrogenase inside the mitochondria utilizes FAD, whereas that in the cytosol uses NAD, resulting in only 2 mol of ATP produced instead of 3 ATP per atom of oxygen. In the malate shuttle used in the kidney, liver, and heart, the malate dehydrogenases on both sides of the mitochondrial membrane use NAD.

239. The answer is b. *(Murray, pp 92–101. Scriver, pp 2297–2326.)* The tricarboxylic acid (citric acid) cycle and fatty acid oxidation are two important pathways localized in mitochondria. Absence of efficient substrate oxidation will diminish levels of NADH, thus diminishing oxidation by the respiratory chain with diminished phosphorylation. Diminished production of ATP impacts tissues like heart and skeletal muscle with high-energy requirements. Children with organic acidemias like methylmalonic acidemia (251000) will tie up their carnitine as methylmalonyl carnitine, thus inhibiting transport of fatty acids into mitochondria (the medium and long chain fatty acids can only traverse the mitochondrial membrane as fatty acyl carnitines). Such children are often asymptomatic if well-fed, but can develop heart failure after fasting and glycogen depletion. Depletion of carnitine also causes accumulation of the organic acid with progressive metabolic acidosis.

240. The answer is c. *(Murray, pp 92–101. Scriver, pp 2367–2424.)* NADH generated from glycolysis must be relieved of an electron to form nicotinamide adenine dinucleotide (NAD^+) so that glycolysis may continue. However, mitochondrial membranes are impermeable to both NADH and NAD^+. The solution to this problem is the transfer of electrons from NADH to molecules that traverse the membrane. These shuttles include dihydroxyacetone phosphate (DHAP) to glycerol-3-phosphate—this shuttle regenerates $NAD^+$when the glycerol-3-phosphate diffuses into mitochondria, is oxidized by FAD back to DHAP, releasing DHAP back to the cytosol. In heart and liver, the more energy-efficient malate-aspartate shuttle moves electrons into mitochondria. Cytoplasmic oxaloacetate is reduced to malate, which diffuses into the mitochondria and is oxidized by NAD^+back to oxaloacetate. The mitochondrial oxaloacetate is converted to aspartate, which diffuses into the cytosol, where it is converted back into cytoplasmic oxaloacetate. The pyruvate dehydrogenase reaction may be reversed under anaerobic conditions when it generates NAD^+ needed for glycolysis.

241. The answer is b. *(Murray, pp 122–129. Scriver, pp 4637–4664.)* Muscle cells are the only cells listed that are capable of utilizing all the energy sources available—glucose, fatty acids, and, during fasting, ketone bodies. Mitochondria are required for metabolism of fatty acids and ketone bodies. Since red blood cells (erythrocytes) do not contain mitochondria, no utilization of these energy sources is possible. Red cells are thus extremely dependent on glycolysis, accounting for anemias caused by deficiency of glycolytic enzymes like hexokinase (235700). Although the brain may utilize glucose and ketone bodies, fatty acids cannot cross the blood-brain barrier. Hepatocytes (liver cells) are the sites of ketone body production, but the mitochondrial enzyme necessary for utilization of ketone bodies is not present in hepatocytes.

Lipid, Amino Acid, and Nucleotide Metabolism

Questions

DIRECTIONS: Each item below contains a question or incomplete statement followed by suggested responses. Select the **one best** response to each question.

242. A child with a large head, multiple fractures, and blue sclerae (whites of the eyes) is evaluated for osteogenesis imperfecta (166200). One study involves labeling of collagen chains in tissue culture to assess their mobility by gel electrophoresis. Amino acids labeled with radioactive carbon 14 are added to the culture dishes in order to label the collagen. Which of the following amino acids would not result in labeled collagen?

a. Serine
b. Glycine
c. Aspartate
d. Glutamate
e. Hydroxyproline

243. Liver aminotransferases, which are also called transaminases, catalyze the transfer of α-amino groups from many different amino acids to α-ketoglutarate. The intermediate produced is deaminated back to α-ketoglutarate with the formation of ammonium ion. The structure of α-ketoglutarate is shown below. Which of the following is the intermediate produced?

a. Aspartate
b. Alanine
c. Oxaloacetate
d. Glutamate
e. Pyruvate

$$^{-}OOC-CH_2-CH_2-\overset{\overset{\displaystyle O}{\|}}{C}-COO^{-}$$

Questions 244–245

244. Children with urea cycle disorders have low tolerance for ingested protein because they cannot excrete nitrogen efficiently. In the urea cycle diagrammed below, which compound is derived from a condensation of CO_2 and NH_4^+?

a. Compound A
b. Compound B
c. Compound C
d. Compound D
e. Compound E

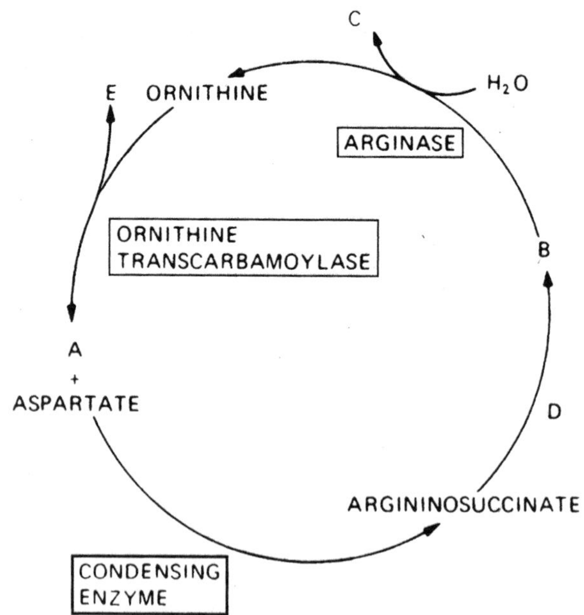

245. Children with urea cycle disorders usually present in the newborn period with lethargy progressing to coma as they are exposed to protein in breast milk or infant formula. The diagnosis is confirmed by finding elevated serum ammonia, often in the thousands with the upper limit of normal of 30–50 mmol/L, depending on the laboratory. Initial therapy consists of giving glucose instead of protein, and "priming" the urea cycle with a compound from the diagram in the above figure. Specific therapy will depend on which step of the cycle is blocked, diagnosed by blood amino acids (e.g., elevated citrulline versus ornithine) and enzyme assays. Which of the compounds in the figure would be most helpful in priming the cycle?

a. Compound A
b. Compound B
c. Compound C
d. Compound D
e. Compound E

246. Certain organic acidemias or fatty acid oxidation disorders will also involve elevated ammonia. This relates to the location of reactions of the urea cycle, occurring in which of the following?

a. In the cytosol
b. In lysosomes
c. In the mitochondrial matrix
d. In the mitochondrial matrix and the cytosol
e. In peroxisomes

247. A newborn becomes progressively lethargic after feeding and increases his respiratory rate. He becomes virtually comatose, responding only to painful stimuli, and exhibits mild respiratory alkalosis. Suspicion of a urea cycle disorder is aroused and evaluation of serum amino acid levels is initiated. In the presence of hyperammonemia, production of which of the following amino acids is always increased?

a. Glycine
b. Arginine
c. Proline
d. Histidine
e. Glutamine

248. A pregnant woman is found to have elevated blood pressure on her check-up at 8 months gestation, and testing by her obstetrician demonstrates anemia with Hemolysis, Elevated Liver enzymes, and Low Platelets that are characteristic of disease represented by the acronym HELLP syndrome. The woman is hospitalized and fetal maturity tests are performed that allow elective premature delivery. The woman quickly recovers but the premature newborn has a dilated heart and elevated liver enzymes that are characteristic of a defect in long chain fatty acid oxidation. The potential enzyme deficiencies are those responsible for sequential oxidation of fatty acids, which include which of the following?

a. Dehydrogenase, hydratase, dehydrogenase, thiolase
b. Transacylase, synthase, reductase
c. Hydratase, reductase, thiesterasel
d. Thioesterase, dehydrogenase, thiolase
e. Dehydrogenase, thiolase, thioesterae

249. A 2-year-old girl has been healthy until the past weekend when she contracted a viral illness at day care with vomiting, diarrhea, and progressive lethargy. She presents to the office on Monday with disorientation, a barely rousable sensorium, cracked lips, sunken eyes, lack of tears, flaccid skin with "tenting" on pinching, weak pulse with low blood pressure, and increased deep tendon reflexes. Laboratory tests show low blood glucose, normal electrolytes, elevated liver enzymes, and (on chest x-ray) a dilated heart. Urinalysis reveals no infection and no ketones. The child is hospitalized and stabilized with 10% glucose infusion, and certain admission laboratories come back 1 week later showing elevated medium chain fatty acyl carnitines in blood and 6–8 carbon dicarboxylic acids in the urine. The most likely disorder in this child involves which of the following?

a. Defect of medium chain coenzyme A dehydrogenase
b. Defect of medium chain fatty acyl synthetase
c. Mitochondrial defect in the electron transport chain
d. Mitochondrial defect in fatty acid transport
e. Carnitine deficiency

250. Which of the following is an important intermediate in the biosynthesis of fatty acids?

a. Carnitine
b. Cholesterol
c. Glucose
d. Malonyl-CoA

251. Which of the following enzymes is most important in regulating lipogenesis?

a. Acetyl-CoA carboxylase
b. Acetyl transacetylase
c. Enoyl reductase
d. Hydratase
e. 3-ketoacyl reductase

252. An adolescent female develops hemiballismus (repetitive throwing motions of the arms) after anesthesia for a routine operation. She is tall and lanky, and it is noted that she and her sister both had previous operations for dislocated lenses of the eyes. The symptoms are suspicious for the disease homocystinuria (236300). Which of the following statements is descriptive of this disease?

a. Patients may be treated with dietary supplements of vitamin B_{12}
b. Patients may be treated with dietary supplements of vitamin C
c. There is deficient excretion of homocysteine
d. There is increased excretion of cysteine
e. There is a defect in the ability to form cystathionine from homocysteine and serine

253. A child from a refugee camp presents with an unusual rash that suggests malnutrition. However, his parents relate that two sibs have had the same rash, and are affected with a disorder called Hartnup disease (234500). In this disorder, patients have a defect in neutral amino acid absorption from the intestine. The physician reads about Hartnup disease and decides the rashes are likely to be pellagra, caused by deficiency of niacin. Which of the following abnormalities in Hartnup disease would account for the niacine deficiency?

a. High fecal levels of tryptophan and indole derivatives
b. Deficiency of phenylalanine
c. Deficiency of alanine
d. Deficiency of leucine
e. Deficiency of glycine
f. Deficiency of isovaline
g. Deficiency of tryptophan

254. Which of the following is the important reactive group of glutathione in its role as an antioxidant?

a. Serine
b. Sulfhydryl
c. Tyrosine
d. Acetyl-CoA
e. Carboxyl

255. Which of the following processes generates the most ATP?

a. Citric acid cycle
b. Fatty acid oxidation
c. Glycolysis
d. Pentose phosphate pathway
e. Glycogenolysis

256. A newborn develops jaundice (yellow skin and yellow sclerae) that is greater than average at its usual peak at 3 days and requires laboratory evaluation. Which of the following porphyrin derivatives is conjugated, reacts directly, and is a major component of bile?

a. Bilirubin diglucuronide
b. Stercobilin
c. Biliverdin
d. Urobilinogen
e. Heme

257. A 40-year-old woman of fair complexion is admitted for evaluation of acute vomiting with abdominal pain. The episode began the night before after a fatty meal, and she has noted her stools are a peculiar grey white color. Abdominal examination is difficult because she is obese, but she exhibits acute tenderness in the right upper quadrant and has pain just below her left shoulder blade. Interference with which aspect of porphyrin metabolism best accounts for the white stools?

a. Sterile gut syndrome with defective bilirubin oxidation
b. Excess oxidation of bilirubin to urobilinogen
c. Heme synthesis defect causing increased bilirubin clearance
d. Bile duct excretion of bilirubin with oxidation to stercobilin
e. Excess reabsorption of urobilinogen with excess Urobilin

258. Chylomicrons, intermediate-density lipoproteins (IDLs), low-density lipoproteins (LDLs), and very-low-density lipoproteins (VLDLs) are all serum lipoproteins. Which of the following is the correct ordering of these particles from the lowest to the highest density?

a. LDLs, IDLs, VLDLs, chylomicrons
b. Chylomicrons, VLDLs, IDLs, LDLs
c. VLDLs, IDLs, LDLs, chylomicrons
d. Chylomicrons, IDLs, VLDLs, LDLs
e. LDLs, VLDLs, IDLs, chylomicrons

259. A 3-year-old child is brought into the ER while you are on duty. She is cold and clammy and is breathing rapidly. She is obviously confused and lethargic. Her mother indicates she has accidentally ingested automobile antifreeze while playing in the garage. Following gastrointestinal lavage and activated charcoal administration, which of the following treatments should you immediately initiate?

a. Intravenous infusion of oxalic acid
b. Nasogastric tube for ethanol administration
c. Flushing out the bladder via a catheter
d. Intramuscular injection of epinephrine
e. Simply waiting and measuring vital signs

260. After finding that infants, particularly those with prematurity, are vulnerable to fatty acid deficiencies, major manufacturers began supplementing their infant formulas with these compounds. Which of the following is a nutritionally essential fatty acid along with its usual dietary source?

a. Eicosapentaenoic acid-plants
b. Linoleic acid-plants
c. Oleic acid-animals
d. Palmitoleic acid-animals
e. Linolenic acid-animals

261. A middle-aged man develops episodes of incoordination and slurred speech. His wife notes that he seems depressed and argumentative. His physician diagnoses multiple sclerosis, which is best described as which of the following?

a. Demyelinating disease with loss of phospholipids and ceramide from brain and spinal cord
b. Lipid storage disease with loss of sphingolipids and ceramide from brain and spinal cord
c. Lipid storage disease with loss of sphingolipids and gangliosides from brain and spinal cord.
d. Demyelinating disease with loss of phospholipids and sphingolipids from brain and spinal cord
e. Lipid storage disease with accumulation of sphingolipids in brain

262. A child with chronic diarrhea and anemia is evaluated and found to have abetalipoproteinemia (200100), a disorder caused by defective transport and deficiency of the apoB protein. Which of the following classes of serum lipids would be expected to be deficient in abetalipoproteinemia?

a. Lipoprotein (a)
b. High density lipoproteins (HDL)
c. Chylomicrons
d. Triglycerides
e. Low density lipoprotein receptor

263. Children with very long or long chain fatty acid oxidation disorders are severely affected from birth, while those with short or medium chain oxidation defects may be asymptomatic until they have an intercurrent illness that causes prolonged fasting. The severe symptoms of longer chain diseases are best explained by which of the following statements?

a. Longer chain fatty acids inhibit gluconeogenesis and deplete serum glucose needed for brain metabolism
b. Glycogen is the main fuel reserve of the body but is quickly depleted with fasting
c. Starch is an important source of glucose and is inhibited by high fatty acid concentrations
d. Triacylglycerols are the main fuel reserve of the body and are needed for energy production in actively metabolizing tissues
e. Longer chain fatty acids from micelles and block synapses

264. A man with chronic alcoholism is admitted with hematochezia (bright red blood in stools) and hematemesis (bloody vomitus). Transfusions and esophageal tube pressure fail to maintain his blood pressure, and he dies from shock and cardiac failure. Autopsy would expect to show which of the following?

a. Normal liver with excess chylomicrons
b. Cirrhotic liver with excess HDL
c. Fatty liver with excess LDL
d. Fatty liver with VLDL
e. Cirrhotic and fatty liver with excess triacylglycerol

265. It has been noted that infants placed on extremely low-fat diets for a variety of reasons often develop skin problems and other symptoms. This is most often due to which of the following?

a. Lactose intolerance
b. Glycogen storage diseases
c. Antibody abnormalities
d. Deficiency of fatty acid desaturase greater than Δ^9
e. Deficiency of chylomicron and VLDL production

266. Which of the following best explains why statin therapy is effective for individuals with hypercholesterolemia?

a. Statins inhibit HMG-CoA reductase, a key regulator of cholesterol synthesis
b. Statins inhibit HMG-CoA synthase, key step for synthesis of mevalonate that inhibits fatty acid synthesis
c. Stains stimulate thiolase, thus making more malonyl CoA for inhibition of the tricarboxylic acid cyle
d. Statins bind to LDL receptor, displacing cholesterol and inhibiting cholesterol synthesis
e. Statins stimulate synthesis of trans-unsaturated fatty acids

267. A child from Nigeria is evaluated for developmental delay. His coloring seems much lighter than that of his family background, and his physician orders a blood amino acid test that demonstrates elevated phenylalanine. A special low phenylalanine formula is begun (Lofenelac) as treatment for phenylketonuria (261600), but the parents refuse to come in for follow-up appointments. A public health evaluation reports that the child is failing to thrive despite apparent adherence to the diet by his parents. The symptoms of decreased skin pigment and later failure to thrive in this child are most likely related to which of the following?

a. Deficiency of alanine
b. Deficiency of tyrosine and melanin
c. Deficiency of tryptophan and niacin
d. Deficiency of leucine and isoleucine
e. Deficiency of phenylalanine

268. Niemann-Pick disease (257220), like other neurolipidoses, present in infancy or childhood with plateauing of development and neurologic regression. The accumulating substance is a phospholipid made in which of the following steps in the figure below?

a. Step A
b. Step B
c. Step C
d. Step D
e. Step E

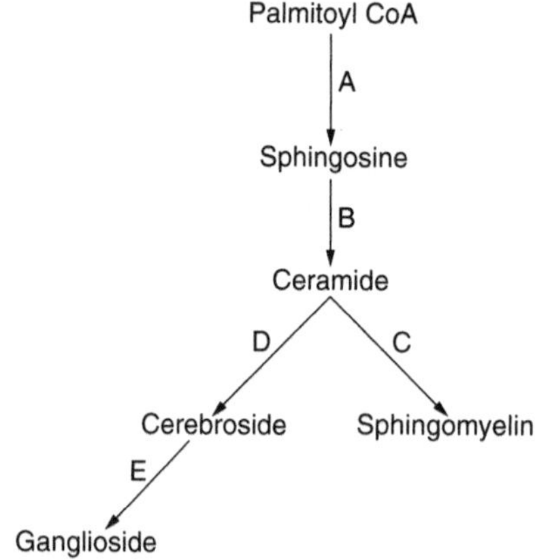

269. A 10-year-old female presents with chest pain and unusual skin patches over her elbows and knees. Her father died of a heart attack at age 35 and her mother is known to have high cholesterol. Her physician suspects familial hypercholesterolemia (144010) in the parents with homozygous severe disease in the daughter. This disease results from mutations in the receptor for low-density lipoprotein (LDL) or the ligand portion of its apoprotein coat, which is which of the following?

a. AI
b. B48
c. CII
d. B100
e. E

270. A 45-year-old man is found to have an elevated serum cholesterol of 300 mg percent measured by standard conditions after a 12-hour fast. Which of the following lipoproteins would contribute to a measurement of plasma cholesterol in a normal person following a 12-hour fast?

a. Very-low-density lipoproteins (VLDL) and low-density lipoproteins (LDL)
b. High-density lipoproteins (HDL) and low-density lipoproteins (LDL)
c. Chylomicrons and very-low-density lipoproteins (VLDL)
d. Chylomicron remnants and very-low-density-lipoproteins (VLDL)
e. Low-density lipoproteins (LDL) and adipocyte lipid droplets

271. A newborn with meconium ileus (plugging of the small intestine with meconium or fetal stool) is found to have air in thè bowel wall (pneumatosis intestinalis) and free air in the abdomen. Antibiotics are begun for suspected peritonitis, and emergency surgery is performed to remove the diseased intestinal segment and heal the intestinal perforation that led to air in the abdomen. Because the gut must be kept at rest for healing, meconium peritonitis was usually fatal until parenteral alimentation solutions were developed. Hyperalimentation consists of essential amino acids and other metabolites that provide a positive calorie balance while keeping the bowel at rest. The alimentation solution must be kept to a minimum of metabolites because of its high osmotic load that necessitates frequent changing of intravenous sites or catherization of a large vein. Which of the following amino acids could be excluded from the alimentation solution?

a. Cysteine
b. Phenylalanine
c. Histidine
d. Methionine
e. Tryptophan

272. A 15-year-old boy has a long history of school problems and is labeled as hyperactive. His tissues are puffy, giving his face a "coarse" appearance. His IQ tests have declined recently and are now markedly below normal. Laboratory studies demonstrate normal amounts of sphingolipids in fibroblast cultures with increased amounts of glycosaminoglycans in urine. Which of the following enzyme deficiencies might explain the boy's phenotype?

a. Hexosaminidase A
b. Glucocerebrosidase
c. α-L-iduronidase
d. α-galactocerebrosidase
e. β-gangliosidase A

273. Leukocyte samples isolated from the blood of a newborn infant are homogenized and incubated with ganglioside GM_2. Approximately 47% of the expected normal amount of *N*-acetylgalactosamine is liberated during the incubation period. These results indicate which of the following regarding this infant?

a. It is a heterozygote (carrier) for Tay-Sachs disease
b. It is homozygous for Tay-Sachs disease
c. It has Tay-Sachs syndrome
d. It will most likely have mental deficiency
e. It has relatively normal β-*N*-acetylhexosaminidase activity

274. Most of the reducing equivalents utilized for synthesis of fatty acids can be generated from which of the following?

a. The pentose phosphate pathway
b. Glycolysis
c. The citric acid cycle
d. Mitochondrial malate dehydrogenase
e. Citrate lyase

275. Which enzyme catalyzes the only step of fatty acid oxidation that requires energy?

a. Acyl-CoA dehydrogenase
b. Acyl-CoA synthetase
c. Δ2-enoyl-CoA hydratase
d. L(+)-3-hydroxyacyl-CoA dehydrogenase
e. Thiolase

276. Which of the following amino acids (1) is the product of reduction from another amino acid, (2) can be transaminated to pyruvate, and (3) accumulates in an inborn error affecting the eyes and kidney?

a. Alanine
b. Cysteine
c. Serine
d. Glycine
e. Hydroxyproline

277. Urea synthesis requires five enzymes. Which of the following enzymes requires two ATPs?

a. Arginase
b. Argininosuccinase
c. Argininosuccinic acid synthase
d. Carbamoyl phosphate synthase I
e. Ornithine carboxylase

278. The citric acid cycle intermediate oxaloacetate is formed by which amino acid?

a. Asparagine
b. Glutamine
c. Proline
d. Serine
e. Theronine

279. Which of the following is not used in the synthesis of fatty acids?

a. ATP
b. Cobalamin (vitamin B_{12})
c. $FADH_2$
d. HCO_3^-
e. NADPH

Questions 280–281. Refer to the figure below for the next two questions.

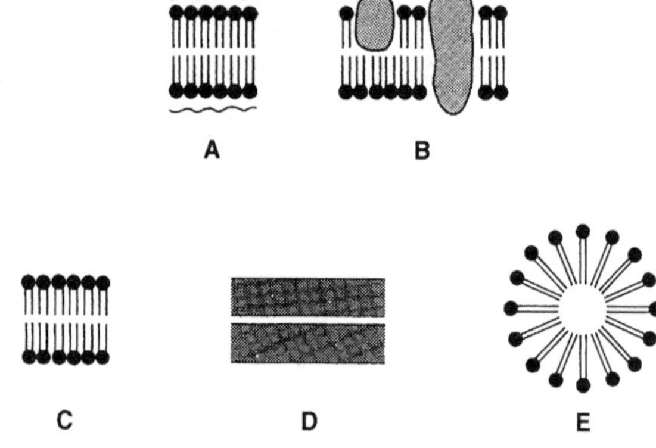

280. Group II signal transduction hormones and growth factors (e.g., insulin, insulin-like growth factors) act at cell membranes, stimulating release of "second messengers" like cyclic AMP that effect cellular responses. Which of the diagrammatic structures in the above figure represents the model of biologic membranes that most successfully accounts for membrane asymmetry?

a. Structure A
b. Structure B
c. Structure C
d. Structure D
e. Structure E

281. Which of the diagrammatic structures shown above most clearly represents a model of the configuration of lipids obtained during the emulsification process that precedes hydrolysis during digestion?

a. Structure A
b. Structure B
c. Structure C
d. Structure D
e. Structure E

282. Coronary artery disease is a multifactorial disorder involving occlusion of the coronary artery with atherosclerotic plaques. Several Mendelian disorders affecting lipid metabolism increase susceptibility for heart attacks, while environmental factors include smoking and high-fat diets. A 45-year-old man has a mild heart attack and is placed on diet and mevastatin therapy. Which of the following will be the most likely result of this therapy?

a. Low blood glucose
b. Low blood LDLs
c. High blood cholesterol
d. High blood glucose
e. Low oxidation of fatty acids

283. A newborn male is evaluated because of inability to breast feed and found to have severe hypotonia (low muscle tone). The child lays in a frog leg posture with minimal spontaneous movements, and the head and legs dangle to the bed when suspended by his stomach. A large anterior fontanel is noted, and initial laboratory tests indicate elevated liver enzymes. The physician suspects Zellweger syndrome (214100), an end phenotype reflecting peroxisome dysfunction that may be caused by mutations in several different peroxisomal membrane protein genes. The diagnosis is confirmed by demonstrating elevated plasma levels of very long chain fatty acids and of erythrocyte plasmalogens. Which of the following compounds is the starting point of ether lipid and plasmalogen synthesis?

a. Acetyl CoA
b. Pyruvate
c. Dihydroxyacetone phosphate
d. Malonyl CoA
e. Palmitoyl CoA

284. A prime diagnostic indicator for the first presentation of diabetes mellitus is the presence of ketonuria and severe acidosis; the acidosis produces exaggerated attempts at respiratory compensation known as Kussmaul breathing. Which of the following are "ketone bodies" that would be elevated in serum and urine from a child with diabetic ketoacidosis?

a. Acetone and ethanol
b. β-hydroxybutyrate and acetoacetate
c. Pyrvuate and lactate
d. Fumarate and succinate
e. Oxaloacetate and pyruvate

285. Gangliosides and receptors for hormones such as glucagon can be found in which of the following structures?

a. Plasma membrane
b. Mitochondria
c. Lysosomes
d. Endoplasmic reticulum
e. Ribosomes

286. Folic acid deficiency may present with megaloblastic anemia or be diagnosed by its effect on certain metabolic pathways. Which of the following amino acids and their catabolic products require folate along with an intermediate that, when elevated in serum, indicates folate deficiency?

a. Serine, glycine, carbon dioxide
b. Cystine, cysteine, mercaptopyruvate
c. Glycine, alanine, pyruvate
d. Threonine, acetaldehyde, acetate
e. Histidine, formaminoglutamate, glutamate

287. Which of the following is the major source of extracellular cholesterol for human tissues?

a. Very-low-density lipoproteins (VLDLs)
b. Low-density lipoproteins (LDLs)
c. High-density lipoproteins (HDLs)
d. Albumin
e. γ-Globulin

288. Arginine can be converted to which citric acid cycle intermediate?

a. Citrate
b. Fumarate
c. α-ketoglutarate
d. Malate
e. Oxaloacetate

289. When the liver is actively synthesizing fatty acids, a concomitant decrease in β-oxidation of fatty acids is due to which of the following?

a. Inhibition of a translocation between cellular compartments
b. Inhibition by an end product
c. Activation of an enzyme
d. Detergent effects
e. Decreases in adipocyte lipolysis

290. A 4-year-old girl presents in the clinic with megaloblastic anemia and failure to thrive. Blood chemistries reveal orotic aciduria (258900). Enzyme measurements of white blood cells reveal a deficiency of the pyrimidine biosynthesis enzyme orotate phosphoribosyltransferase and abnormally high activity of the enzyme aspartate transcarbamoylase. Which of the following treatments will reverse all symptoms if carried out chronically?

a. Blood transfusion
b. White blood cell transfusion
c. Dietary supplements of phosphoribosylpyrophosphate (PRPP)
d. Oral thymidine
e. Oral uridine

291. A 1-year-old male has a normal birth and infantile history except for delay in sitting up, crawling, and standing (delayed motor milestones). He begins the unusual habit of chewing on his fingers and lips, and in one instance bites through the lip and leaves a large wound. His physician documents an elevated serum uric acid and suspects Lesch-Nyhan syndrome (300322). In considering potential therapy, the physician reads that purines are overproduced in gout and Lesch-Nyhan syndrome, causing hyperuricemia, yet the hypoxanthine analogue allopurinol is only effective in gout. Allopurinol does not treat the neurologic symptoms of Lesch-Nyhan syndrome because it does not do which the following?

a. Decrease de novo purine synthesis
b. Decrease de novo pyrimidine synthesis
c. Diminish urate synthesis
d. Increase phosphoribosylpyrophosphate (PRPP) levels
e. Inhibit xanthine oxidase

292. Which of the following would make hyperuricemia very unlikely in a patient?

a. Lesch-Nyhan syndrome
b. Gout
c. Xanthine oxidase hyperactivity
d. Carbamoyl phosphate synthase deficiency
e. Purine overproduction secondary to von Gierke's disease

293. Which of the following contributes nitrogen atoms to both purine and pyrimidine rings?

a. Aspartate
b. Carbamoyl phosphate
c. Carbon dioxide
d. Glutamine
e. Tetrahydrofolate

294. A woman consults her physician because of occasional periods of confusion and lethargy, usually after a meal. The physician suspects a deficiency in an enzyme of the urea cycle, which in this case would most likely be which of the following?

a. Arginase
b. Argininosuccinase
c. Argininosuccinic acid synthase
d. Carbamoyl phosphate synthase I
e. Ornithine transcarbamylase deficiency

295. A 35-year-old man presents to the emergency room with an acute abdomen (severe abdominal pain with tightness of muscles, decreased bowel sounds, and vomiting and/or diarrhea). He has been drinking, and a urine sample is unusual because it has a port-wine color. Past history indicates several prior evaluations for abdominal pain, including an appendectomy. The physician notes unusual neurologic symptoms with partial paralysis of his arms and legs. At first concerned about food poisons like botulism, the physician recalls that acute intermittent porphyria may cause these symptoms (176000) and consults a gastroenterologist. Elevation of which of the following urinary metabolites would support a diagnosis of porphyria?

a. Urobilinogen and bilirubin
b. Delta-aminolevulinic acid and porphobilinogen
c. Biliverdin and stercobilin
d. Urobilin and urobilinogen
e. Delta-aminolevulinic acid and urobilinogen

296. Gout is an inflammatory reaction due to uric acid crystallization in soft tissues and joints. One defect responsible for this is in which enzyme of purine biosynthesis?

a. Adenylosuccinase
b. Formyltransferase
c. IMP cyclohydrolase
d. PRPP glutamyl amidotransferase
e. PRPP synthetase

297. Hyperuricemia in Lesch-Nyhan syndrome is due to a defect in which of the following pathways?

a. Purine biosynthesis
b. Pyrimidine biosynthesis
c. Purine salvage
d. Pyrimidine salvage

298. Which of the following is the rate-controlling step of pyrimidine synthesis that exhibits allosteric inhibition by cytidine triphosphate (CTP)?

a. Aspartate transcarbamoylase
b. Hypoxanthine-guanine phosphoribosyl transferase (HGPRT)
c. Thymidylate synthase
d. Ribose-phosphate pyrophosphokinase
e. Xanthine oxidase

299. Which of the following compounds is a required substrate for purine biosynthesis?

a. 5-methyl thymidine
b. Ara C
c. Ribose phosphate
d. 5-phosphoribosylpyrophosphate (PRPP)
e. 5-FU

300. Which of the following compounds is an analogue of hypoxanthine?

a. Ara C
b. Allopurinol
c. Ribose phosphate
d. 5-phosphoribosylpyrophosphate (PRPP)
e. 5-FU

301. Which of the following compounds is joined with nicotinamide to form NAD and NADP, components that are deficient in niacin deficiency?

a. Cytosine monophosphate
b. Inosine diphosphate
c. Thymidine monophosphate
d. Hypoxanthine monophosphate
e. Adenosine diphosphate

302. Which of the following nucleotides is associated with activated sugars in galactose, glycogen, and glycoprotein?

a. Adenosine diphosphate
b. Guanosine diphosphate
c. Thymidine diphosphate
d. Cytosine diphosphate
e. Uridine diphosphate

Lipid, Amino Acid, and Nucleotide Metabolism

Answers

242. The answer is e. *(Murray, pp 38–39, 535–539. Scriver, pp 5241–5286.)* Collagen has an unusual amino acid composition in that approximately one-third of collagen molecules are glycine. The amino acid proline is also present in a much greater amount than in other proteins. In addition, two somewhat unusual amino acids, 4-hydroxyproline and 5-hydroxylysine, are found in collagen. Hydroxyproline and hydroxylysine per se are not incorporated during the synthesis of collagen. Proline and lysine are hydroxylated by specific hydroxylases after collagen is synthesized. A reducing agent such as ascorbate (vitamin C) is needed for the hydroxylation reaction to occur. In its absence, the disease known as scurvy occurs. Only proline or lysine residues located on the amino side of glycine residues are hydroxylated. Because hydroxylation of proline and lysine occurs after collagen is synthesized, addition of labeled hydroxyproline to the tissue culture will not result in labeled collagen.

243. The answer is d. *(Murray, pp 242–263. Scriver, pp 1667–1724.)* Amino acid degradation ultimately leads to the formation of ammonium ion (NH_4^+), which is toxic in significant amounts. In the liver of humans, as in most terrestrial vertebrates, NH_4^+ is produced and converted into urea for excretion. For many amino acids, the conversion of α-amino groups into ammonium ion and then into urea is carried out by two groups of enzymes. Transaminases (aminotransferases) transfer α-amino groups to α-ketoglutarate to form glutamate, which is then oxidatively deaminated by glutamate dehydrogenase to release free ammonium ions that can be converted to urea.

244. The answer is e. *(Murray, pp 242–248. Scriver, pp 1909–1964.)* In the liver, the urea cycle converts excess NH_4^+ to a form amenable to excretion by the kidneys. Free NH_4^+ condenses with CO_2 to form carbamoyl phosphate in a reaction catalyzed by carbamoyl phosphate synthetase. This is an energy-expensive, essentially irreversible reaction requiring two molecules of ATP. Carbamoyl phosphate (compound E in the urea cycle diagram) then combines with ornithine to produce citrulline in the first step of the urea cycle proper. The second nitrogen of urea is derived from the amino acid aspartate, which condenses with citrulline to form arginosuccinase in the second step of the cycle. This step is catalyzed by arginosuccinase synthetase and also requires a molecule of ATP.

245. The answer is b. *(Murray, pp 242–248. Scriver, pp 1909–1964.)* In humans and other land mammals, excess NH_4^+ is converted into urea (compound C in the urea cycle diagram of Fig. 35) in the liver for excretion by the kidneys. Malfunctions of the urea cycle can lead to hyperammonemia and result in brain damage. Compound C is arginine, the next to last step in the cycle and available as an intravenous solution. Adding arginine bypasses the most severe urea cycle defects—carbamoyl phosphate synthetase deficiency (formation of compound E, 237300), ornithine transcarbamylase deficiency (compound E to A, 311250), citrullinemia (A to argininosuccinate, 215700), argininosuccinic aciduria (argininosuccinate to arginine (compound B-209700)—and increases the substrate concentration for the last enzyme defect, argininemia (208700). Note that nitrogen is excreted in the form of urea with its two nitrogen and one carbonyl group. The first nitrogen is derived from free NH_4^+ (condensed with CO_2 to form carbamoyl phosphate—compound E) and the second nitrogen from the amino group of aspartate.

246. The answer is d. *(Murray, pp 242–248. Scriver, pp 1909–1964.)* The steps of the urea cycle are divided between the mitochondrial matrix and cytosol of liver cells in mammals. The formation of ammonia, its reaction with carbon dioxide to produce carbamoyl phosphate, and the conversion to citrulline occur in the matrix of mitochondria. Citrulline diffuses out of the mitochondria, and the next three steps of the cycle, which result in the formation of urea, all take place in the cytosol. Fatty acid oxidation and some reactions of organic acid degradation also occur in the mitochondria. Peroxisomes have single membranes, in contrast to the double membranes of mitochondria. They house catalase and enzymes for medium- to long-chain fatty acid oxidation.

247. The answer is e. *(Murray, pp 242–248. Scriver, pp 1909–1964.)* Deficiencies of urea cycle enzymes cause symptoms ranging from confusion and fatigue after a high-protein meal to neonatal lethargy, vomiting, coma, and death. Female carriers for ornithine transcarbamylase (OTC) deficiency (300461) and some mild urea cycle mutations have hyperammonemia with confusion and lethargy after a high protein meal (e.g., hamburgers) and develop aversions to such foods. On the other side of the spectrum, severe urea cycle blocks are incompatible with life. A major reason for the toxicity is the severe depletion of ATP levels caused by the siphoning off of α-ketoglutarate from the citric acid cycle in an attempt to consume ammonia. Glutamate dehydrogenase and glutamine synthetase, respectively, catalyze the following reaction:

$$\alpha\text{-ketoglutarate} + NH_4^+ \rightarrow \text{glutamate} + NH_4^+ \rightarrow \text{glutamine}$$

As can be seen, this is the reverse order of steps whereby glutamine is successively deaminated first to glutamate and then to α-ketoglutarate by the enzymes glutaminase and glutamate dehydrogenase, respectively. It is thought that the high level of ammonia ions shifts the equilibrium of the dehydrogenase in favor of the formation of glutamate. Depending on the step in the urea cycle that is blocked, levels of arginine may be decreased.

248. The answer is a. *(Murray, pp 122–129, 173–179. Scriver, pp 2297–2326.)* Fatty acids are bound to coenzyme A as thiol esters for synthesis or degradation, each proceeding in two-carbon steps. The serially repeated steps in fatty acid oxidation involve (1) removal of two hydrogens to form a double bond between the carbons adjacent to the acid group (acyl-CoA dehydrogenase), (2) addition of water to the double bond so that a hydroxyl is on the second carbon (enoyl-CoA hydratase), oxidation of the hydroxyl group to a ketone (3-hydroxyacylCoA dehydrogenase), and removal of acetyl CoA (thiolase) to leave a fatty acyl CoA that is two carbons shorter. At least three groups of these sequentially acting enzymes are present in the mitochondrion, specific for very long or long chain, medium chain, or short chain fatty acids. Children with very long or long chain oxidation enzyme deficiencies, e.g. very long chain fatty acyl CoA dehydrogenase deficiency (VLCAD, 201475) accumulate fat in their heart and liver and have energy deficits in heart and muscle due to inadequate fat oxidation. Severely affected children often die of cardiac failure in the newborn period, and their enzyme deficiency combined with the maternal heterozygote state may cause HELLP syndrome in the last trimester of pregnancy, a variant of toxemia or preeclampsia that can be fatal. Premature delivery may be necessary for maternal health, and therapy with low-fat diets, frequent feeding (to minimize need for fat oxidation), and carnitine (to maximize transport of fatty acyl CoAs into mitochondria) may be attempted with the affected child.

249. The answer is a. *(Murray, pp 122–129, 173–179. Scriver, pp 2297–2326.)* Fatty acid oxidation is a major source of energy after glycogen is depleted during fasting. Fatty acids are first coupled with coenzyme A, transferred for mitochondrial import as acylcarnitines, and degraded in steps that remove two carbons. The fatty acyl CoA dehydrogenases, enoyl hydratases, hydroyacyl CoA dehydrogenases, and thiolases that carry out each oxidation step are present in three groups with specifities for very long/long, medium, and short chain fatty acyl esters. As would be expected, deficiencies of long-chain oxidizing enzymes have more severe consequences than those for short chains since they impair many more cycles of two-carbon removal. Long chain deficiencies may be lethal in the newborn period, while medium or short chain deficiencies may be undetected until a child goes without food for a prolonged time and must resort to extensive fatty acid oxidation for energy. Medium chain coenzyme A dehydrogenase (MCAD) deficiency (201450) can be fatal if not recognized, and sometimes presents as Sudden Unexplained Death Syndrome (SUDS—usually at older ages than Sudden Infant Death Syndrome—SIDS—that is mostly from respiratory problems). The deficit of acetyl CoA from fatty acid oxidation impacts gluconeogenesis with hypoglycemia, and the energy deficit leads to heart, liver, and muscle disease that may be lethal. Unlike most causes of hypoglycemia, the impaired fatty acid oxidation does not produce ketones (nonketotic hypoglycemia). Carnitine is tied up as medium chain acylcarnitines and is secondarily deficient in fatty acid oxidation disorders. Rare primary carnitine deficiencies (as in answer option e) impair oxidation of all fatty acids because they cannot be imported into mitochondria.

250. The answer is d. *(Murray, pp 173–179; Scriver, pp 2327–2356.)* Acetyl-CoA is carboxylated to form malonyl CoA through the addition of carbon dioxide by acetyl-CoA carboxylase. The acetyl and malonyl-CoA groups are added to sulfydryl groups of fatty acid synthase multienzyme complex (one on each subunit) through transacylation reactions. Condensation forms acetoacetyl-S-enzyme on one subunit and a free sulfydryl group of the other subunit—a sequence of enzyme reactions then converst the acetoacetyl-S-enzyme to acyl (acetyl) enzyme. A second round of two-carbon addition begins as another malonyl CoA residue displaces the acyl-S-enzyme to the other sulfhydryl group, then condenses to extend the acyl group by two carbons. Fatty acid synthesis then proceeds by successive addition of malonyl CoA residues with condensation, causing the acyl chain to grow by two carbons with each cycle.

251. The answer is a. *(Murray, pp 173–179. Scriver, pp 2327–2356.)* Acetyl-CoA carboxylase catalyzes the first step of lipogenesis in which acetyl-CoA is linked to malonyl-CoA. This enzyme is activated by citrate. Acetyl-CoA does not readily cross the mitochondrial membrane. Instead, citrate translocates to the cytosol where it is cleaved to acetyl-CoA and oxaloacetate by ATP-citrate lyase. Citrate increases in the fed state and indicates an abundant supply of acetyl-CoA for lipogenesis.

252. The answer is e. *(Murray, pp 249–269. Scriver, pp 2007–2056.)* In the synthesis of cysteine, the following sequence of steps occurs, where SAM is S-adenosylmethionine, cys is cysteine, and α-KG is α-ketoglutarate:

$$\text{methionine} \rightarrow \text{SAM} \rightarrow \text{homocysteine} + \text{adenosine}$$

$$\text{homocysteine} + \text{serine} \rightarrow \text{cystathionine} \rightarrow \text{cys} + \alpha\text{-KG} + NH_4^+$$

Cystathionine synthetase, a pyridoxal phosphate (vitamin B_6) enzyme, catalyzes the condensation of serine and homocysteine to form cystathionine. A deficiency of this enzyme leads to a buildup of homocysteine, which oxidizes to form homocysteine. This may result in mental retardation, but sometimes causes dislocated lenses and a tall, asthenic build reminiscent of Marfan syndrome. Patients with homocystinuria also have a clotting diathesis, requiring care to avoid dehydration during anesthesia. Their cysteine deficiency must be made up from dietary sources. In some cases, dietary intake of vitamin B_6 (pyrixodal phosphate) may alleviate symptoms because of its requirement by the crucial enzymes.

253. The answer is g. *(Murray, pp 249–263,490. Scriver, pp 2079–2108.)* Hartnup disease (234500) is caused by defective neutral amino acid transport in the intestinal and/or kidney. Neutral aminoaciduria is observed as well as increased fecal excretion of indole derivations due to bacterial conversion of unabsorbed dietary tryptophan. The disorder is very rare in industrialized countries with good diets, since deficiency of tryptophan as a precursor for niacin synthesis causes the most severe symptoms. Niacin deficiency is called pellagra and produces skin rashes, psychiatric symptoms, and neurologic problems like ataxia (wobbly gait) or diplopia (double vision). Deficiencies of the other mentioned amino acids are not recognized as clinical syndromes, although excess of phenylalanine in phenylketonuria (PKU—261600) or of leucine or isovaline in maple syrup urine disease is associated with severe symptoms if untreated.

254. The answer is b. *(Murray, pp 611–613. Scriver, pp 2205–2216.)* The antioxidant activity of glutathione is dependent on maintenance of its reduced state. The enzyme glutathione reductase transfers electrons from NADPH via FAD to oxidized glutathione. Oxidized glutathione is composed of two glutathione molecules held together by a disulfide bridge. Reduced glutathione is a tripeptide with a free sulfhydryl group. It is the presence of the free sulfhydryl group that is of importance to the antioxidant activity of glutathione. In red blood cells, the function of cysteine residues of hemoglobin and other proteins is maintained by the reducing power of glutathione.

255. The answer is b. *(Murray, pp 130–144, 163–172, 180–189. Scriver, pp 4517–4554.)* The pentose phosphate pathway does not generate any ATP but instead forms NADPH and ribose phosphate. Glycolysis produces a net two ATP molecules per glucose. The citric acid cycle produces a net 12 ATP per turn of the cycle. Fatty acid oxidation of palmitate results in a total of 129 ATP. Electron transport in the respiratory chain results in 5 ATP for each of the first 7 acetyl-CoA produced by the oxidation of palmitate for a total of 35 ATP. Each of the 8 acetyl-CoA molecules produced from palmitate results in 12 ATP from the citric acid cycle for 96 total ATP. This gives a total of 131 ATP per palmitate oxidized, minus 2 ATP for the initial activation of palmitate for a grand total of 129 ATP per palmitate.

256. The answer is a. *(Murray, pp 270–285. Scriver, pp 2961–3104.)* Jaundice refers to the yellow color of the skin and eyes caused by increased levels of bilirubin in the blood. It has many causes, including increased production of bilirubin due to hemolytic anemia or malaria, blockage in the excretion of bilirubin due to liver damage, or obstruction of the bile duct.

In newborns, jaundice is normal (physiologic) because of liver immaturity. Only excess jaundice is evaluated (bilirubin over 10–12 at age 3–4 days) based on the age of the infant. High levels of bilirubin in serum (indirect bilirubin) points toward hemolysis from maternofetal blood group incompatibility, whereas high levels of bilirubin diglucuronide (one of several conjugated bilirubins tested as direct bilirubin) suggest liver/gastrointestinal disease.

Reticuloendothelial cells degrade red blood cells following approximately 120 days in the circulation. The steps in the degradation of heme include (1) formation of the green pigment biliverdin by the cleavage of the porphyrin ring of heme; (2) formation of the red-orange pigment bilirubin by the reduction of biliverdin, (3) uptake of bilirubin by the liver and the formation of bilirubin diglucuronide, and (4) active excretion of bilirubin into bile and eventually into the stool. The change in color of a bruise from bluish-green to reddish-orange reflects the heme degradation and the change in color of the bile pigments biliverdin and bilirubin. Bilirubin, which is quite insoluble, is transported to the liver attached to albumin. In the liver, bilirubin is conjugated to two glucuronic acid molecules to form bilirubin diglucuronide. Bilirubin diglucuronide is transported against a concentration gradient into the bile. If bilirubin is not conjugated, it is not excreted.

257. The answer is d. *(Murray, pp 270–285. Scriver, pp 2961–3104.)* Once bile is excreted into the gut, bilirubin diglucuronide is hydrolyzed and reduced by bacteria to form urobilinogen, which is colorless. Much of the urobilinogen of the stools is further oxidized by intestinal bacteria to stercobilin, which gives stools their characteristic brown color. Some urobilinogen is reabsorbed by the gut into the portal blood, transported to the kidney, and converted and excreted as urobilin, which gives urine its characteristic yellow color. The woman has usual risk factors for cholecystitis (inflammation of the gall bladder) remembered as fair, fat, and forty. The inflammation can block excretion of conjugated bilirubin into the intestine, reducing oxidation to stercobilin and producing white (acholic) stools.

258. The answer is b. *(Murray, pp 205–218. Scriver, pp 2705–2716.)* Chylomicrons are triglyceride-rich transport particles containing dietary lipids. Very-low-density lipoproteins (VLDLs) are triglyceride- and cholesterol-containing particles from the liver that contain endogenously packaged lipids. Delipidation of triglycerides from VLDLs leads to formation of intermediate forms (IDLs) and finally to a cholesterol-enriched small particle, the low-density lipoprotein (LDL). Thus, VLDL → IDL → LDL. The following table summarizes the characteristics of these plasma lipoproteins.

259. The answer is b. *(Scriver, pp 2297–2326, 121–138, 287–320.)* Untreated ethylene glycol of antifreeze can be converted to the kidney toxin oxalate crystals. This occurs by oxidation of ethylene glycol. The first committed step in this process is the oxidation of ethylene glycol to an aldehyde by alcohol dehydrogenase. This is normally the route for converting ethanol (drinking alcohol) to acetate. Patients who have ingested ethylene glycol or wood alcohol (methanol) are placed on a nearly intoxicating dose of ethanol by a nasogastric tube together with intravenous saline and sodium bicarbonate. This treatment is carried out intermittently along with hemodialysis until no traces of ethylene glycol are seen in the blood. Ethanol acts as a competitive inhibitor of alcohol dehydrogenase with respect to ethylene glycol or methanol metabolism.

260. The answer is b. *(Murray, pp 190–196.)* Linoleic and α-linolenic acid are nutritionally essential in that they cannot be made by most animals and are instead made only by plants. Oleic acid and palmitoleic acid can be produced by introduction of a double bond at the Δ^9 position of a saturated fatty acid. These essential unsaturated fatty acids are required for synthesis of prostaglandin, thromboxane, leukotriene, and lipoxin.

261. The answer is d. *(Murray, pp 197–204. Scriver, pp 5875–5902.)* Ceramide is an important signaling molecule for apoptosis and is a precursor for glycosphingolipids and gangliosides. Sphingolipids and phospholipids are structural lipids in membranes. Multiple sclerosis is a demyelinating disease in which both phospholipid and sphingolipid levels are decreased, unlike lipid storage diseases, which affect sphingolipid levels. The cause of multiple sclerosis is unknown, but it exhibits multifactorial determination with autoimmune characteristics.

262. The answer is c. *(Murray, pp 205–218. Scriver, pp 2705–2716.)* Apo B is the major protein of chylomicrons, very-low-density lipoproteins (VLDL), and low-density lipoproteins (LDL); these serum lipids are reduced in the lipoprotein electrophoretic patterns of children with abetalipoproteinmia (200100). The disorder is benefited by administration of fat-soluble vitamins like E that are malabsorbed. Chylomicrons are one of four major groups of lipoproteins and are responsible for transport of lipids from digestion and absorption. The other groups of lipoproteins are very-low-density lipoproteins (VLDL), which are responsible for transport of triacylglycerol from the liver, low-density lipoproteins (LDL), which deliver cholesterol, and high-density lipoproteins (HDL), which remove cholesterol from tissues.

263. The answer is d. *(Murray, pp 205–218.)* Triacylglycerol is the major fuel reserve in the body and is mainly stored and hydrolyzed in adipose tissue. Triglyceride and fatty acid metabolism become active during fasting after glycogen stores are depleted in 3–4 hours. However, stores of triglycerides in heart and muscle are needed for energy even with adequate feeding. Longer chain fatty acids will contain many more two-carbon units for oxidation than shorter chains, accounting for disproportionate energy depletion and severe cardiac and skeletal disease in children with longer chain enzyme deficiencies. Glucose is important as a brain nutrient but will not be depleted by fatty acid oxidation. Glycogen (in animals) and starch (in plants) are glucose storage molecules. Glycogen is depleted with fasting but is not the major fuel reserve in mammals.

264. The answer is e. *(Murray, pp 205–218.)* Fatty liver is associated with a buildup of triacylglycerol due either to an inability to produce enough VLDL or an inability to produce plasma lipoproteins. Under normal conditions, VLDL is responsible for the transport of triacylglycerol from the liver to extrahepatic tissues. Alcoholism causes chronic injury to liver cells, producing increased fat retention in early stages and scarring due to cell death (cirrhosis) at later stages.

265. The answer is d. *(Murray, pp 190–196. Scriver, pp 2705–2716.)* Infants placed on chronic low-fat formula diets often develop skin problems, impaired lipid transport, and eventually poor growth. This can be overcome by including linoleic acid to make up 1–2% of the total caloric requirement. Essential fatty acids are required because humans have only Δ^4, Δ^5, Δ^6, and Δ^9 fatty acid desaturase. Only plants have desaturase greater than Δ^9. Consequently, certain fatty acids such as arachidonic acid cannot be made "from scratch" (de novo) in humans and other mammals.

However, linoleic acid, which plants make, can be converted to arachidonic acid. Arachidonate and eicosapentaenoate are 20-carbon prostanoic acids that are the starting point of the synthesis of prostaglandins, thromboxanes, and leukotrienes.

266. The answer is a. *(Murray, pp 219–230. Scriver, pp 2863–2914.)* Cholesterol is formed in five steps. The first step, biosynthesis of mevalonate, is catalyzed by three enzymes—acetyl CoA thiolase, HMG-CoA synthase, and HMG-CoA reductase. Thiolase catalyzes the condensation of two molecules of acetyl-CoA to form acetoacetyl-CoA. HMG-CoA synthase catalyzes the addition of a third molecule of acetyl-CoA to form HMG-CoA. This compound is reduced to mevalonate by HMG-CoA reductase. This enzyme is the principal regulatory step in the pathway. In the second step of cholesterol synthesis, mevalonate is phosphorylated and decarboxylated to produce isopentyl diphosphate. Six of these isoprenoid units are condensed to form squalene in the third step. Lanosterol is formed in the fourth step and is subsequently converted to cholesterol.

Malonyl CoA is a three-carbon acyl CoA that condenses with acetyl CoA to initiate fatty acid synthesis. Malonate does inhibit the Krebs tricarboxylic acid cycle at the step from succinate to fumarate and may have an important role in diabetes mellitus.

267. The answer is b. *(Murray, pp 237–241. Scriver, pp 1667–1724.)* Phenylalanine is an essential amino acid that is converted to tyrosine by phenylalanine hydroxylase. Tyrosine is metabolized to various dopamine metabolites as well as melanin. Children with phenylketonuria (PKU-261600) have deficient phenylalanine hydroxylase and develop elevated phenylalanine with severe mental deficiency that is perhaps related to brain dopamine pathways. Dietary treatment of PKU is effective if begun before age 2–3 months (hence neonatal screening that may not be done in underdeveloped countries), but it must be monitored because phenylalanine cannot be completely excluded from the diet. Complete absence of phenylalanine will cause protein malnutrition and failure to grow. Tyrosine is a precursor to melanin, so deficient tyrosine synthesis in children with PKU often causes a lighter hair and skin color than usual for their family. Phenylalanine and tyrosine levels must be monitored every 3–4 months in children on low phenylalanine diets to ensure balance between accumulation and deficiency.

268. The answer is c. *(Murray, pp 197–204. Scriver, pp 2297–2326.)* Ceramide is the basic unit composing all sphingolipids, which include sphingomyelin and gangliosides. Sphingomyelin, which usually contains phosphocholine as a polar head group, is the only phospholipid that does not have a glycerol backbone. In contrast, gangliosides have complex oligosaccharide head groups. The defect in Niemann-Pick disease is in the enzyme sphingomyelinase, resulting in accumulation of ceramide-phosphocholine (sphingomyelin).

269. The answer is d. *(Murray, pp 205–218. Scriver, pp 2863–2914.)* The shell of apoproteins coating blood transport lipoproteins is important in the physiologic function of the lipoproteins. Some of the apoproteins contain signals that target the movement of the lipoproteins in and out of specific tissues. B48 and E seem to be important in targeting chylomicron remnants to be taken up by liver. B100 is synthesized as the coat protein of VLDLs and marks their end product, LDLs, for uptake by peripheral tissues. Other apoproteins are important for the solubilization and movement of lipids and cholesterol in and out of the particles. CII is a lipoprotein lipase activator that VLDLs and chylomicrons receive from HDLs. The A apoproteins are found in HDLs and are involved in lecithin–cholesterol acyl transferase (LCAT) regulation. Familial hypercholesterolemia (144010) causes early heart attacks in heterozygotes, particularly in males, and childhood disease in rare homozygotes. The daughter's chest pain was likely angina due to coronary artery occlusion and her skin patches were fatty deposits known as xanthomata.

270. The answer is b. *(Murray, pp 205–230. Scriver, pp 2863–2914.)* In the postabsorptional (postprandial) state, plasma contains all the lipoproteins: chylomicrons derived from dietary lipids packaged in the intestinal epithelial cells and their remnants; very-low-density lipoproteins (VLDLs), which contain endogenous lipids and cholesterol packaged in the liver; low-density lipoproteins (LDLs), which are end products of delipidation of VLDLs; and high-density lipoproteins (HDLs), which are synthesized in the liver. HDLs are in part catalytic, since transfer of their CII apolipoprotein to VLDLs or chylomicrons activates lipoprotein lipase. In normal patients, only LDLs and HDLs remain in plasma following a 12 hour fast, since both chylomicrons and VLDLs have been delipidated. Most of the cholesterol measured in blood plasma at this time is present in the cholesterol-rich LDLs. However, HDL cholesterol also contributes to the measurement. In addition to total plasma cholesterol, the ratio of HDL (good) to LDL (bad) cholesterol is also useful for predicting heart attack risks.

271. The answer is a. *(Murray, pp 237–241. Scriver, pp 1667–2108.)* Cysteine can be formed from the essential amino acid methionine, one of nine essential amino acids (histidine, isoleucine, luecine, lysine, methionine, phenylalanine, threonine, tryptophan, valine) and one semiessential amino acid (arginine) that is needed for growth. Tyrosine can be made from phenylalanine, proline or glutamine from glutamate, asparagines from aspartate. Other metabolites like 3-phosphoglycerate (serine), glyoxylate (glycine), pyruvate (alanine) can be converted to amino acids at reasonable rates, rendering them nonessential. Hydroxylysine, hydroxyproline, and selenocysteine are converted from parent amino acids after incorporation into protein. Hyperalimentation solutions required years of research to define essential nutrients, which include unsaturated fatty acids, vitamins, and trace elements. Though effective for healing and growth, hyperalimentation still has unexplained side effects like liver disease that can arise during or after therapy.

272. The answer is c. *(Murray, p 546. Scriver, pp 3421–3452.)* The two major groups of lysosomal storage disease are sphingolipidoses and mucopolysaccharidoses. An absence of α-L-iduronidase, as in Hurler's syndrome (252800) and Scheie syndrome (252800), leads to accumulations of dermatan sulfate and heparan sulfate. Scheie's syndrome is less severe, with corneal clouding, joint degeneration, and increased heart disease. Hurler's syndrome has the same symptoms plus mental and physical retardation leading to early death. The later onset in this child is compatible with a diagnosis of Scheie's syndrome. Note that Hurler's and Scheie's syndromes result from mutations at the same locus—hence their identical McKusick numbers. The reasons for the differences in disease severity are unknown. All of the other enzyme deficiencies listed lead to the lack of proper breakdown of sphingolipids and their accumulation as gangliosides, glucocerebrosides, and sphingomyelins. Symptoms of lipidoses may include organ enlargement, mental retardation, and early death.

273. The answer is a. *(Murray, p 203. Scriver, pp 3827–3876. 121–138. 287–320.)* Gangliosides are continually synthesized and broken down. The specific hydrolases that degrade gangliosides by sequentially removing terminal sugars are found in lysosomes. In the lipid storage disease known as Tay-Sachs disease (272800), ganglioside GM_2 accumulates because of a deficiency of β-*N*-acetylhexosaminidase, a lysosomal enzyme that removes the terminal *N*-acetylgalactosamine residue. Homozygotes produce virtually no functional enzyme and suffer weakness, retardation, and blindness. Death usually occurs before infants are 3 years old. Carriers (heterozygotes) of the autosomal recessive disease produce approximately 50% of the normal levels of enzyme but show no ill effects. In high-risk populations, such as Ashkenazi Jews, screening for carrier status may be performed.

274. The answer is a. *(Murray, pp 122–129, 163–172. Scriver, pp 2297–2326.)* The sources of NADPH for synthesis of fatty acids are the pentose phosphate pathway and cytosolic malate formed during the transfer of acetyl groups to the cytosol as citrate. The enzyme citrate lyase splits citrate into acetyl CoA and oxaloacetate. The oxaloacetate is reduced to malate by NADH. NADP-linked malate enzyme catalyzes the oxidative decarboxylation of malate to pyruvate and carbon dioxide. Thus, the diffusion of excess citrate from the mitochondria to the cytoplasm of cells not only provides acetyl CoA for synthesis of fatty acids but NADPH as well. One NADPH is produced for each acetyl CoA produced. However, most of the NADPHs needed for synthesis of fatty acids are derived from the pentose phosphate pathway. For this reason, adipose tissue has an extremely active pentose phosphate pathway.

275. The answer is b. *(Murray, pp 180–189.)* The first step of fatty acid oxidation requires activation of the fatty acid to an acyl-CoA. This reaction is catalyzed by the enzyme acyl-CoA synthetase and requires one ATP. In subsequent reactions, two carbons are removed at a time from the carboxyl end to form acetyl-CoA.

276. The answer is b. *(Murray, pp 242–248.)* Most amino acids except lysine, threonine, proline, and hydroxyproline can undergo transamination to convert α-amino acids and α-keto acids. Transamination reactions can contribute amino groups to the urea cycle for urea biosynthesis or initiate catabolism of the amino acid. Six amino acids (listed as answer options) are degraded to pyruvate, joining another six (tyrosine, phenylalanine, lysine, hydroxylysine, tryptophan, methionine) that are in part converted to acetyl-CoA. Cysteine can be made from cystine (essentially a cysteine dimer with disulfide linkage) by cystine reductase. The inborn error cystinosis (219800) results from mutations in a lysosomal membrane transporter, causing cystine accumulation in lysosomes with crystals in the lens of the eye and renal proximal tubules. Children with cystinosis present in early childhood with short stature, photophobia, and progressive renal disease. The synthetic compound cysteamine can complex with cystine and allow egress from lysosomes, slowing the progression of renal failure.

277. The answer is d. *(Murray, pp 242–248. Scriver, pp 1909–1964.)* Carbamoyl phosphate synthase I catalyzes the first reaction of urea biosynthesis and is the rate-limiting step. Formation of carbamoyl phosphate requires 2 ATP, one as a phosphate donor and the other to provide the driving force for synthesis of the amide bond and the mixed acid anhydride bond. Argininosuccinic acid synthase also requires 1 ATP.

278. The answer is a. *(Murray, pp 249–263.)* Asparagine is converted to aspartate by the enzyme asparaginase. A transaminase subsequently converts aspartate to oxaloacetate. The amino group from aspartate is used to convert pyruvate to alanine. Likewise, glutamine is converted to glutamate and then α-ketoglutarate by glutaminase and a transaminase.

279. The answer is c. *(Murray, pp 173–179. Scriver, pp 2297–2326.)* Two major enzyme complexes are involved in the synthesis of fatty acids. The first is acetyl-CoA carboxylase, which synthesizes malonyl CoA by the steps shown below for the synthesis of palmitate:

$$7\text{ acetyl-CoA} + 7\ HCO_3^- + 7\text{ ATP} \rightarrow 7\text{ malonyl-CoA} + 7\text{ ADP} + 7\ P_i$$

Using the malonyl-CoA, palmitate is then synthesized by seven cycles of the fatty acid synthetase complex, whose stoichiometry is summarized below:

$$\text{acetyl-CoA} + 7\text{ malonyl-CoA} + 14\text{ NADPH} \rightarrow \text{palmitate} + 7\ CO_2 + 14\ NAD^+ + 8\text{ CoA} + 6\ H_2O$$

As can be seen from the equations above, the necessary amount of malonyl-CoA is synthesized. Palmitate is subsequently synthesized from malonyl-CoA and one initial acetyl-CoA. Thus, acetyl-CoA, NADPH, ATP, and HCO_3^- are all necessary in this process. In contrast, $FADH_2$ is not utilized in fatty acid synthesis, but is one of the products of fatty acid oxidation. Vitamin B_{12} is required for conversion of propionic acid to methylmalonic acid, a step in the β-oxidation of odd-numbered fatty acid chains.

280. The answer is b. *(Murray, pp 415–433. Scriver, pp 2297–2326.)* The fluid mosaic model of membrane structure shown in the question describes plasma membranes as a mosaic of globular proteins in a phospholipid bilayer. The lipids as well as the proteins are in a fluid and dynamic state capable of translational (side-to-side) movement, but not "flip-flop"-type movements. Hence, both the phospholipid and protein components are amphipathic, with a highly polar end in contact with the aqueous phase and hydrophobic residues buried within the membrane. Integral proteins may be embedded in the membrane or exposed on only one side or they may extend completely through the membrane with different portions of the proteins exposed to opposite sides of the membrane. In contrast to the fluid mosaic model, the models of a protein-coated bimolecular layer of lipid diagrammed in A and the unit membrane "railroad track" shown in D (which is based on osmium tetroxide fixed membranes) suggest that membranes are simply bimolecular layers of lipid coated with protein that does not penetrate the lipid. A simple bimolecular layer of lipid is shown in C, and a micelle of lipids is diagrammatically illustrated in E.

281. The answer is e. *(Murray, pp 415–433. Scriver, pp 2297–2326.)* The process of emulsification of hydrophobic fat globules by the detergent action of phospholipids and bile acids in the gut breaks the globules down to mixed micelles. The formation of small micelles from large fat globules greatly increases the surface area available for the action of hydrolytic lipases in the gut. Mixed micelle formation is dependent on the amphipathic properties of bile acids and phospholipids that allow them to act as detergents. Simply put, the hydrophobic moieties (fatty acid chains) of phospholipids are inserted into the hydrophobic fat globules and the hydrophilic polar head groups interact with and face the water, in essence forming a monomolecular layer around the fat (triacylglycerides). This successful strategy of mixed micelles is used to solve many potential problems, including the transport of blood lipoproteins.

282. The answer is b. *(Murray, pp 219–230. Scriver, pp 2863–2914.)* Mevastatin, an analogue of mevalonic acid, acts as a feedback inhibitor of

3′-hydroxy-3′-methylglutaryl CoA (HMG-CoA) reductase, the regulated enzyme of cholesterol synthesis. Effective treatment with mevastatin, along with a low-fat diet, decreases levels of blood cholesterol. The lowering of cholesterol also lowers the amounts of the lipoprotein that transports cholesterol to the peripheral tissues, low-density lipoprotein (LDL). Because lipids like cholesterol and triglycerides are insoluble in water, they must be associated with lipoproteins for transport and salvage between their major site of synthesis (liver) and the peripheral tissues. Those lipoproteins associated with more insoluble lipids thus have lower density during centrifugation (see the table in answer 258), a technique that separates the lowest-density chylomicrons from very-low-density lipoproteins (VLDLs with pre-β-lipoproteins), low-density lipoproteins (LDLs with β-lipoproteins), intermediate-density lipoproteins (IDLs), and high-density lipoproteins (HDLs with α-lipoproteins). Each type of lipoprotein has typical apolipoproteins such as the apo B100 and apo B48 (translated from the same messenger RNA) in LDL. LDL is involved in transporting cholesterol from the liver to peripheral tissues, whereas HDL is a scavenger of cholesterol. The ratio of HDL to LDL is thus a predictor of cholesterol deposition in blood vessels, the cause of myocardial infarctions (heart attacks). The higher the HDL/LDL ratio, the lower the rate of heart attacks.

283. The answer is c. *(Murray, pp 173–179. Scriver, pp 3181–3218.)* Triacylglycerols are assembled from glycerol and saturated fatty acids that are synthesized from condensation of malonyl and acetyl CoA through the fatty acyl synthase complex. Plasmalogens and certain signaling agents like platelet activating factor are ether lipids, distinguished by an ether (C-O-C) bond at carbon 1 of glycerol. Ether lipid synthesis is initiated by placing an acyl group on carbon 1 of dihydroxyacetone phosphate (DHAP) using DHAP acyltransferase. The acyl side chain is then exchanged with an alcohol to form an ether linkage by an acylDHAP synthase—the acyltransferase and synthase plus other enzymes of ether lipid synthesis are localized in peroxisomes. Subsequent additions of phosphocholine yield ether/acyl glycerols analogous to lecithins (including platelet activating factor), and addition of a phosphoethanolamine to carbon 3 of ether (alkyl) glycerols forms plasmalogens. Acetyl and palmitoyl CoA can contribute to these ether lipid modifications after the core carbon 1 ether linkage has produced an alkylglycerol. Disruption of peroxisome structure by mutations in various peroxisomal membrane proteins ablates DHAP acyltransferase and other enzymes for ether lipid/plasmalogen synthesis, causing deficienty of brain lipids, severe neurologic disease, hypotonia, and liver failure—the most severe phenotype of which is Zellweger syndrome (214100).

284. The answer is b. *(Murray, pp 153–162. Scriver, pp 1471–1488, 2327–2356.)* The ketone bodies, β-hydroxybutyrate and acetoacetate, are synthesized in liver mitochondria from acetyl CoA. The liver produces ketone bodies under conditions of fasting associated with high rates of fatty acid oxidation. The inability to get glucose into extrahepatic cells because of insulin deficiency in diabetes also increases fatty acid oxidation and ketogenesis. The acid groups of β-hydroxybutyrate and acetoacetate cause acidosis and an anion gap (sum of serum sodium and potassium minus the sum of chloride and bicarbonate) that is greater than normal (over 8–15). In the case of diabetes, the "hidden anions" that add to bicarbonate in balancing the cations can be recognized as ketones through urine ketostix testing. In metabolic disorders like methylmalonic aciduria (251000) or fatty acid acid oxidation defects, there are scanty abnormal or no ketones (if fat cannot be oxidized) so the hidden anions must be identified by plasma acylcarnitine or urine organic acid profiles. Acetone is a ketone body produced in diabetes that produces an acrid breath during ketoacidosis.

285. The answer is a. *(Murray, pp 415–433. Scriver, pp 2297–2326.)* Plasma membranes are unique as compared to intracellular membranes in that their composition contains cholesterol, glycoproteins, and glycolipids known as gangliosides. Plasma membranes of the cells of different tissues are distinguished from each other because of the properties that make them unique. Hormone receptors allow each cell type to respond to systemic stimulation appropriately. All chronic hormone receptors are localized to plasma membranes and upon stimulation release a second messenger into the interior of the cell. Glucagon, like epinephrine and norepinephrine, stimulates adenylate cyclase to produce cyclic AMP. Glucagon is found on the plasma membranes of liver and adipose tissue cells.

286. The answer is e. *(Murray, pp 130–135, 249–263. Scriver, pp 3897–3944.)* Of the indicated amino acids and catabolic intermediates—the serine to glycine, glycine to carbon dioxide and ammonia, and formaminoglutamate (figlu—from histidine) to glutamate reactions—all require tetrahydrofolate as a cofactor. In folate deficiency, the figlu accumulates abnormally and is an unusual metabolite that serves as a diagnostic marker. Methyltetrahydrofolate and vitamin B_{12} (cobalamin) are required for conversion of homocysteine to methionine (with accompanying conversion of methyl- to tetrahydrofolate, so vitamin B_{12} deficiency can "trap" folate reserves as methyltetrahydrofolate and cause secondary folate deficiency. Mutations in the converting enzyme methionine synthase can cause one form of homocystinuria (236200) with connective tissue disease resembling Marfan syndrome. Certain of these mutations can be ameliorated by folate and B_{12} supplementation to augment residual enzyme activity.

287. The answer is b. *(Murray, pp 205–230. Scriver, pp 2705–2716.)* The uptake of exogenous cholesterol by cells results in a marked suppression of endogenous cholesterol synthesis. Low-density human lipoprotein not only contains the greatest ratio of bound cholesterol to protein but also has the greatest potency in suppressing endogenous cholesterogenesis. LDLs normally suppress cholesterol synthesis by binding to a specific membrane receptor that mediates inhibition of hydroxymethylglutaryl (HMG) coenzyme A reductase. In familial hypercholesterolemia (143890), the LDL receptor is dysfunctional, with the result that cholesterol synthesis is less responsive to plasma cholesterol levels. Suppression of HMG CoA reductase is attained using inhibitors (statins) that mimic the structure of mevalonic acid, the natural feedback inhibitor of the enzyme.

288. The answer is c. *(Murray, pp 130–135, 249–263 Scriver, pp 1909–1964.)* Arginase catalyzes the conversion of arginine to ornithine, which is subsequently converted to α-ketoglutarate. The guanido group of arginine is converted to urea. Both proline and histidine can also be converted to α-ketoglutarate.

289. The answer is a. *(Murray, pp 173–189. Scriver, pp 2297–2326.)* Under conditions of active synthesis of fatty acids in the cytosol of hepatocytes, levels of malonyl-CoA are high. Malonyl CoA is the activated source of two carbon units for fatty acid synthesis. Malonyl CoA inhibits carnitine acyltransferase I, which is located on the cytosolic face of the inner mitochondrial membrane. Thus, long-chain fatty acyl-CoA units cannot be transported into mitochondria where β oxidation occurs, and translocation from cytosol to mitochondrial matrix is prevented. In this situation compartmentalization of membranes as well as inhibition of enzymes comes into play.

290. The answer is e. *(Murray, pp 293–302. Scriver, pp 2663–2704.)* Orotic aciduria (258900) is the buildup of orotic acid due to a deficiency in one or both of the enzymes that convert it to UMP. Either orotate phosphoribosyltransferase and orotidylate decarboxylase are both defective, or the decarboxylase alone is defective. UMP is the precursor of UTP, CTP, and TMP. All of these end products normally act in some way to feedback-inhibit the initial reactions of pyrimidine synthesis. Specifically, the lack of CTP inhibition allows aspartate transcarbamoylase to remain highly active and ultimately results in a buildup of orotic acid and the resultant orotic aciduria. The lack of CTP, TMP, and UTP leads to a decreased erythrocyte formation and megaloblastic anemia. Uridine treatment is effective because uridine can easily be converted to UMP by omnipresent tissue kinases, thus allowing UTP, CTP, and TMP to be synthesized and feedback-inhibit further orotic acid production.

291. The answer is a. *(Murray, pp 293–302. Scriver, pp 2537–2570.)* Most forms of gout are probably X-linked recessive with deficiencies in phosphoribosyl pyrophosphate (PRPP) synthase, the first step of purine synthesis (e.g., 311850). Some patients may have a partial deficiency of hypoxanthine-guanine phosphoribosyl transferase (HGPRTase), which salvages hypoxanthine and guanine by transferring the purine ribonucleotide of PRPP to the bases and forming inosinate and guanylate, respectively. In all of these patients, the hypoxanthine analogue allopurinol has two actions: (1) it inhibits xanthine oxidase, which catalyzes the oxidation of hypoxanthine to xanthine and then to uric acid stones and tissue deposits; and (2) it forms an inactive allopurinol ribonucleotide from PRPP in a reaction catalyzed by HGPRTase, thereby decreasing the rate of purine synthesis. In contrast, because of the total loss of HGPRTase activity in Lesch-Nyhan patients, the allopurinol ribonucleotide cannot be formed. Thus, PRPP levels are not decreased and de novo purine synthesis continues unabated. The gouty arthritis caused by urate crystal formation is relieved in Lesch-Nyhan patients, but their neurological symptoms (mental deficiency, self-mutilation with compulsive chewing of fingers and lips) are not.

292. The answer is d. *(Murray, pp 163–172, 293–302. Scriver, pp 2513–2570.)* Carbamoyl phosphate (CAP) synthase I is found in mitochondrial matrix and is the first step in urea synthesis, condensing CO_2 and NH_4^+. Hyperammonemia occurs when CAP is deficient. CAP synthase II forms CAP as the first step in pyrimidine synthesis. Its complete deficiency would probably be a lethal mutation. When its activity is decreased, purine catabolism to uric acid is decreased, decreasing the possibility of hyperuricemia. In contrast, gout, Lesch-Nyhan syndrome, high xanthine oxidase activity, and von Gierke's disease [glycogen storage disease type la (232200)] all lead to increased urate production and excretion.

293. The answer is a. *(Murray, pp 293–302. Scriver, pp 2513–2570.)* During purine ring biosynthesis, the amino acid glycine is completely incorporated to provide C4, C5, and N7. Glutamine contributes N3 and N9, aspartate provides N1, and derivatives of tetrahydrofolate furnish C2 and C8. Carbon dioxide is the source of C6. In pyrimidine ring synthesis, C2 and N3 are derived from carbamoyl phosphate, while N1, C4, C5, and C6 come from aspartate.

294. The answer is e. *(Murray, pp 242–248. Scriver, pp 2513–2570.)* Although defects in any of these enzymes will result in a buildup of ammonia in the bloodstream and ammonia intoxication, blocks at carbamoyl phosphate synthase I and ornithine transcarbamylase are usually more severe. Ornithine transcarbamylase deficiency (300461) is an X-linked recessive disorder, allowing for mild manifestations in female carriers; deficiencies in the other four enzymes are autosomal recessive traits. Gene therapy approaches to treatment are being tested, but resulted in the death of one patient due to suspected reaction to the adenovirus vector.

295. The answer is b. *(Murray, pp 237–241. Scriver, pp 2961–3062.)* The porphyrias are a group of inborn errors that affect synthesis of porphyrins, the precursors of heme in hemoglobin. Defective synthesis of heme would not elevate heme breakdown products of the heme catabolic pathway, including bilirubin to conjugated bilirubin diglucuronide (in liver), bilirubin diglucuronide to urobilinogen and stercobilin (by bacteria in stool), and reabsorption of urobilinogen to be excreted in urine as urobilin. Delta-aminolevulinic acid (ALA) is synthesized from succinyl CoA and glycine followed by condensation of two ALA molecules to form porphobilinogen (PBG) with a 5-member pyrrole ring. Four molecules of PBG are converted to the four-ring uroporphyrin by hydroxymethylbilane synthase, the primary defect in acute intermittent porphyria (176000). Deficiencies in other enzymes of the pathway from ALA to heme cause symptoms varying from anemia to photosensitivity to the well-known but rarely encountered presentation with abdominal pain and neuropsychiatric symptoms.

296. The answer is e. *(Murray, pp 293–302.)* PRPP synthetase catalyzes the first reaction in purine biosynthesis from ribose-5-phosphate. This enzyme is normally subject to feedback inhibition. Defects in this enzyme or its regulation can result in overproduction and overexcretion of purine catabolites, leading to gout.

297. The answer is c. *(Murray, pp 293–302. Scriver, pp 2537–2570.)* Purine salvage reactions convert purines, purine ribonucleosides, and purine deoxyribonucleoside to mononucleotides. Such salvage reactions require much less energy than de novo synthesis. The liver is the major site of purine nucleotide biosynthesis and provides excess purines for other tissues that cannot synthesize purines. A defect in hypoxanthine-guanine phosphoribosyl transferase, one of the enzymes of purine salvage, is responsible for purine overproduction and subsequent hyperuricemia observed in Lesch-Nyhan syndrome.

298. The answer is a. *(Murray, pp 75, 293–302. Scriver, pp 2513–2570.)* Aspartate transcarbamoylase catalyzes the first reaction unique to pyrimidine biosynthesis. This enzyme is inhibited by CTP but activated by ATP. Both ATP and CTP bind at a different site from either substrate. Aspartate transcarbamoylase consists of multiple catalytic and regulatory subunits. Each regulatory subunit contains at least two CTP binding sites.

299. The answer is d. *(Murray, pp 293–302. Scriver, pp 2513–2570.)* 5′-phosphoribosyl-1-pyrophosphate (PRPP) donates the ribose phosphate unit of nucleotides and is absolutely required for the beginning of the synthesis of purines. In fact, the enzymes regulating the synthesis of PRPP and the subsequent synthesis of phosphoribosylamine from PRPP are all end product–inhibited by inosine monophosphate (IMP), adenosine monophosphate (AMP), and guanosine monophosphate (GMP), the products of this reaction pathway.

300. The answer is b. *(Murray, pp 286–302. Scriver, pp 2513–2570.)* The degradation of purines to urate can lead to gout when an elevated level of urate is present in serum, causing the precipitation of sodium urate crystals in joints. The excessive production of urate in many patients seems to be connected to a partial deficiency of hypoxanthine-guanine phosphoribosyl transferase (HGPRT). Allopurinol, an analogue of hypoxanthine, is a drug used to correct gout. It accomplishes this by inhibiting the production of urate from hypoxanthine and in doing so undergoes suicide inhibition of xanthine oxidase. Ribose phosphate and PRPP are required for purine synthesis. 5-fluorouracil (5-FU) and cytosine arabinoside (Ara C) are cancer chemotherapy agents, the former being an analogue of thymine that inhibits thymidylate synthetase and the latter an inhibitor of RNA synthesis.

301. The answer is e. *(Murray, pp 286–292. Scriver, pp 2513–2570.)* Adenosine diphosphate (adenylate) is joined to nicotinamide to form nicotinamide adenine dinucleotide (NAD), further phosphorylated at the 3' position of ribose to form NADP. Niacin can be synthesized from tryptophan and is not strictly a vitamin. Deficiency of tryptophan and niacin can occur from diet or with diseases that increase requirements, causing pellagra (photosensitivity, dermatitis, psychosis).

Ribonucleosides consist of a base at the 1' position of ribose, while ribonuceotides have 5′-phosphate groups. Guanosine (G) and adenosine (A) contain purine bases, cytosine (C), uridine (U), and thymidine (T) pyrimidine bases. Ribonucleotides (adenylate, guanidylate, cytidylate, uridylate) have a phosphate ester on the 5′-hydroxyl of ribose (note that the ribo-prefix is usually omitted). Deoxyribonucleotides have a phosphate ester on the 5′-hydroxyl of deoxyribose (deoxyadenylate, deoxyguanidylate, deoxycytidylate, and thymidylate).The ribonucleosides A, G, C, and U can be incorporated into RNA, while the deoxyribonucleosides A, G, C, and T join with deoxyribose (lacking a hydroxyl at the 2' carbon) and are incorporated into DNA. Uridine occurs only as the ribonucleoside, thymidine as the deoxyribonucleotide (actually as thymidylate deoxyribonucleotide synthesized from uridylate by thymidylate synthetase. Hypoxanthine and inosine are precursors of purine A, G synthesis.

302. The answer is e. *(Murray, pp 145–152, 293–302. Scriver, pp 2513–2536.)* The activated form of glucose utilized for the synthesis of glycogen and galactose is UDP-glucose, which is formed from the reaction of glucose-1-phosphate and UTP. The conversion of galactose to glucose is at the UDP-sugar level, and is deficient in galactosemia (230400). UDP derivatives of glucose and galactose and of sugar amines (glucosamine,

N-acetylmannosamine or neuraminic/sialic acids) are key precursors for synthesis of derivative polysaccharide chains including cerebrosides and gangliosides. A group of neurolipidoses with developmental regression and neurodegeneration result from deficiencies in enzymes that degrade complex polysaccharides (glycosphingolipids).

Nutrition

Vitamins and Minerals

Questions

DIRECTIONS: Each item below contains a question or incomplete statement followed by suggested responses. Select the **one best** response to each question.

303. A middle-aged man presents with congestive heart failure with elevated liver enzymes. His skin has a grayish pigmentation. The levels of liver enzymes are higher than those usually seen in congestive heart failure, suggesting an inflammatory process (hepatitis) with scarring (cirrhosis) of the liver. A liver biopsy discloses a marked increase in iron storage. In humans, molecular iron (Fe) is which of the following?

a. Stored primarily in the spleen
b. Stored in combination with ferritin
c. Excreted in the urine as Fe^{2+}
d. Absorbed in the intestine by albumin
e. Absorbed in the ferric (Fe^{3+}) form

304. Intestinal bowel resections are necessary for autoimmune inflammatory diseases like Crohn disease and for congenital anomalies like malrotation or volvulus (twisted intestine with impaired blood supply). Once the absorptive intestinal mucosa falls below a certain length, oral or parenteral alimentation must be instituted to maintain nutrition. In such solutions, which of the following nutrients is most dispensable?

a. Protein
b. Iodine
c. Carbohydrates
d. Lipids
e. Calcium

305. Which of the following disorders is associated with a deficiency of vitamin B_{12}?

a. Cheilosis
b. Beriberi
c. Pernicious anemia
d. Scurvy
e. Rickets

306. In adults, a severe deficiency of vitamin D causes which of the following disorders?

a. Night blindness
b. Osteomalacia
c. Rickets
d. Osteogenesis imperfecta
e. Osteopetrosis

307. Which of the following vitamins would most likely become deficient in a person who develops a completely carnivorous lifestyle?

a. Thiamine
b. Niacin
c. Cobalamin
d. Pantothenic acid
e. Vitamin C

308. Children with autism and other disorders with mental disability are often put on megavitamin supplements despite no scientific evidence of benefit. Although most vitamins are harmless in excess, merely being excreted in urine, vitamin A can be toxic. Which of the following statements regarding vitamin A is true?

a. It is not an essential vitamin
b. It is related to tocopherol
c. It is a component of rhodopsin
d. It is derived from ethanol
e. It is also known as opsin

309. Fully activated pyruvate carboxylase depends on the presence of which of the following substances?

a. Malate and niacin
b. Acetyl-CoA and biotin
c. Acetyl-CoA and thiamine pyrophosphate
d. Oxaloacetate and biotin
e. Oxaloacetate and niacin

310. A group of neurodegenerative diseases with onset ranging from neonates to adults have been found to involve deficiency of pantothenic acid kinase (e.g., Hallavorden-Spatz disease, 234200). The correlation between defective pantothenic acid activation and loss of myelin to cause neurodegenerative disease relates to its role in which of the following?

a. Decarboxylation reactions
b. Acetylation and acyl group metabolism
c. Dehydrogenation and redox reactions
d. Phosphorylation reactions
e. Methyl transfer reactions

311. Mothers taking warfarin for anticoagulation during pregnancy may have children with fetal warfarin syndrome involving very short nose and skeletal changes. Studies of the actions of the anticoagulants dicumarol and warfarin (the latter also a hemorrhagic rat poison)—have revealed which of the following?

a. Vitamin C is necessary for the synthesis of fibrinogen
b. Vitamin C activates fibrinogen
c. Vitamin K is a clotting factor
d. Vitamin K is essential for γ-carboxylation of glutamate
e. The action of vitamin E is antagonized by these compounds

312. A child presents with hair loss, skin, rashes, and exaggerated acidosis after infections. The child is found to have deficiency of biotinidase (253260), and improves dramatically with biotin therapy. Biotin is involved in which of the following types of reactions?

a. Hydroxylations
b. Carboxylations
c. Decarboxylations
d. Dehydrations
e. Deaminations

313. Which of the following vitamins is the precursor of CoA?

a. Riboflavin
b. Pantothenate
c. Thiamine
d. Cobamide
e. Pyridoxamine

314. In the Far East, beriberi is a serious health problem. It is characterized by neurologic and cardiac symptoms. Beriberi is caused by a deficiency of which of the following vitamins?

a. Choline
b. Ethanolamine
c. Thiamine
d. Serine
e. Glycine

315. Both acyl carrier protein (ACP) of fatty acid synthetase and coenzyme A (CoA):

a. Contain reactive phosphorylated tyrosine groups
b. Contain thymidine
c. Contain phosphopantetheine-reactive groups
d. Contain cystine-reactive groups
e. Carry folate groups

316. Chronic alcoholics are at risk to develop lactic acidosis and neurologic symptoms, one example of which is the Wernicke-Korsakoff syndrome (277730). This complex of symptoms includes nerve problems like nystagmus (oscillating eyes), ophthalmoplegia (deviated or weak eye), peripheral numbness/tingling and cerebral problems like confusion, delirium, coma, and memory loss in survivors. Explanation of why certain alcoholics get Wernicke-Korsakoff encephalopathy was suggested when altered transketolase (an important enzyme in the pentose phosphate pathway) was found in these individuals. Which of the following is most likely to be important in the development of lactic acidosis and/or Wernicke-Korsakoff susceptibility in alcoholics?

a. Thiamine pyrophosphate
b. Lipoamide
c. ATP
d. NADH
e. FADH

317. Which of the following cofactors must be utilized during the conversion of acetyl-CoA to malonyl-CoA?

a. Thiamine pyrophosphate
b. Acyl carrier protein (ACP)
c. NAD_1
d. Biotin
e. FAD

318. Tryptophan deficiency in diet or disease can cause pellagra, a condition with skin rash on sunlight exposure (photosensitivity), diarrhea, and death. Tryptophan can be a precursor for one part of a compound that is an enzyme cofactor and donor of ADP-ribose that is added to certain histones and DNA repair enzymes (topoisomerases). Which of the following components can be derived from tryptophan, along with its active compound?

a. Biotin, carboxybiotin
b. Intrinsic factor, cobalamin
c. Pantothenic acid, coenzyme A
d. Nicotinamide, nicotinamide adenine dinucleotide
e. Pyridoxine, pyridoxal phosphate

319. One of the first chemotherapeutic agents was methotrexate, a compound that was effective in killing rapidly dividing cells like those of leukemias. This compound would be expected to elevate concentrations of which of the following compounds?

a. Homocysteine and dUMP
b. Thymine and choline
c. Serine and methionine
d. Glycine and methionine
e. Homocysteine and thymine

320. One of many roles for vitamins is their use as a reactive agent at the active sites of enzymes. Since these are catalytic reactions, the vitamin is not consumed in the reaction and is required in small amounts. Knowledge of this common mechanism should discourage use of megavitamin supplements that are promoted as cures for autism, cancer, and colds, but an unfortunate 30% of the American public admit to taking such supplements. Which of the following enzymes uses a vitamin-derived cofactor that is reoxidized by but different from NAD^+?

a. Lactate dehydrogenase
b. Glutamate dehydrogenase
c. Pyruvate dehydrogenase
d. Malate dehydrogenase
e. Glyceraldehyde-3-phosphate dehydrogenase

321. Which of the following foods should be emphasized for individuals with peripheral neuritis, insomnia, mouth and skin irritation, and diarrhea?

a. Human and cow (not goat) milk, uncooked fruits, vegetables
b. Milk, eggs, meats, fruits
c. Vegetables, cereals, fruits
d. Liver, poultry, eggs
e. Egg yolks, fish oils, leafy vegetables

322. Which of the following foods should be emphasized for individuals with dry eyes and decreased vision in dim light?

a. Human and cow (not goat) milk, uncooked fruits, vegetables
b. Milk, eggs, meats, fruits
c. Vegetables, cereals, fruits
d. Liver, poultry, eggs
e. Egg yolks, fish oils, leafy vegetables

323. Among the following compounds that may be affected by an inborn error of metabolism, which is a coenzyme?

a. Glucose-6-phosphate
b. Glucose-1-phosphate
c. Ornithine
d. Lipoic acid
e. UDP-galactose

324. Which one of the following is definitely associated with a human disease when deficient?

a. Arsenic
b. Lead
c. Zinc
d. Antimony
e. Vanadium

325. A 10-day-old child arriving in the United States from a refugee camp is found to have large areas of bruising on the skin (purpura) with oozing of blood from his umbilicus. Which of the following statements regarding his likely vitamin deficiency and its mechanism are true?

a. The vitamin is broken down by intestinal bacteria and facilitates synthesis of clotting factors
b. The vitamin is antagonized by heparin and faciliates glycosylation of clotting factors
c. The vitamin is obtained by eating egg yolk and liver but not green vegetables
d. The vitamin is antagonized by a rat poison, is active in glutamate carboxylation, and facilitates calcium chelation
e. The vitamin was discovered by studying hemorrhagic disease of the newborn

326. A 1-year-old child recently emigrated from Africa exhibits intermittent diarrhea, pallor (pale skin), extreme tenderness of the bones, "rosary" of lumps along the ribs, nose bleeds, bruising over the eyelids, and blood in the urine. Which of the following is the most likely cause?

a. Deficiency of vitamin C due to a citrus-poor diet during pregnancy
b. Hypervitaminosis A due to ingestion of beef liver during pregnancy
c. Deficiency of vitamin C because of reliance on a milk only diet
d. Deficiency of vitamin K because of neonatal deficiency and continued poor nutrition
e. Deficiency of vitamin D due to darker skin pigmentation and poor sun exposure

327. Which of the following statements regarding vitamin A is true?

a. Vitamin A promotes maintenance of epithelial tissue
b. Vitamin A is necessary for hearing but not for vision
c. Vitamin A is synthesized in skin
d. All vitamin A derivatives are safe to use during pregnancy
e. Vitamin A is a form of calciferol

328. Which of the following conditions most rapidly produces a functional deficiency of vitamin K?

a. Coumadin therapy to prevent thrombosis in patients prone to clot formation
b. Broad-spectrum antibiotic therapy
c. Lack of red meat in the diet
d. Lack of citrus fruits in the diet
e. Premature birth

329. A 3-month-old boy presents with poor feeding and growth, low muscle tone (hypotonia), elevation of blood lactic acid (lactic acidemia), and mild acidosis (blood pH 7.3 to 7.35). The ratio of pyruvate to lactate in serum is elevated, and there is decreased conversion of pyruvate to acetyl coenzyme A in fibroblasts. Which of the following compounds should be considered for therapy?

a. Pyridoxine
b. Thiamine
c. Free fatty acids
d. Biotin
e. Ascorbic acid

330. A homeless person is brought into the emergency room with psychotic imagery and alcohol on his breath. Which of the following compounds is most important to administer?

a. Glucose
b. Niacin
c. Nicotinic acid
d. Thiamine
e. Riboflavin

331. Which of the following vitamins becomes a major electron acceptor, aiding in the oxidation of numerous substrates?

a. Vitamin B_6
b. Niacin
c. Riboflavin
d. Thiamine
e. Vitamin B_1

332. Which of the following vitamins would most likely be deficient in an adult who avoids bright light, has sore eyes, mouth, and tongue, feels tired and confused?

a. Riboflavin
b. Retinol
c. Niacin
d. Thiamine
e. Pyridoxine

333. A 2-year-old child presents with neonatal meconium ileus, chronic cough and bronchitis, growth failure, and chronic diarrhea with light-colored, foul-smelling stools. A deficiency of which of the following vitamins should be considered?

a. Vitamin A
b. Vitamin C
c. Vitamin B_1
d. Vitamin B_2
e. Vitamin B_6

334. Pantothenic acid is important for which of the following steps or pathways?

a. Pyruvate carboxylase
b. Fatty acid synthesis
c. Pyruvate carboxykinase
d. Gluconeogenesis
e. Glycolysis

335. Which of the following enzymes requires a vitamin that is rarely deficient except in those eating fad diets with excess raw egg white?

a. Pyruvate carboxylase
b. Pyruvate dehydrogenase
c. Phosphoenolpyruvate carboxykinase
d. Glucokinase
e. Fructokinase

336. Neural tube defects such as anencephaly and spina bifida have higher frequencies in certain populations like those of Celtic origin and in certain regions like South Texas. This suggestion of environmental cause produced research showing that deficiency of which of the following vitamins is associated with the occurrence of neural tube defects (anencephaly and spina bifida)?

a. Ascorbic acid (vitamin C)
b. Thiamine (vitamin B_1)
c. Riboflavin (vitamin B_2)
d. Niacin (vitamin B_3)
e. Folic acid

337. An African American infant presents with prominent forehead, bowing of the limbs, broad and tender wrists, swellings at the costochondral junctions of the ribs, and irritability. The head is deformable, able to be depressed like a ping-pong ball, while palpation of the joints is very painful. Which of the following treatments is recommended?

a. Lotions containing retinoic acid
b. Diet of baby food containing leafy vegetables
c. Diet of baby food containing liver and ground beef
d. Milk and sunlight exposure
e. Removal of eggs from diet

Vitamins and Minerals

Answers

303. The answer is b. *(Murray, pp 580–597. Scriver, pp 3127–3162.)* Ferrous iron (Fe^{2+}) is the form absorbed in the intestine by ferritin, transported in plasma by transferrin, and stored in the liver in combination with ferritin or as hemosiderin. There is no known excretory pathway for iron, either in the ferric or ferrous form. For this reason, excessive iron uptake over a period of many years may cause hemochromatosis (235200), the likely diagnosis for this man. This is a condition of extensive hemosiderin deposition in the liver, myocardium, pancreas, and adrenals. The resulting symptoms include liver cirrhosis, congestive heart failure, diabetes mellitus, and changes in skin pigmentation.

304. The answer is c. *(Murray, pp 474–480. Scriver, pp 1623–1650.)* Certain amino acids and lipids are dietary necessities because humans cannot synthesize them. The energy usually obtained from carbohydrates can be obtained from lipids and the conversion of some amino acids to intermediates of the citric acid cycle. These alternative substrates can thus provide fuel for oxidation and energy plus reduce equivalents for biosynthesis. Iodine is important for thyroid hormone synthesis, whereas calcium is essential for muscle contraction and bone metabolism.

305. The answer is c. *(Murray, pp 481–497. Scriver, pp 3897–3964.)* The absorption of vitamin B_{12} from the intestine is very complex, involving a binding protein called intrinsic factor with other transcobalamin proteins that also carry it in blood. Intrinsic factor is secreted by the gastric mucosa, and pernicious anemia results from gastric atrophy at older ages or more rarely, from mutations affecting the intrinsic factor itself that present with cobalamin deficiency in childhood (e.g., 261000). Inability to absorb vitamin B_{12} from the gastrointestinal tract causes more severe deficiency than nutritional deprivation in vegetarian diets or small bowel disease. Intrinsic factor may also be diminished by autoantibodies in autoimmune diseases like diabetes mellitus or Graves disease (hyperthyroidism). When the symptoms of cobalamin deficiency go beyond megaloblastic anemia to neurologic symptoms like numbness and weakness in the extremities, poor coordination, dementia they are called "pernicious" because of potential irreversibility and death. Clinical signs of pernicious anemia may not appear until 3 to 5 years following the onset of vitamin B_{12} deficiency and the neurologic signs may occur without obvious anemia.

Cheilosis is dryness and scaling of the lips that is characteristic of riboflavin (vitamin B_2) deficiency. Scurvy is caused by vitamin C deficiency and is characterized by bleeding gums and bone disease. Rickets is softening and deformation of the bones due to vitamin D deficiency or defects in vitamin D processing. The word beriberi is Singhalese for "I cannot," referring to muscular atrophy and paralysis caused by the inflammation of multiple nerves (polyneuritis). Beriberi is caused by thiamine (vitamin B_1) deficiency and is common in Asians who subsist on a diet of polished white rice.

306. The answer is b. *(Murray, pp 481–497. Scriver, pp 3897–3964.)* Osteomalacia is the name given to the disease of bone seen in adults with vitamin D deficiency. It is analogous to rickets, which is seen in children with the same deficiency. Both disorders are manifestations of defective bone formation. The osteogenesis imperfectas are a group of genetic bone disorders caused by collagen gene mutations. Osteopetrosis is a hardening of the bones that occurs in certain hereditary conditions. Night blindness is associated with vitamin A deficiency.

307. The answer is e. *(Murray, pp 481–497. Scriver, pp 3897–3964.)* Ascorbic acid (vitamin C) is found in fresh fruits and vegetables. Deficiency of ascorbic acid produces scurvy, the "sailor's disease." Ascorbic acid is necessary for the hydroxylation of proline to hydroxyproline in collagen, a process required in the formation and maintenance of connective tissue. The failure of mesenchymal cells to form collagen causes the skeletal, dental, and connective tissue deterioration seen in scurvy. Thiamine, niacin, cobalamin, and pantothenic acid can all be obtained from fish or meat products. The nomenclature of vitamins began by classifying fat-soluble vitamins as A (followed by subsequent letters of the alphabet such as D, E, and K) and water-soluble vitamins as B. Components of the B vitamin fraction were then given subscripts, e.g., thiamine (B_1), riboflavin (B_2), niacin [nicotinic acid (B_3)], panthothenic acid (B_5), pyridoxine (B_6), and cobalamin (B_{12}). The water-soluble vitamins C, biotin, and folic acid do not follow the B nomenclature.

308. The answer is c. *(Murray, pp 481–497. Scriver, pp 3897–3964.)* The retinal pigment rhodopsin is composed of the 11-cis-retinal form of vitamin A coupled to opsin. Light isomerizes 11-cis-retinal to all-trans-retinal, which is hydrolyzed to free all-trans-retinal and opsin. In order for regeneration of rhodopsin to occur, 11-cis-retinal must be regenerated. This dark reaction involves the isomerization of all-trans-retinal to 11-cis-retinal, which combines with opsin to reform rhodopsin. A deficiency of vitamin A, which is often derived from the β-carotene of plants, results in night blindness. Excess of vitamin A (hypervitaminosis A) is toxic, causing cerebral edema and other problems.

309. The answer is b. *(Murray, pp 130–135, 153–162. Scriver, pp 3897–3964.)* Pyruvate carboxylase catalyzes the conversion of pyruvate to oxaloacetate in gluconeogenesis:

$$\text{pyruvate} + HCO_3^- + \text{ATP} \rightarrow \text{oxaloacetate} + \text{ADP} + P_i$$

In order for pyruvate carboxylase to be ready to function, it requires biotin, Mg^{2+}, and Mn^{2+}. It is allosterically activated by acetyl-CoA. The biotin is not carboxylated until acetyl-CoA binds the enzyme. By this means, high levels of acetyl-CoA signal the need for more oxaloacetate. When ATP levels are high, the oxaloacetate is consumed in gluconeogenesis. When ATP levels are low, the oxaloacetate enters the citric acid cycle. Gluconeogenesis only occurs in the liver and kidneys.

310. The answer is b. *(Murray, pp 481–497. Scriver, pp 3897–3964, 121–138, 287–320.)* Pantothenic acid combines with the amino acid cysteine to become the pentetheine sulfhydryl component of coenzyme A (CoA) and acyl carrier protein (important for fatty acid synthesis). Acetyl-CoA is the activated form of acetate employed in acetylation reactions, including the citric acid cycle and lipid metabolism. Loss of myelin in Hallavorden-Spatz disease correlates with a role for activated pantothenic acid as a cofactor for fatty acid synthesis and as a carrier of acyl chains (which must be added to glycerol to form triacylglycerols, alkylacylglycerols (ether lipids), and (by acyl addition to sphingosine) cerebrosides, sphingomyelin, and gangliosides.

Mutations with severe impact on panthothenic acid kinase (mediating activation by its phosphorylation) present with neurologic signs in infancy (e.g., infantile neuroaxonal dystrophy—256600) while those with less impact present in the second or third decades with cognitive decline, dementia, and psychiatric symptoms (e.g., Hallavorden-Spatz disease, 234200). Nutritional deficiencies of pantothenic acid have not been described except in artificial studies, perhaps because they would limit CoA and have deadly consequences in mammals. However, because it is common in foodstuffs, there is little evidence of pantothenic acid deficiency in humans.

311. The answer is d. *(Murray, pp 481–497. Scriver, pp 3897–3964.)* In order to be converted to thrombin during clot formation, prothrombin must bind Ca^{2+}, which allows it to anchor to platelet membranes produced by injury. Prothrombin's affinity for Ca^{2+} is dependent on the presence of 10 γ-carboxyglutamate residues found in the first 35 amino acid residues of its amino terminal region. The vitamin K–dependent γ-carboxylation of prothrombin is a posttranslational modification that occurs as nascent prothrombin is synthesized on liver rough endoplasmic reticulum and passes into the lumen of the reticulum. The anticoagulants warfarin and dicumarol are structural analogues that block the γ-carboxylation of prothrombin by substituting for vitamin K. Hence, the prothrombin produced has a weak affinity for Ca^{2+} and cannot properly bind to platelet membranes in order to be converted to thrombin. Exposure of the fetus to warfarin during maternal therapy can produce a syndrome involving small, "fleur-de lys" nose and skeletal defects.

312. The answer is b. *(Murray, pp 481–497. Scriver, pp 3935–3964.)* The vitamin biotin is the cofactor required by carboxylating enzymes such as acetyl-CoA, pyruvate, and propionyl-CoA carboxylases. The fixation of CO_2 by these biotin-dependent enzymes occurs in two stages. In the first, bicarbonate ion reacts with adenosine triphosphate (ATP) and the biotin carrier protein moiety of the enzyme; in the second, the "active CO_2" reacts with the substrate—e.g., acetyl-CoA.

313. The answer is b. *(Murray, pp 481–497. Scriver, pp 3897–3964.)* Pantothenate is the precursor of CoA, which participates in numerous reactions throughout the metabolic scheme. CoA is a central molecule of metabolism involved in acetylation reactions. Thus a deficiency of pantothenic acid would have severe consequences. There is no documented deficiency state for pantothenate, however, because this vitamin is common in foodstuffs.

314. The answer is c. *(Murray, pp 481–497. Scriver, pp 3897–3964.)* In the Far East, rice is a staple of the diet. When rice is unsupplemented, beriberi can be manifest, because rice is low in vitamin B_1 (thiamine). Thiamine pyrophosphate is the necessary prosthetic group of enzymes that transfers activated aldehyde units. Such enzymes include transketolase, pyruvate dehydrogenase, and α-ketoglutarate dehydrogenase. Beriberi is a wasting disease whose symptoms include pain in the limbs induced by peripheral neuropathy, weak musculature, and heart enlargement. Yeast products, whole grains, nuts, and pork are rich in thiamine. Choline, ethanolamine, and serine are polar head groups of phospholipids. Glycine is a common amino acid.

315. The answer is c. *(Murray, pp 173–179. Scriver, pp 2297–2356.)* The almost universal carrier of acyl groups is coenzyme A (CoA). However, acyl carrier protein (ACP) also functions as a carrier of acyl groups. In fatty acid synthesis, ACP carries the acyl intermediates. The reactive prosthetic group of both ACP and CoA is a phosphopantetheine sulfhydryl. In ACP, the phosphopantetheine group is attached to the 77-residue polypeptide chain via a serine hydroxyl. In CoA, the phosphopantetheine is linked to the 5′-phosphate of adenosine that is phosphorylated in its 3′-hydroxyl.

316. The answer is a. *(Murray, pp 481–497. Scriver, pp 3897–3964.)* Thiamine (vitamin B_1) activated as its pyrophosphate is a cofactor for pyruvate dehydrogenase, α-ketoglutarate dehydrogenase of the citric acid cycle, branched chain keto-acid dehydrogenase that metabolizes leucine/isoleucine/valine, and transketolase of the pentose phosphate pathway. Deficiency of thiamine causes beri beri and exacerbates encephalopathy in alcoholics, having impact on the nervous system in both diseases. Since pyruvate dehydrogenase commits pyruvate from glycolysis to acetyl CoA in the citric acid cycle, its impairment will increase lactate (lactic acidosis), deplete energy (by impacting the citric acid cycle and the first steps of oxidative phosphorylation), and impair glucose metabolism—all key to neural function. Impairment of transketolase and the pentose phosphate shunt would reduce NADPH production, key to glutathione maintenance and reduction of oxidants in brain. Certain mutations in transketolase may thus increase susceptibility to Wernicke-Korsakoff syndrome (277730), a nice example of a Mendelian enzyme alteration brought out by environment (alcohol dependency) to cause a multifactorial disease (encephalopathy).

Lipoamide is also a cofactor in pyruvate dehydrogenase, transferring the acetyl group in pyruvate to coenzyme A. Lipoamide becomes acetyllipoamide and then dihydro-lipoamide as it first accepts and then transfers an acyl group. This reaction and the regeneration of lipoamide are catalyzed by different parts of the dehydrogenase enzyme complex. ATP transfers phosphoryl groups, thiamine pyrophosphate transfers aldehyde groups, NADH and FADH transfer protons. Mutations in the multipeptide pyruvate dehydrogenase complex occur in Leigh disease (256000), an end phenotype of many mutations that simulate the lactic acidosis and encephalopathy accompanying acute forms of thiamine deficiency (beri beri).

317. The answer is d. *(Murray, pp 173–179. Scriver, pp 2297–2326.)* The key enzymatic step of fatty acid synthesis is the carboxylation of acetyl-CoA to form malonyl-CoA. The carboxyl of biotin is covalently attached to an ε-amino acid group of a lysine residue of acetyl-CoA carboxylase. The reaction occurs in two stages. In the first step, a carboxybiotin is formed:

$$HCO_3^- + \text{biotin-enzyme} + \text{ATP} \rightarrow CO_2\text{-biotin-enzyme} + \text{ADP} + P_i$$

In the second step, the CO_2 is transferred to acetyl-CoA to produce malonyl-CoA:

$$CO_2\text{-biotin-enzyme} + \text{acetyl CoA} \rightarrow \text{malonyl-CoA} + \text{biotin-enzyme}$$

None of the other cofactors listed are involved in this reaction.

318. The answer is d. *(Murray, pp 481–497. Scriver, pp 3897–3964.)* The component that can be produced from tryptophan is nicotinamide, which is joined with adenosine diphosphate to form the important cofactor and ADP-ribose donor, nicotinamide adenine dinucleotide (NAD). Nicotinamide and nicotinic acid were discovered as the essential nutrient niacin that could be used to treat pellagra. Niacin is not strictly a vitamin because it can be derived from tryptophan, but its dietary deficiency contributes to pellagra along with deficiencies of riboflavin (vitamin B_2) and pyridoxine (vitamin B_6) that are involved in the biosynthesis of niacin from tryptophan. NAD^+ is a cofactor required by all dehydrogenases and NADPH, produced by the pentose phosphate shunt is utilized in reductive synthesis of compounds such as fatty acids. Since photosensitivity is common in DNA repair disorders like xeroderma pigmentosum (278730), it is possible that deficient ADP-ribosylation of DNA repair topoisomerases relates to the photosensitivity of pellagra.

Pantothenic acid and coenzyme A are involved in acetylation and acyl-transfer reactions important in fatty acid metabolism, biotin and carboxy-biotin in carboxylation reactions like those deficient in multiple carboxylase deficiency (253270). Intrinsic factor is a protein secreted by the gastric mucosa that is important for binding and absorption of cobalamin (vitamin B_{12}). Pyridoxal phosphate also is involved in amino acid metabolism (transamination), muscle glycogen breakdown (glycogen phosphorylase), and steroid hormone action (removes hormone-receptor complexes from DNA, terminating their action.)

319. The answer is a. *(Murray, pp 481–497. Scriver, pp 3897–3964.)* The vitamin folic acid is provided commercially and pharmaceutically as the stable 5-formyltetrahydrofolate known as folinic acid or its synthetic analogue leucovorin. Addition of folate to foods (bread) and encouragement of preconceptional vitamins with folate was prompted by its ability to lower the incidence of neural tube defects by two- to threefold. Folic acid is biologically active as the interconvertible forms tetrahydrofolate (THF), methylTHF, and other methylated forms (methylene THF, N5, N10-methylene THF) that are important for one-carbon (methyl) transfers and interconversions (glycine-serine, formate-formylmethinone, formate-CO_2 homocysteine-methionine, uracil-thymine). THF is required in two steps of purine synthesis and thus required in the de novo synthesis of ATP and GTP. Although de novo synthesis of the pyrimidine ring does not require tetrahydrofolate, the methylation of deoxyuridine monophosphate (dUMP) to form thymine from uracil does. In this thymidylate synthetase reaction, methylene THF donates a methyl group and is converted to dihydrofolate which requires action of dihydrofolate reductase to regenerate THF. Methotrexate inhibits dihydrofolate reductase, depletes THF pools, and thus would elevate substrates of enzymes dependent on this cofactor like dUMP. THF is also a cofactor for methionine synthase that coverts homocysteine to methionine, an enzyme deficient in one form of homocystinuria (236200).

320. The answer is c. *(Murray, pp 481–497. Scriver, pp 3897–3964.)* The vitamin riboflavin (vitamin B_2) is a precursor of two cofactors involved in electron transport systems, riboflavin 5′-phosphate, also known as flavin mononucleotide (FMN), and flavin adenine dinucleotide (FAD). Strictly speaking, these compounds are not nucleotides, as they contain the sugar alcohol ribitol, not ribose. The cofactors are strongly bound to their apoenzymes and function as dehydrogenation catalysts. Pyruvate dehydrogenase is a multienzyme complex and contains the enzyme dihydrolipoyl dehydrogenase, which has as its prosthetic group two molecules of FAD per molecule of enzyme. In the overall reaction, the reduced FAD is reoxidized by NAD^+. Mutations at several loci encoding the components of pyruvate dehydrogenase cause the clinical phenotype of Leigh syndrome (256000) with seizures, low tone, neurodegeneration, and lactic acidosis. Succinate dehydrogenase also contains tightly bound FAD, one molecule per molecule of enzyme. Glutamate, lactate, malate, and glyceraldehyde-3-phosphate dehydrogenases all use nicotinamide dinucleotide cofactors and do not contain FAD as a prosthetic group.

321. The answer is c. *(Murray, pp 481–497. Scriver, pp 3897–3964.)* Pyridoxine (vitamin B_6) deficiency usually occurs concurrently with deficiency of other B vitamins or in association with drug therapy in individuals who are slow-metabolizers for the antituberculosis drug isoniazid and others like penicillamine or sulfa antibiotics (243400). Pyridoxine is present in many foods, particularly vegetables, cereals, and fruits. Niacin (precursor to nicotinamide adenine dinucleotide) is abundant in liver, poultry, and eggs; tetrahydrofolate in human and cow (not goat) milk, uncooked fruits, and vegetables; riboflavin (vitamin B_2—precursor to flavin adenine mononucleotide) in milk, eggs, meats, and fruits; retinoic acid (vitamin A) in animal tissues like egg yolks, fish oils with other carotenoids in leafy vegetables.

The coenzyme pyridoxal phosphate is a versatile compound that aids in amino acid transaminations, deaminations, decarboxylations, and transulfurations. It is also important for operation of glycogen phosphorylase. A common feature of these reactions is formation of a Schiff-base intermediate with a specific lysine group at the active site of the appropriate enzymes.

322. The answer is e. *(Murray, pp 481–497. Scriver, pp 3897–3964.)* Vitamin A is a fat-soluble vitamin that can be deficient in combination with thiamine and riboflavin deficiencies in dry climates with food shortages, with other fat-soluble vitamins (D, E, K) in disorders associated with intestinal malabsorption, and in hypothyroidism where there is defective conversion of carotene to vitamin A. Carotenes and carotenoids in plants (yellow corn, carrots, sweet potatoes, leafy vegetables, green peas) are converted to retinaldehyde in the intestinal mucosa (then to retinol), while retinol is found in animal tissues like egg yolks, fish oils, butter, liver, kidney. The first symptoms of vitamin A deficiency are dryness of the eyes (xerophthalmia) with decreased vision in dim light (night blindness), followed by photophobia, corneal irritation, ulceration, and destruction of the eye. Dry skin and rashes also occur. The importance of eggs in people with restricted diets was vividly portrayed in James Clavell's novel, *King Rat*, where they were prized for prevention of blindness.

Pyridoxine is present in vegetables, cereals, and fruits, niacin in liver, poultry, and eggs; tetrahydrofolate in milk, uncooked fruits, and vegetables; and riboflavin in milk, eggs, meats, and fruits.

323. The answer is d. *(Murray, pp 49–59. Scriver, pp 3897–3964.)* A coenzyme is a nonprotein organic molecule that binds to an enzyme to aid in its catalytic function. Usually it is involved in the transfer of a specific functional group. A coenzyme usually binds loosely and can be separated from the enzyme. When a coenzyme binds tightly to an enzyme, it is spoken of as a prosthetic group of the enzyme. Coenzymes can be viewed as a second substrate for the enzyme, often undergoing chemical changes that counterbalance those of the substrate. Lipoic acid is a short-chain fatty acid with two sulfhydryl groups that is a coenzyme for the pyruvate dehydrogenase reaction that commits pyruvate to the citric acid cycle by converting it to acetyl CoA rather than lactate. Mutations affecting the pyruvate dehydrogenase enzyme complex cause Leigh syndrome of lactic acidosis and neurologic disease (256000), those affecting glucose-6-phosphate dehydrogenase produce anemia (305900), those affecting glucose-1-phosphate incorporation into glucose and glycogen cause type I glycogen storage disease (232200), those affecting ornithine conversion to citrulline in the urea cycle (ornithine transcarbamylase deficiency—311250) cause hyperammonemia and coma, and those affecting conversion of UDP-galactose to UDP-glucose cause the severe form of galactosemia (230400).

324. The answer is c. *(Murray, pp 481–497. Scriver, pp 3897–3964.)* Selected minerals are important cofactors for enzyme reactions; cofactors are distinguished from coenzymes because cofactors do not function in group transfer and do not undergo chemical reactions (other than changes in valence due to oxidation/reduction). Cofactors are usually metallic ions rather than organic molecules, including cobalt, copper, iron, molybdenum, selenium, and zinc. Examples include copper in cytochrome oxidase, iron in all the cytochromes, magnesium for all enzymes utilizing ATP, and zinc in lactate dehydrogenase. Zinc deficiency causes a clinical syndrome called acrodermatitis enterohepatica (201100) with growth failure, diarrhea, loss of hair, eyelashes, and eyebrows, and skin rashes with redness and scaling on the extremities (acrodermatitis). Arsenic, lead, and antimony cause disease when present in excess while vanadium (along with silicon, nickel, and tin) is known to be essential from experimental nutritiion studies but its role is not defined. Fluoride (preventing dental caries) and lithium (a therapy for depression) have effects on humans but are not known to be essential nutrients.

325. The answer is d. *(Murray, pp 481–497. Scriver, pp 4293–4326.)* The major role of vitamin K is in the synthesis of prothrombin and other clotting factors (e.g., VII, IX, and X). Vitamin K acts on the inactive precursor molecules of these proteins, allowing carboxylation of glutamic acid residues to γ-carboxyglutamate. Once carboxylated, the factors bind calcium through these groups and are able to attach to cell membranes as part of clot formation. A true vitamin K deficiency in adults is unusual because vitamin K is found in a variety of foods and can be produced by intestinal bacteria. Liver, egg yolk, spinach, cauliflower, and cabbage are some of the sources of vitamin K. Poor fat metabolism, decreased liver function (reduced clotting factor synthesis), sterile gut with reduced bacterial metabolism (to produce menadiones) and decreased bile excretion in newborns renders them susceptible to vitamin K deficiency and hemorrhagic disease of the newborn, prevented by routine vitamin K injection in industrialized countries. Disorders with increased coagulation are treated with analogues of vitamin K that inhibit its conversion from dietary phylloquinone to hydroquine, epoxide, and quinone. Such inhibitors include coumadin and warfarin, a substance used as rat poison. Heparin is a complex polysaccharide that potentiates antithrombin III and inhibits clotting without effects on vitamin K.

326. The answer is c. *(Murray, pp 481–497. Scriver, pp 3897–3964.)* Prolonged vitamin C deficiency (scurvy) usually occurs with severe malnutrition (famine, prisoners of war, alcoholism, extreme food fadism). Exclusive feeding of cow's milk, as may occur in areas of famine with poor supplies of maternal milk, can result in infantile scurvy with the symptoms described in the question. X-rays of the limbs are helpful in diagnosing scurvy, with a white line at the metaphysis and occasional subperiosteal hemorrhage. These radiologic features may be seen in copper deficiency associated with hyperalimentation, emphasizing the role of ascorbic acid (vitamin C) as a coenzyme for proline/lysine hydroxylases that modify collagen and also require copper.

The causes of hemorrhagic disease of the newborn are desribed in the previous answer, and vitamin K deficiency is almost never seen after the newborn period because of wide dietary availability. Deficiencies of the fat-soluble vitamins A, E, and D can occur with intestinal malabsorption, but avid fetal uptake during pregnancy usually prevents infantile symptoms. Vitamin D deficiency (rickets) can also cause a series of rib lumps (rosary) and is more likely with darker skin pigmentation but has other symptoms. Hypervitaminosis A can cause liver toxicity but not bleeding, and deficiency of vitamin E can be associated with anemia in prematures but is unknown in older children and adults.

327. The answer is a. *(Murray, pp 481–497. Scriver, pp 3897–3964.)* Vitamin A is essential for the normal differentiation of epithelial tissue as well as normal reproduction. Yellow and dark green vegetables as well as fruits are good sources of carotenes, which serve as precursors of vitamin A. However, egg yolk, butter, cream, and liver and kidneys are good sources of preformed vitamin A. Vitamin A is necessary for vision, not hearing. The visual pigment rhodopsin is formed from the protein opsin and 11-cis-retinal. During the photobleaching of rhodopsin, all-trans-retinal plus opsin is formed from dissociated rhodopsin, causing an impulse that is transmitted by the optic nerve to the brain. 11-cis-retinal is isomerized from trans-retinal, which spontaneously combines with opsin to reform rhodopsin, making it ready for another photochemical cycle. All trans-retinoic acid (tretinoin) has been found to be effective for topical treatment of psoriasis. Another form of vitamin A is 13-cis-retinoic acid (Accutane), which has been found to be effective in the treatment of severe cases of acne. Accutane causes birth defects of the face and brain if taken during the first trimester of pregnancy. Vitamin A is not synthesized in the skin. Vitamin D (derivatives of calciferol) can be synthesized in the skin under the influence of sunlight from 7-dehydrocholesterol, an intermediate in cholesterol synthesis.

328. The answer is a. *(Murray, pp 481–497. Scriver, pp 3897–3964, 121–138, 287–320.)* Vitamin K is essential for the posttranscriptional modification of prothrombin by γ-carboxylation of glutamate residues. A functional deficiency exists in patients treated with analogues of vitamin K such as the Coumadin derivatives. The analogues act as anticoagulants by competing with vitamin K and preventing the production of functional prothrombin. By administration of vitamin K, hemorrhage can be prevented in such patients. Vitamin K is normally obtained from green, leafy vegetables in the diet (not from citrus fruits or red meat). Intestinal bacteria also synthesize the vitamin, but even broad-spectrum antibiotic therapy does not completely sterilize the intestine. A deficiency of vitamin K can cause hemorrhagic disease in newborn infants because their intestines do not have the bacteria that produce vitamin K and because vitamin K does not cross the placenta. The neonatal deficiency occurs in term or premature infants.

329. The answer is b. *(Murray, pp 481–497. Scriver, pp 2275–2296.)* An elevation of pyruvate and a deficiency of acetyl-CoA suggest a deficiency of pyruvate dehydrogenase (PDH). This multisubunit enzyme assembly contains pyruvate dehydrogenase, dihydrolipoyl transacetylase, dihydrolipoyl dehydrogenase, and two enzymes involved in regulation of the overall enzymatic activity of the complex. PDH requires thiamine pyrophosphate as a coenzyme, dihydrolipoyl transacetylase requires lipoic acid and CoA, and dihydrolipoyl dehydrogenase has an FAD prosthetic group that is reoxidized by NAD^+. Biotin, pyridoxine, and ascorbic acid are not coenzymes for PDH. An ATP-dependent protein kinase can phosphorylate PDH to decrease activity, and a phosphatase can activate PDH. Increases of ATP, acetyl-CoA, or NADH (increased energy charge) and of fatty acid oxidation increase phosphorylation of PDH and decrease its activity. PDH is less active during starvation, increasing pyruvate, decreasing glycolysis, and sparing carbohydrates. Free fatty acids decrease PDH activity and would not be appropriate therapy for PDH deficiency. PDH deficiency (246900, 312170) exhibits genetic heterogeneity, as would be expected from its multiple subunits, with autosomal and X-linked recessive forms. The infant also could be classified as having Leigh's disease (266150), a heterogenous group of disorders with hypotonia and lactic acidemia that can include PDH deficiency.

330. The answer is d. *(Murray, pp 481–497. Scriver, pp 3897–3964.)* Chronic alcoholics are at risk for thiamine deficiency, which is thought to play a role in the incoordination (ataxia) and psychosis that can become chronic (Wernicke-Korsakoff syndrome). The thiamine deficiency produces relative deficiency of the pyruvate dehydrogenase complex. The administration of glucose without checking glucose levels can therefore be dangerous, since excess glucose is converted to pyruvate by glycolysis. The low rate of pyruvate dehydrogenase conversion of pyruvate to coenzyme A (and entry into the citric acid cycle) causes pyruvate to be converted to lactate (through lactate dehydrogenase). Lactic acidosis can be fatal. Chronic alcoholics can be deficient in the other vitamins mentioned, but thiamine is most likely to help the neurologic symptoms.

331. The answer is b. *(Murray, pp 481–497. Scriver, pp 3897–3964.)* Nicotinamide adenine dinucleotide (NAD^+) is the functional coenzyme derivative of niacin. It is the major electron acceptor in the oxidation of molecules, generating NADH, which is the major electron donor for reduction reactions. Thiamine (also known as vitamin B_1) occurs functionally as thiamine pyrophosphate and is a coenzyme for enzymes such as pyruvate dehydrogenase. Riboflavin (vitamin B_2) functions in the coenzyme forms of flavin mononucleotide (FMN) or flavin adenine dinucleotide (FAD). When concentrated, both have a yellow color due to the riboflavin they contain. Both function as prosthetic groups of oxidation-reduction enzymes or flavoproteins. Flavoproteins are active in selected oxidation reactions and in electron transport, but they do not have the ubiquitous role of NAD^+.

332. The answer is a. *(Murray, pp 481–497. Scriver, pp 3897–3964.)* Riboflavin deficiency involves the insidious onset of photophobia, a burning sensation in the eyes, sore mouth (stomatitis) and tongue (glossitis), oily skin with rash (seborrheic dermatitis), and weight loss, confusion, dizziness, headache, and weakness. Retinol deficiency would cause night blindness and dry eyes that could be part of the described disorder, niacin deficiency rash (pellagra) with neurologic symptoms, thiamine deficiency heart failure and neurologic symptoms if acute (beri beri) or more chronic neuritis, pyridoxine deficiency infantile convulsions or peripheral neuritis (numbness and tingling, more common in slow metabolizers of drugs like isoniazid).

333. The answer is a. *(Murray, pp 481–497. Scriver, pp 5121–5138.)* Vitamins A, D, E, and K are all fat-soluble. The physical characteristics of fat-soluble vitamins derive from the hydrophobic nature of the aliphatic chains composing them. The other vitamins listed are water-soluble, efficiently administered orally, and rapidly absorbed from the intestine. Fat-soluble vitamins must be administered intramuscularly or as oral emulsions (mixtures of oil and water). In intestinal disorders such as chronic diarrhea or malabsorption due to deficient digestive enzymes, fat-soluble vitamins are poorly absorbed and can become deficient. Supplementation of fat-soluble vitamins is thus routine in disorders like cystic fibrosis (219700), a cause of respiratory and intestinal disease that is the likely diagnosis in this child.

334. The answer is b. *(Murray, pp 481–497. Scriver, pp 3897–3964.)* Pantothenic acid is phosphorylated and complexed with the amino acid cysteine to form 4-phosphopantetheine, the precursor for coenzyme A (CoA) and the acyl carrier protein (ACP) that participates in fatty acid synthesis. The thiol group of 4-phosphopantetheine is a carrier of acyl groups in CoA (A stands for acetylation or acetyl group) and ACP (fatty acyl groups). CoA is one of the major molecules in metabolism, carrying a pantetheine group bound to adenosine ribonucleotide-3′-phosphate via a 5′-diphosphate (pyrophosphate). Acetyl groups are linked to the reactive terminal sulfhydryl group to produce acetyl-CoA, which has a high acetyl transfer potential. CoA carries and transfers acetyl groups in much the same way as ATP transfers activated phosphoryl groups. CoA is involved in fatty acid synthesis, fatty acid β-oxidation, and the citric acid cycle; it is not involved in glycolysis or gluconeogenesis, where acetyl transfer does not occur.

Gluconeogenesis generates glucose by converting pyruvate to oxaloacetate (via pyruvate carboxylase) to phosphoenopyruvate (via phosphoenopyruvate carboxykinase) to fructose-1,6-bisphosphate (through reversal of glycolytic enzymes) to fructose-6-phosphate (via fructose-1, 6-bisphosphatase) to glucose-6-phosphate (through reversal of phosphohexose isomerase) to glucose (through glucose-6-phosphatase). Special enzymes are required at steps where reversal of glycolysis is not energetically feasible.

335. The answer is a. *(Murray, pp 481–497. Scriver, pp 3935–3964.)* Biotin functions to transfer carbon dioxide to substrates, adding a carboxyl group. Pyruvate carboxylase and enzymes of the holocarboxylase complex that degrade organic acids (propionate, metabolites of leucine) require biotin to transfer an activated carbonyl group. Biotin may be depleted by a deficiency of the enzyme biotinidase (253260), rendering the mentioned carboxylases less active and producing accumulation of the mentioned organic acids with severe acidosis. Nutritional deficiency of biotin is virtually unknown, but can be induced with raw egg white which contains avidin, a biotin-binding protein. Biotin deficiency causes skin rashes and hair loss, symptoms also seen in biotinidase enzyme deficiency. Thiamine is required for the reactions catalyzed by pyruvate dehydrogenase, transketolases, and α-ketoglutarate dehydrogenase. Kinases such as those in glycolysis require ATP as a cofactor.

336. The answer is e. *(Murray, pp 481–497. Scriver, pp 3897–3964.)* Spina bifida, or myelomeningocele, is a defect of the lower neural tube that produces an exposed spinal cord in the thoracic or sacral regions. Exposure of the spinal cord usually causes nerve damage that results in paralysis of the lower limbs and urinary bladder. Anencephaly is a defect of the anterior neural tube that results in lethal brain anomalies and skull defects. Folic acid is necessary for the development of the neural tube in the first few weeks of embryonic life, and the children of women with nutritional deficiencies have higher rates of neural tube defects. Because neural tube closure occurs at a time when many women are not aware that they are pregnant, it is essential that all women of childbearing age take a folic acid supplement of approximately 0.4 mg per day. Frank folic acid deficiency can also cause megaloblastic anemia because of a decreased synthesis of the purines and pyrimidines needed for cells to make DNA and divide. Deficiencies of thiamine in chronic alcoholics are related to Wernicke-Korsakoff syndrome, which is characterized by loss of memory, lackadaisical behavior, and a continuous rhythmic movement of the eyeballs. Thiamine dietary deficiency from excess of polished rice can cause beriberi. Niacin deficiency leads to pellagra, a disorder that produces skin rash (dermatitis), weight loss, and neurologic changes including depression and dementia. Riboflavin deficiency leads to mouth ulcers (stomatitis), cheilosis (dry, scaly lips), scaly skin (seborrhea), and photophobia. Because biotin is widely distributed in foods and is synthesized by intestinal bacteria, biotin deficiency is rare. However, the heat-labile molecule avidin, found in raw egg whites, binds biotin tightly and blocks its absorption, causing dermatitis, dehydration, and lethargy. Lactic acidosis results as a buildup of lactate due to the lack of functional pyruvate carboxylase when biotin is missing. Vitamin C deficiency leads to scurvy, which causes bleeding gums and bone disease.

Vitamin B_{12} can be deficient due to a lack of intrinsic factor, which is a glycoprotein secreted by gastric parietal cells. A lack of intrinsic factor or a dietary deficiency of cobalamin can cause pernicious anemia and neuropsychiatric symptoms. The only known treatment for intrinsic factor deficiency (vitamin B_{12} deficiency) is intramuscular injection of cyanocobalamin throughout the patient's life.

337. The answer is d. *(Murray, pp 481–497. Scriver, pp 4223–4240.)* People with bowed legs and other bone malformations were quite common in the northeastern United States following the industrial revolution. This was caused by childhood diets lacking foods with vitamin D and by minimal exposure to sunlight due to the dawn-to-dusk working conditions of the textile mills. Vitamin D is essential for the metabolism of calcium and phosphorus. Soft and malformed bones result from its absence. Liver, fish oil, and egg yolks contain vitamin D, and milk is supplemented with vitamin D by law. In adults, lack of sunlight and a diet poor in vitamin D lead to osteomalacia (soft bones). Dark-skinned peoples are more susceptible to vitamin D deficiency.

Biotin deficiency can be caused by diets with excess egg white, leading to dehydration and acidosis from accumulation of carboxylic and lactic acids. Retinoic acid is a vitamin A derivative that can be helpful in treating acne but not vitamin D deficiency. Leafy vegetables are a source of B vitamins such as niacin and cobalamin.

Hormones and Integrated Metabolism

Questions

DIRECTIONS: Each item below contains a question or incomplete statement followed by suggested responses. Select the **one best** response to each question.

338. A teenage female presenting with lack of menstruation (amennorhea) is found to have a 46,XY karyotype, and DNA testing shows a dysfunctional testosterone receptor characteristic of testicular feminization or androgen insensitivity syndrome (300068). Which of the following statements accurately describes sex hormones such as testosterone?

a. They bind specific membrane receptors
b. They interact with DNA directly
c. They cause release of a proteinaceous second messenger from the cell membrane
d. They enhance transcription when bound to receptors
e. They inhibit translation through specific cytoplasmic proteins

339. After a meal and clearance of carbohydrates/chyomicrons from the blood stream, blood glucose is initially maintained by liver glycogenolysis then sustained by fat mobilization from adipose tissue. Children with glycogen storage disorders have immediate problems with glucose maintenance while those with fatty acid oxidation disorders have later problems after glycogen is depleted. Which of the following mechanisms best explains the coordinate stimulation of glycogenolysis and lipolysis?

a. The type I hormone cortisol, a glucocorticoid, alters transcription in liver and adipocytes
b. The type II hormone cortisol, a glucocorticoid, binds to liver and adipose plasma membrane receptors to increase cAMP
c. The type II hormone epinephrine diffuses into the cytosol of liver and adipose cells, activating phosphorylase kinase and triglyceride lipase by allosteric mechanisms
d. Adenosine 3′,5′-cyclic monophosphate (cyclic AMP) is the second messenger in adipocytes, but not in the liver
e. The type II hormone epinephrine acts through the second messenger cAMP and protein kinases to stimulate glycogen phosphorylase and triglyceride lipase activities

340. Which of the following is noted in Cushing syndrome, a disease of the adrenal cortex?

a. Decreased production of epinephrine
b. Excessive production of epinephrine
c. Excessive production of vasopressin
d. Excessive production of cortisol
e. Decreased production of cortisol

341. A child with holoprosencephaly, a severe forebrain malformation, is hospitalized because of decreased urine output, hypernatremia (high serum sodium concentration), and cardiac arrythmia. Which of the following hormones is implicated?

a. Cortisol
b. Insulin
c. Vasopressin
d. Glucagon
e. Aldosterone

342. Patients with Addison disease (103230) have muscle weakness and fatigue due to adrenal insufficiency. Lack of glucocorticoids and mineralocorticoids might be a consequence of which of the following defects in the adrenal cortex?

a. Androstenedione deficiency
b. 17α-hydroxyprogesterone deficiency
c. Estrone deficiency
d. C-21-hydroxylase deficiency
e. Testosterone deficiency

343. A patient presents with a complaint of muscle weakness following exercise. Neurological examination reveals that the muscles supplied by cranial nerves are most affected. You suspect myasthenia gravis. Your diagnosis is confirmed when lab tests indicate antibodies against which of the following in the patient's blood?

a. Acetylcholinesterase
b. Muscle endplates
c. Cranial nerve synaptic membranes
d. Cranial nerve presynaptic membranes
e. Acetylcholine receptors

344. Several skeletal dysplasia (disproportionate skeletal growth or dwarfism) and craniosynostosis (premature fusion of the cranial sutures) syndromes are caused by mutations in fibroblast growth factor or its receptor. Fibroblast growth factor belongs to which of the following hormone groups?

a. Group I hormones interacting with nuclear receptors
b. Group I hormones interacting with cytoplasmic receptors
c. Group II hormones acting through calcium/phosphatidyl inositols
d. Group II hormones acting through cAMP/cGMP
e. Group II hormones acting through kinase cascades

345. Which of the following statements correctly describes insulin?

a. It is an anabolic signal to cells that glucose is scarce
b. It is converted from proinsulin to insulin primarily following secretion from β-cells
c. It does not have a prohormone form
d. It is a small polypeptide composed of a single chain bridged by disulfide groups
e. Its action is antagonistic to that of glucagon

346. Some individuals with diabetes mellitus are susceptible to rapid drops in blood sugar (hypoglycemia) with lethargy and potential seizures or coma. Such diabetics are called "brittle" and require careful monitoring of glucose levels as proper insulin doses are titrated. Of the many actions of insulin, decrease in which of the following cellular activities best accounts for "brittleness" of certain diabetics?

a. Plasma membrane transfer of glucose
b. Glucose oxidation
c. Gluconeogenesis
d. Lipogenesis
e. Formation of ATP, DNA, and RNA

347. A middle-aged man presents to his physician because of anxiety attacks accompanied by profuse sweating and heart palpitations. His physician documents a high blood pressure of 175/110 (hypertension) and orders ultrasound studies that show an adrenal tumor called pheochromocytoma. The man has also noted weight loss and fatigue over the past month when the attacks began. Knowing that pheochromocytoma releases epinephrine from the adrenal medulla, alteration of which of the following metabolic processes best explains symptoms of decreased energy and weight loss?

a. Glycolysis
b. Lipolysis
c. Gluconeogenesis
d. Glycogenolysis
e. Ketogenesis

348. Which of the following statements about prostaglandins is true?

a. They are precursors to arachidonic acid
b. They release arachidonic acid from membranes through the action of phospholipase A
c. They were first observed to cause uterine contraction and lowering of blood pressure
d. Although found in many organs, they are synthesized only in the prostate and seminal vesicles
e. They may be converted to leukotrienes by lipoxygenase

349. A male college student presents to his physician complaining of fatigue, weight loss, inability to concentrate, and occasional fainting spells. He also has noted a slight brown pigmentation to his skin despite no sun exposure. His physician suspects Addison disease, a multifactorial disorder that causes dysfunction of the adrenal cortex. Which of the following hormones is most likely deficient in Addison disease?

a. ACTH
b. Norepinephrine
c. Aldosterone
d. Testosterone
e. Epinephrine

350. The absorption of glucose from the gut into intestinal mucosal cells is coupled to Na^+, K^+-ATPase. In contrast, the movement of glucose from the intestinal epithelial cells into the submucosal bloodstream occurs through passive transport. Given these facts, which of the following statements can be true at one time or another?

a. Cytosolic levels of glucose in intestinal mucosal cells are regulated by levels of glucose in skeletal muscle cells
b. Free glucose levels in the lumen of the intestine can never be higher than levels in intestinal cells
c. Plasma glucose levels are much higher than intestinal cell cytosolic levels of glucose
d. Levels of glucose in the intestinal lumen are always higher than those in the cytosol of intestinal epithelial cells
e. Levels of plasma glucose are approximately equal to levels in the cytosol of intestinal epithelial cells

351. Which of the following proteins is responsible for secretion of pancreatic juice into the intestine?

a. Cholecystokinin
b. Gastrin
c. Insulin
d. Intrinsic factor
e. Secretin

352. Anti-inflammatory steroids are a mainstay for treatments of disorders ranging from asthma to severe poison ivy. Recent advances have avoided the side-effects of chronic steroid therapy (obesity, hypertension, shock susceptibility) by using short bursts of oral therapy or inhaled steroids that affect nasal/bronchial membranes without systemic absorption. Which step in the diagram below is thought to be responsible for the effect of anti-inflammatory steroids?

a. Step A
b. Step B
c. Step C
d. Step D
e. Step E

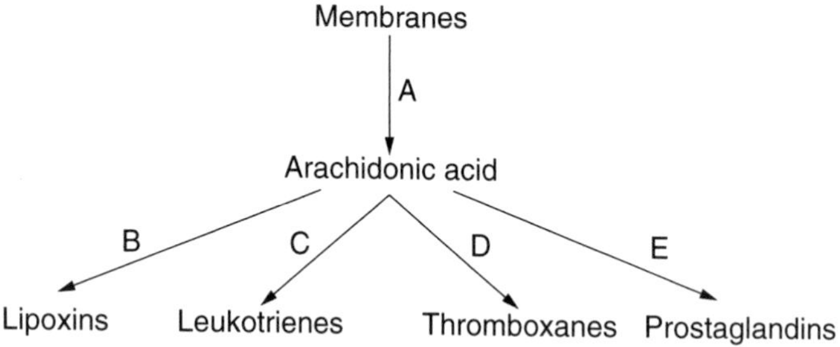

353. An infant presents with prolongation of usual neonatal jaundice and is found to have atypical elevation of direct-reacting, conjugated bilirubin. Further investigation indicates that the infant has liver disease with simultaneous elevation of liver transaminases. A sibling died with similar symptoms, and an inborn error of bile acid metabolism is suspected (e.g., intrahepatic cholestasis with defective conversion of trihydroxycoprostanic bile acid to cholic acid—214950). Which of the following compounds is normally used to conjugate bile acids?

a. Acetate
b. Glucuronic acid
c. Glutathione
d. Sulfate
e. Glycine

354. Several weight-loss diets are based on decreased carbohydrate intake to prevent stimulation of insulin secretion; insulin drives the feeling of hunger and also inhibits lipolysis. The suggested way of monitoring the success of low carbohydrate intake during fasting reflects the greatest increase in plasma concentration of which of the following?

a. Free fatty acids
b. Glucose
c. Glycogen
d. Ketone bodies
e. Triacylglycerols

355. Congestive heart failure can be caused by intrinsic defects of the heart muscle/valves or by pumping against increased pressure as with prolonged hypertension. Which of the following effects of the steroid digitalis is observed after treatment of congestive heart failure?

a. Decrease in cytosolic sodium levels
b. Inhibition of Na^+, K^+-ATPase
c. Decrease in the force of heart muscle contraction
d. Stimulation of the plasma membrane ion pump
e. Decrease in cytosolic calcium

356. Defects in the ability to oxidize fatty acids can be asymptomatic in the presence of frequent feeding, a therapy applied to all but the most severe long chain fatty acid oxidation disorders that are frequently lethal. In asymptomatic children with medium or short chain fatty acid oxidation defects, unintentional fasting due to intercurrent infections can produce lethargy and even coma after 4–6 hours without food. A deficit in which of the following compounds in serum most likely causes these neurologic symptoms?

a. Pyruvate and lactate
b. Free fatty acids
c. Propionate and methylmalonate
d. Glucose and ketone bodies
e. Triacylglycerols

357. A teenage girl is evaluated in the emergency room and noted to have increased respiration (tachypnea), vomiting, and confusion. She bleeds from puncture sites during withdrawal of blood for testing, and a urine toxicology screen reveals increased amounts of acetosalicylic acid, ibuprofen, and acetaminophen. She has a past history of depression and suicide attempts. Which of the following enzymes are likely to be inhibited?

a. Lipoprotein lipase
b. Lipoxygenase
c. Cyclooxygenase
d. Phospholipase D
e. Phospholipase A_2

358. Which of the following processes cannot provide arachidonic acid in mammals?

a. Dietary vegetable oils
b. Chain elongation and desaturation from linoleic acid
c. Cleavage of 2'-linoleic acid as the linoleoyl CoA from membrane triacylglycerols with chain elongation/desaturation
d. Biosynthesis of linoleic acid by fatty acid synthase followed by elongation/desaturation
e. Dietary animal fats

359. A patient stung by a bee is rushed into the emergency room with a variety of symptoms including increasing difficulty in breathing due to nasal and bronchial constriction. Although your subsequent treatment is to block the effects of histamine and other acute-phase reactants released by most cells, you must also block the slow-reacting substance of anaphylaxis (SRS-A), which is the most potent constrictor of the muscles enveloping the bronchial passages. An SRS-A is composed of which of the following?

a. Thromboxanes
b. Interleukins
c. Complement
d. Leukotrienes
e. Prostaglandins

360. Which of the following is an essential fatty acid?

a. Palmitic acid
b. Linoleic acid
c. Arachidonic acid
d. Oleic acid
e. Eicosatetraenoic acid

361. The central ring structure shown below is found in which of the following compounds?

a. Adrenocorticotropin
b. Aldosterone
c. Geranyl phosphate
d. Prostaglandin
e. Vitamin C

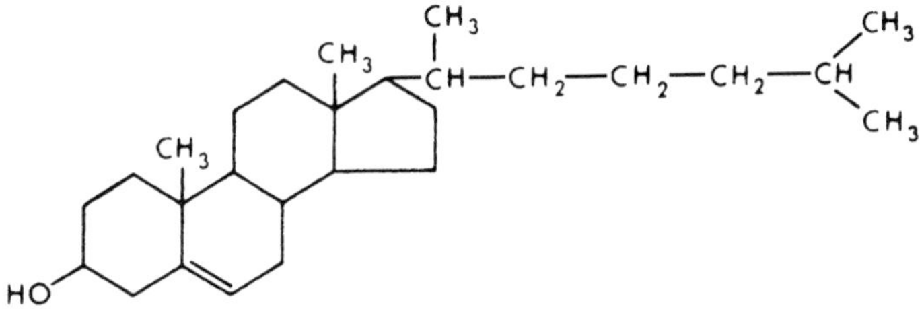

362. Which of the following compounds serves as a primary link between the citric acid cycle and the urea cycle?

a. Malate
b. Succinate
c. Isocitrate
d. Citrate
e. Fumarate

363. Which of the following can be converted to an intermediate of either the citric acid cycle or the urea cycle?

a. Tyrosine
b. Lysine
c. Leucine
d. Tryptophan
e. Aspartate

364. Most major metabolic pathways are considered to be either mainly anabolic or catabolic. Which of the following pathways is most correctly considered to be amphibolic (anabolic or catabolic)?

a. Lipolysis
b. Glycolysis
c. β-Oxidation of fatty acids
d. Citric acid cycle
e. Gluconeogenesis

365. Which of the following aspects of protein metabolism will contribute most directly to gluconeogenesis during starvation?

a. Entry of ornithine into the urea cycle
b. Transamination of amino acids
c. Carboxylation of amino acids
d. Peptide absorption from the gut
e. Ubiquitin binding to cytosolic proteins

366. Which of the following is a correct statement about the regulation and sequence of reactions in metabolic pathways?

a. The initial step in many pathways is a major determinant of control
b. The sequence of steps in catabolic pathways is usually the exact reverse of the biosynthetic sequence
c. Enzymes found in an anabolic pathway are rarely found in the corresponding catabolic pathway
d. A small set of large precursors serves as the starting point for most biosynthetic processes in energy metabolism
e. Steps in both anabolic and catabolic pathways are usually irreversible

367. Which of the following statements is correct regarding the well-fed state?

a. NADPH production by the hexose monophosphate shunt is decreased
b. Acetoacetate is the major fuel for muscle
c. Glucose transport into adipose tissue is decreased
d. The major fuel used by the brain is glucose
e. Amino acids are utilized for glucose production

368. During an overnight fast, which of the following is the major source of blood glucose?

a. Dietary glucose from the intestine
b. Hepatic glycogenolysis
c. Gluconeogenesis
d. Muscle glycogenolysis
e. Glycerol from lipolysis

369. The jinga bean, found in the jungles of Brazil, is unique in that it is composed almost exclusively of protein. Studies have shown that, immediately following a meal composed exclusively of jinga beans, which of the following occurs?

a. A decreased release of epinephrine
b. A complete absence of liver glycogen
c. Hypoglycemia
d. An increased release of insulin
e. Ketosis caused by the metabolism of ketogenic amino acids

370. Approximately 3 hours following a well-balanced meal, blood levels of which of the following are elevated?

a. Fatty acids
b. Glucagon
c. Glycerol
d. Epinephrine
e. Chylomicrons

371. If a homogenate of liver cells is centrifuged to remove all cell membranes and organelles, which of the following enzyme activities will remain in the supernatant?

a. Glucose-6-phosphate dehydrogenase
b. Glycogen synthetase
c. Aconitase
d. Acyl CoA hydratase
e. Hydroxybutyrate dehydrogenase

372. Which of the following descriptions of calcium is correct?

a. Calcium is abundant in the body as deposits of calcium sulfate
b. Calcium ion is required as a cofactor for many reactions
c. Calcium freely diffuses across the endoplasmic reticulum of muscle cells
d. Calcium is most highly concentrated in muscle
e. Calcium is mostly excreted by the kidney

373. Which of the following enzymes is active in adipocytes following a heavy meal?

a. Glycogen phosphorylase
b. Glycerol kinase
c. Hormone-sensitive triacylglyceride lipase
d. Glucose-6-phosphatase
e. Phosphatidate phosphatase

374. Which of the following tissues is capable of contributing to blood glucose?

a. Skeletal muscle
b. Adipose tissues
c. Cardiac muscle
d. Duodenal epithelium
e. Cartilage

375. Which of the following statements correctly apply to energy metabolism?

a. Fatty acids can be precursors of glucose
b. High energy levels turn on glycolysis
c. Pyruvate is committed to the citric acid cycle by acetylation through pyruvate dehydrogenase
d. Phosphorylation activates enzymes that store fat and glycogen
e. Guanosine triphosphate (GTP) is the major donor for enzyme phosphorylation

376. Which of the following is appropriate for a patient with renal failure?

a. High-carbohydrate diet
b. High-protein diet
c. Low-fat diet
d. High-fiber diet
e. Free water of at least 3 L/d

377. An unfortunate complication of long-term diabetes mellitus is the occurrence of heart attacks and gangrene of the extremities. Which of the following is the most likely cause?

a. Decreased glucose availability to liver cells
b. Decreased glucose availability to extrahepatic tissues
c. Increased catecholamine synthesis
d. Decreased catecholamine synthesis
e. Decreased glucose concentrations in vascular epithelium

378. An adolescent presents with abdominal discomfort, abdominal fullness, excess gas, and weight loss. Blood glucose, cholesterol, and alkaline phosphatase levels are normal. There is no jaundice or elevations. The stool tests positive for reducing substances. Which of the following is the most likely diagnosis?

a. Diabetes mellitus
b. Starvation
c. Nontropical sprue
d. Milk intolerance
e. Gallstones

379. Which of the following diseases reflects the loss of ability to move specific molecules between membrane-separated cellular compartments?

a. McArdle's phosphorylase disease
b. Carnitine deficiency
c. Methanol poisoning
d. Ethylene glycol poisoning
e. Diphtheria

380. Which of the following sets of blood values most closely correlates with a patient who has conducted a hunger strike for 1 month? (The blood levels listed by option a. represent the immediate postprandial state, and other options list blood levels after the hunger strike relative to a.)

	CONCENTRATION OF BLOOD FUELS (mM)			
	Glucose	**Free Fatty Acids**	**Ketone Bodies**	**Amino Acids**
a.	4.5	0.5	0.02	4.5
b.	Twofold decreased	Sixfold higher	100-fold higher	Slightly increased
c.	Threefold higher	Threefold higher	100-fold higher	Slightly increased
d.	Same	Twofold decreased	Same	Same
e.	Same	Sixfold higher	100-fold higher	Slightly decreased

Hormones and Integrated Metabolism

Answers

338. The answer is d. *(Murray, pp 434–473. Scriver, pp 4117–4146.)* All steroid hormones, including the sex hormones estrogen, testosterone, and progesterone, can be classified as group I hormones, meaning that they act by binding specific cytoplasmic receptors that enter the nucleus and stimulate transcription by specific DNA binding. Most nonsteroidal hormones, for example epinephrine, are group II hormones that interact with the cell membrane and produce a second-messenger effect. The group II hormones, in contrast to steroids, act in minutes while steroid hormones require hours for a biologic effect. Recent studies have indicated that specific cytoplasmic receptors for steroid hormones have an extraordinarily high affinity for the hormones. In addition, the receptors contain a DNA-binding region that is rich in amino acid residues that form metal binding fingers. Likewise, thyroid hormone receptors contain DNA-binding domains with metal-binding fingers. Like steroid hormones, thyroid hormones are transcriptional enhancers.

339. The answer is e. *(Murray, pp 180–189, 434–473. Scriver, pp 2297–2226.)* Type I hormones like the glucocorticoids are lipophilic, allowing them to diffuse into the cytosol, form ligand-receptor complexes, and mediate action in the cytosol or nucleus. Type II hormones like epinephrine interact with membrane receptors, often activating G protein complexes, elevating cytosolic levels of adenosine 3′,5′-cyclic monophosphate (cyclic AMP), and modifying protein kinases. Epinephrine (as well as glucagon) in liver stimulates adenylate cyclase and a kinase cascade ending with glycogen phosphorylase to initiate glycogenolysis. In adipose tissue, epinephrine more directly activates cyclic AMP, protein kinase, and triglyceride lipase to initiate lipolysis of stored triacylglycerides. Failure of glycogenolysis in glycogen storage diseases transmits a continuous signal of low glucose and enhanced fatty acid metabolism, causing high cholesterol and triglycerides. Normal glycogenolysis and failure of fat oxidation in fatty acid oxidation disorders causes later hypoglycemia without hyperlipidemia, but deficient energy yield from fat burning causes more lethal liver and heart failure.

340. The answer is d. *(Murray, pp 434–473. Scriver, pp 4029–4240.)* A tumor of the adrenal cortex would be expected to affect the production of adrenal steroid hormone. Cortisol and aldosterone are synthesized in the cortex. In Cushing syndrome, hypersecretion of cortisol occurs. Cortisol is a type I hormone and glucocorticoid that has the effect of encouraging metabolism of proteins, lipids, and carbohydrates. Because the multiple clinical effects of Cushing syndrome (truncal obesity, fat pad below neck or "buffalo hump," striae or stretch marks) can be related to the single cause of cortisol excess, Cushing disease is the preferred term. Cushing disease is multifactorial, caused by various factors like excessive production of ACTH by pituitary tumors or even specific mutations in G proteins that modulate the cortisol response (see 219080). Diseases affecting the adrenal medulla might be expected to disrupt or potentiate production of epinephrine in some way. Epinephrine (adrenalin) is synthesized in the medulla.

341. The answer is c. *(Murray, pp 434–473. Scriver, pp 4029–4240.)* Vasopressin, which is also called antidiuretic hormone, increases the permeability of the collecting ducts and distal convoluted tubules of the kidney and thus allows passage of water. Vasopressin is secreted by the posterior pituitary (neurohypophysis), which may undergo altered development in concert with brain malformations like holoprosencephaly. Like the mineralocorticoid aldosterone, vasopressin results in an expansion of blood volume. However, the mode of action of aldosterone is different; it causes sodium reabsorption, not water reabsorption. Sodium reabsorption indirectly leads to increased plasma osmolality and thus water retention in the blood. Cortisol is a glucocorticoid that potentiates catabolic metabolism chronically. Epinephrine stimulates catabolic metabolism acutely. Insulin acutely favors anabolic metabolism, in large part by allowing glucose and amino acid transport into cells.

342. The answer is d. *(Murray, pp 434–473. Scriver, pp 4029–4240.)* Both cortisol and aldosterone contain C-21-hydroxyl groups. Both are also derived from progesterone in the adrenal cortex. Addison disease is produced by adrenal insufficiency, with consequent potassium loss, muscle weakness, tendency to faint due to hypotension. In contrast, the sex hormones are synthesized in the ovaries and testicular interstitial cells. In the synthesis of sex hormones, progesterone is converted to 17α-hydroxyprogesterone and then androstenedione, which may either become estrone or testosterone. Testosterone gives rise to estradiol in the ovaries, while progesterone is produced by the corpus luteum that persists in the ovary after conception.

343. The answer is e. *(Murray, pp 556–579. Scriver, pp 5493–5524.)* The major problem in myasthenia gravis is a marked reduction of acetylcholine receptors on the motor endplate where cranial nerves form a neuromuscular junction with muscles. In these patients, autoantibodies against the acetylcholine receptors effectively reduce receptor numbers. Normally, acetylcholine molecules released by the nerve terminal bind to receptors on the muscle endplate, resulting in a stimulation of contraction by depolarizing the muscle membrane. The condition is improved with drugs that inhibit acetylcholinesterase.

344. The answer is e. *(Murray, pp 434–473. Scriver, pp 4029–4240.)* Group I hormones (most steroid hormones like gluco- and mineralocorticoids, sex steroids) freely enter cells and form receptor complexes that act in the cytosol or nucleus. Group II hormones are water soluble and cannot cross cell membranes. Group II hormones act at the plasma membrane, binding to membrane receptors and activating second messengers. These can involve G protein complexes and cAMP or cGMP through adenyl or guanyl cyclases (e.g., epinephrine, glucagons, nitric oxide), calcium-phosphatidyl inositols (e.g., angiotensin II, vasopressin), or protein kinase cascades as with fibroblast growth factor (FGFs), epidermal growth factor (EGF), insulin-like growth factors (IGFs), platelet-derived growth factors (PDGFs), as well as growth hormone and insulin. Growth and insulin factors are thus easily matched with group II kinase messenger mechanisms with the exception that platelet derived growth factors may also use calcium/phosphatidyl inositol second messengers.

345. The answer is e. *(Murray, pp 456–473. Scriver, pp 1471–1488.)* The action of insulin is antagonistic to that of glucagon, which is a catabolic hormone secreted by the α-cells of the pancreas. The anabolic hormone called insulin is synthesized on the endoplasmic reticulum of pancreatic β-cells as a nascent polypeptide chain called preproinsulin. Immediately following synthesis, the amino terminal signal sequence of 16 residues is cleaved off to form proinsulin. Proinsulin is composed of one continuous polypeptide that contains in sequence an A chain of 21 residues, a connecting peptide (C peptide) of about 30 residues, and a B chain of 30 residues. The molecule is folded so that two disulfide bridges span the A and B chains. The proinsulin molecule is transported from the lumen of the endoplasmic reticulum to the Golgi apparatus, where it is packaged into storage granules. In the Golgi apparatus and in the storage granules, proteolysis of the C peptide occurs. Exocytosis of the granules releases insulin as well as C peptides into the bloodstream. Neither proinsulin nor the C peptide is biologically active.

346. The answer is c. *(Murray, pp 456–473. Scriver, pp 1471–1488.)* Gluconeogenesis is a catabolic process for the synthesis of glucose, mainly from the amino acids of degraded proteins. Gluconeogenesis is the adaptive response of the organism to low blood levels of glucose and is, therefore, diminished by insulin. Insulin regulates the disposition and utilization of glucose, particularly exogenous glucose. Glucose can enter liver and pancreatic β-cells freely, and high blood glucose signals the latter cells to secrete insulin. The group II hormone acts through various protein kinase cascades to stimulate entry of glucose and amino acids into certain extrahepatic tissues that include muscle and fat cells. The presence of glucose stimulates synthesis of glucose oxidation, lipogenesis, and macromolecular precursors such as nucleotides. Chronic insulin therapy as with type I (juvenile onset, insulin-dependent) diabetes may stimulate extrahepatic glucose entry under conditions of inhibited gluconeogenesis, potentiating hypoglycemia while suppressing its correction.

347. The answer is a. *(Murray, pp 434–473. Scriver, pp 4029–4240.)* The β-adrenergic catecholamines like epinephrine are type II hormones that act at cell membranes, stimulating second messengers including cAMP and protein kinases. These hormones are secreted by the adrenal medulla in keeping with its neural crest derivation and response to neural stimulation (e.g., anxiety, fight or flight response). The actions of epinephrine (adrenaline) and norepinephrine are catabolic; that is, these catecholamines are antagonistic to the anabolic functions of insulin and, like glucagon, are secreted in response to low blood glucose or during "fight or flight" stress. Glycolysis is an anabolic process that is decreased in the presence of elevated catecholamines. Unlike glucagon, which only acts on the liver, the catecholamines affect most tissues, including liver and muscle. The catabolic processes increased by secretion of epinephrine and norepinephrine include glycogenolysis, gluconeogenesis, lipolysis, and ketogenesis. Thus, products that increase blood sugar or spare it, such as ketone bodies and fatty acids, are increased. Prolonged synthesis of adrenergic hormones causes a "hypermetabolic" or catabolic state, inhibiting anabolism and favoring energy expenditure/depletion (fatigue) and weight loss rather than inactivity and weight gain.

348. The answer is c. *(Murray, pp 190–196. Scriver, pp 4029–4240.)* Although prostaglandins were originally isolated from prostate glands, seminal vesicles, and semen, their synthesis in other organs has been amply documented; indeed, few organs have failed to demonstrate prostaglandin release. Prostaglandins cause platelet aggregation, smooth-muscle contraction, vasodilation, and uterine contraction. Prostaglandins are synthesized from arachidonic acid, a 20-carbon fatty acid with interspersed carbon double bonds. Signals such as angiotensin II, bradykinin, epinephrine, and thrombin can activate phospholipase A_2 and release arachidonic acid from membrane lipids. The arachidonic acid is cyclized by cyclooxygenase to form prostaglandins. Arachidonic acid can also be oxidized to leukotrienes by the action of lipoxygenases.

349. The answer is c. *(Murray, pp 434–473. Scriver, pp 4029–4240.)* Glucocortidoids (e.g., cortisol) and mineralocorticoids (e.g., aldosterone) are secreted by zona glomerulosa cells at the outer layer of the adrenal cortex. Sex steroids like testosterone are secreted in part by the adrenal cortex but also by the gonads. Adrenergic hormones like norepinephrine are secreted by the adrenal medulla as would be expected by their synergy with neural tissues. ACTH-releasing hormone (adrenocorticotropin) is one of several pituitary hormones that regulate secondary hormone release from target endocrine organs or tissues (e.g., thyroid stimulating hormone, growth hormone). Lower adrenal hormone action in Addison's disease would be associated with higher rather than deficient ACTH secretion. Addison's disease has many causes and, like other autoimmune disorders—diabetes mellitus, Hashimoto thyroiditis—shows familial aggregation typical of multifactorial determination. As with these diseases, rare cases show simple Mendelian inheritance, as with a type of Addison disease (240200) that is probably due to a defect in cortisol synthesis.

350. The answer is e. (*Murray, pp 153–162. Scriver, pp 4263–4274.*) The plasma membranes of intestinal epithelial cells contain a sodium gradient that drives the active transport of glucose. The rate and amount of glucose transported depend on the sodium gradient maintained across the plasma membrane. Sodium ions entering the cell in the company of glucose are pumped out again by Na^+,K^+-ATPase. Once in the cytosol of the intestinal cell, the glucose moves across the cell and diffuses out of the cell into the interstitial fluid of the submucosa and then into the plasma of the capillaries underlying the intestinal epithelium. This occurs for the following reason: while glucose is maintained in blood plasma at an approximately constant level, it is always slowly moving out of the plasma into the cells of tissue that use it. Given that the diffusion from the intestinal cells into the plasma is passive, the intestinal cells and the plasma try to maintain an equilibrium. Thus, plasma glucose levels are always approximately equal to or slightly less than levels in the intestinal cells. Because of the passive maintenance of this equilibrium, it is highly unlikely that the concentration of glucose in the plasma can get much higher than that in the intestinal cell cytosol. It is also unlikely that the levels of glucose in other tissues of the body (for example, muscle) will have any bearing on those found in the intestinal cells.

351. The answer is e. (*Murray, pp 434–473. Scriver, pp 4029–4240.*) Secretin, a circulatory hormone liberated in response to peptides or acid in the duodenum, stimulates the flow of pancreatic juice. Gastrin governs acid production by the stomach, and cholecystokinin causes the gallbladder to contract. Cholecystokinin stimulates this contraction after it is released by the duodenum into the circulation, with subsequent emptying of bile into the intestine. The C-terminal octapeptide of cholecystokinin is more than five times as potent as the parent hormone, and its C-terminal pentapeptide is identical to gastrin. Gastrin, produced in specialized cells of the antral mucosa of the stomach, stimulates parietal cells to produce HCl (approximately 0.16 M) and KCl (0.007 M); it also stimulates secretion of glucagon and insulin. Production of gastrin is inhibited by secretin.

352. The answer is a. (*Murray, pp 190–196, 434–473. Scriver, pp 4029–4240.*) The evidence indicates that anti-inflammatory steroids inhibit phospholipase A_2, which is responsible for hydrolyzing arachidonate off of membrane phospholipids. Corticosteroids and their manufactured derivatives are thought to cause induction of the phospholipase A_2–inhibitory protein lipocortin. In this manner, production of all of the derivatives of arachidonic acid (lipoxins, leukotrienes, thromboxanes, and prostaglandins) is shut off. In contrast, nonsteroidal anti-inflammatory agents such as aspirin, indomethacin, and ibuprofen act by inhibiting the cyclooxygenase component of prostaglandin synthase. The synthase is responsible for the first step in the production of prostaglandins (step E) and thromboxanes (step D) from arachidonic acid. The lipoxygenase pathway leads to the synthesis of lipoxins (step B) and leukotrienes (step C).

353. The answer is e. *(Murray, pp 219–230. Scriver, pp 2981–2960.)* Bile acids often are conjugated with glycine to form glycocholic acid and with taurine to form taurocholic acid. In human bile, glycocholic acid is by far the more common. The presence of the charged carboxyl group of glycine or the charged sulfate of taurine adds to the hydrophilic nature of the bile acids, thereby increasing their ability to emulsify lipids during the digestive process. Glucuronic acid is used to conjugate bilirubin and many xenobiotics (foreign chemicals), such as polychlorinated biphenyls (PCBs) and insecticides. A hydroxyl group is added to the xenobiotic by the cytochrome P450 system and then conjugated with glucuronide, sulfate, acetate, or glutathione to make it water-soluble for excretion in urine. A group of rare inborn errors affect the enzymes of bile acid synthesis, resulting in accumulation of toxic acids in liver. Patients with these disorders may have lethal accumulation of abnormal bile acids and conjugated bilirubin in liver due to cholestasis (abnormal concentration of bile acids in gall bladder), illustrated by infants with defective cholic acid synthesis (214950) that live 4–6 months on average.

354. The answer is d. *(Murray, pp 180–189.)* Under fed conditions, glucose is the preferred fuel for most tissues. However, under starvation conditions, glucose must be reserved for use by the central nervous system. There is a small initial decrease in plasma glucose upon starvation but the concentration levels off after a time because of conversion of glycogen in the liver. Under starvation conditions, ketone bodies are made in the liver and provide a major metabolic fuel source for skeletal and heart muscle and can serve to meet some of the brain's energy needs. Urine ketone measurements by Ketostix were recommended for monitoring of success in limiting carbohydrate intake. Another effect of starvation and carbohydrate limitation is accelerated lipogenesis and elevated serum cholesterol/triglycerides, which was exaggerated by substituting fat (meat, eggs) in one famous low-carbohydrate diet. These effects may have contributed to the sudden collapse and death of the diet's founder, although post-mortem studies were refused by heirs. Low-fat, heart-friendly low carbohydrate diets have since been promoted.

355. The answer is b. *(Murray, pp 434–473. Scriver, pp 5433–5452.)* Treatment of patients with congestive heart failure is often based on the use of cardiotonic steroids such as digitalis. Digitalis is derived from the foxglove plant and has been used as an herbal treatment for heart problems since ancient times. Digitalis and ouabain are cardiotonic steroids that inhibit the Na^+,K^+-ATPase pump located in the plasma membrane of cardiac muscle cells. They specifically inhibit the dephosphorylation reaction of the ATPase when the cardiotonic steroid is bound to the extracellular face of the membrane. Because of inhibition of the pump, higher levels of sodium are left inside the cell, leading to a diminished sodium gradient. This results in a slower exchange of calcium by the sodium-calcium exchanger. Subsequently, intracellular levels of calcium are maintained at a higher level and greatly enhance the force of contraction of cardiac muscle.

356. The answer is d. *(Murray, pp 180–189. Scriver, pp 2297–2326.)* The brain uses glucose as its major energy source but can also use ketone bodies to provide up to 20% of its energy needs. Glucose is the preferred metabolic fuel for most tissues. However, extrahepatic tissues such as heart prefer ketone bodies and fatty acids as energy sources over glucose. Children with medium or short chain fatty acid oxidation defects can breakdown glycogen over the first 1–3 hours of fasting to maintain glucose, but have deficient fat breakdown when glycogen is depleted. They have normal lipases and can mobilize triacylglycerols but cannot metabolize the fatty acid side chains. Some abnormal ketones are produced as expected from sequential breakdown of fatty acyl CoAs in two-carbon steps—dehydrogenase to make β-double bond, enolase to make β-hydroxyl, dehydrogenase to make β-ketone, thiolase to cleave off acetyl CoA and an acyl CoA two carbons shorter. A block like that in medium chain CoA dehydrogenase (MCAD) deficiency (201450) will cause accumulation of 8–12 carbon β-hydroxyl and ketone β-compounds, but these will have much less serum concentrations and metabolic efficiency than the normal

4-carbon acetoacetate, β-hydroxybutyrate, and 2-carbon acetone. Even greater deficiency of ketone bodies with long chain oxidation defects may explain their early and lethal cardiac failure. Lactate but not pyruvate will be deficient in mitochondrial pyruvate dehydrogenase deficiency (e.g., 300502), while propionate and methylmalonate will accumulate in disorders like methylmalonic aciduria (251000).

357. The answer is c. *(Murray, pp 190–196, 598–608. Scriver, pp 4029–4240.)* Eicosanoids consist of C20 unsaturated fatty acids that include prostaglandins, thromboxanes, leukotrienes, and lipoxins. They can be synthesized from essential linoleic and linolenic (C18) fatty acids in the diet or from (C20) arachidonic acid. Arachidonate can also come from diet or from elongation of linolenic acid released from the 2′ position of membrane acyltriglyceride phospholipids by the action of phospholipase A_2. The lipoxygenase pathway that produces leukotrienes/lipoxins competes with the cyclooxygenase (prostaglandin synthetase) pathway for available arachidonate. Aspirin (acetosalicylic acid) inhibits the cyclooxygenase, while nonsteroidal anti-inflammatory drugs (NSAIDS) like ibuprofen and indomethacin compete for arachidonate and influence both pathways. Additional effects of aspirin in toxic doses include uncoupling of oxidative phosphorylation and inhibition of the tricarboxylic acid cycle, creating metabolic acidosis with compensatory increases in respiration. Although aspirin and ibuprofen overdoses can be treated effectively, acetaminophen (Tylenol) causes irreversible liver damage and failure above certain levels and requires liver transplant.

358. The answer is d. *(Murray, pp 190–196. Scriver, pp 4029–4240.)* In mammals, arachidonic (5,8,11,15-eicosatetraenoic) acid can be synthesized from dietary essential fatty acids (linoleic—9,12-octadecadienoic or C18 with 2 double bonds, lenolenic—9,12,15-octadecatrienoic or C18 with 3 double bonds). These fatty acids are essential because the fatty acid synthase system in mammals lacks desaturases to produce the requisite fatty acyl double bonds. Arachidonic acid occurs in vegetable oils and animal fats with linoleic and linolenic acids, and can also be synthesized from linoleic acid following liberation from membrane phospholipids by phospholipase A_2 cleavage at the 2′-carbon of glycerol. Oleic, palmitic, and stearic acids are all nonessential fatty acids that can be manufactured by the fatty acid synthase system but cannot be desaturated or elongated to produce arachidonate.

359. The answer is d. *(Murray, pp 190–196. Scriver, pp 4029–4240.)* Leukotrienes C_4, D_4, and E_4 together compose the slow-reacting substance of anaphylaxis (SRS-A), which is thought to be the cause of asphyxiation in individuals not treated rapidly enough following an anaphylactic shock. SRS-A is up to 1000 times more effective than histamines in causing bronchial muscle constriction. Anti-inflammatory steroids are usually given intravenously to end chronic bronchoconstriction and hypotension following a shock. The steroids block phospholipase A_2 action, preventing the synthesis of leukotrienes from arachidonic acid. Acute treatment involves epinephrine injected subcutaneously initially and then intravenously. Antihistamines such as diphenhydramine are administered intravenously or intramuscularly.

360. The answer is b. *(Murray, pp 173–179. Scriver, pp 2297–2326.)* The essential fatty acid linoleic acid (C-18:2-$\Delta^{9,12}$), with 18 carbons and two double bonds at carbons 9 and 18, is desaturated to form α-linolenic acid (C-18:3-$\Delta^{6,9,12}$), which is sequentially elongated and desaturated to form eicosatrienoic acid (C-20:3-$\Delta^{8,11,14}$) and arachidonic acid (C-20:4-$\Delta^{5,8,11,14}$). Many of the eicosanoids (20-carbon compounds)—prostaglandins, thromboxanes, and leukotrienes—are derived from arachidonic acid. The scientific name of arachidonic acid is eicosatetraenoic acid. Arachidonic acid can only be synthesized from essential fatty acids obtained from the diet. Palmitic acid (C-16:0) and oleic acid (C-18:1-Δ^{9}) can be synthesized by the tissues.

361. The answer is b. *(Murray, pp 434–473. Scriver, pp 4029–4240.)* Steroid hormones such as aldosterone are ultimate derivatives of cholesterol. The compound illustrated in the question is cholesterol, one of a large group of steroids. Cholesterol, which can be derived from the diet as well as synthesized de novo, is the precursor of all steroids involved in mammalian metabolism. These include the bile acids, the steroid hormones, and vitamin D. Cholesterol cannot be metabolized to carbon dioxide and water in humans. It must be excreted as a component of bile. Adrenocorticotropin (ACTH) is a peptide hormone of the adenohypophysis that influences the secretion of corticosteroid hormones. Prostaglandins are eicosanoid derivatives that are also made up of isoprene units. Geranyl phosphate is a 2-isoprenoid unit precursor in cholesterol synthesis.

362. The answer is e. *(Murray, pp 130–135, 242–248. Scriver, pp 1909–1964.)* All the compounds listed are intermediates of the citric acid cycle. However, only fumarate is an intermediate of both the citric acid and urea cycles. It and arginine are produced from argininosuccinate. Once produced by the urea cycle, fumarate enters the citric acid cycle and is converted to malate and then oxidized to oxaloacetate. Depending upon the organism's needs, oxaloacetate can either enter gluconeogenesis or react with acetyl CoA to form citrate.

363. The answer is e. *(Murray, pp 130–135, 242–248. Scriver, pp 1909–1964.)* Aspartate is a glucogenic amino acid that is also used to carry NH_4^+ into the urea cycle. Aspartate aminotransferase catalyzes the direct transamination of aspartate to oxaloacetate:

$$\text{aspartate} + \alpha\text{-ketoglutarate} \rightarrow \text{oxaloacetate} + \text{glutamate}$$

Oxaloacetate may either be utilized in the citric acid cycle or undergo gluconeogenesis. Argininosuccinate synthetase catalyzes the condensation of citrulline and aspartate to form argininosuccinate:

$$\text{citrulline} + \text{asparate} + \text{ATP} \rightarrow \text{argininosuccinate} + \text{AMP} + \text{PP}_i$$

In this manner, one of the two nitrogens of urea is introduced into the urea cycle.

364. The answer is d. *(Murray, pp 130–135. Scriver, pp 1327–1406.)* In general, the corresponding pathways of catabolism and anabolism are not identical (glycolysis versus gluconeogenesis, lipolysis, and β-oxidation of fatty acids versus fatty acid synthesis and lipogenesis, glycogenolysis versus glycogenesis). However, the citric acid cycle is a central pathway from which anabolic precursors of biosynthetic reactions may derive or into which the complete catabolism of small molecules to carbon dioxide and water may occur. For these reasons, the citric acid cycle is often called an amphibolic pathway.

365. The answer is b. *(Murray, pp 242–248. Scriver, pp 1327–1406.)* During the early phases of starvation, the catabolism of proteins is at its highest level. Anabolic enzymes, which are not utilized during starvation, are targeted for degradation (with ubiquitin) and their synthesis repressed. The transamination of amino acids is a first step in amino acid degradation and also yields ketoacids for gluconeogenesis. The protein and amino acid degradation with ketogenesis results in a negative nitrogen balance, increasing ammonia and urea levels in the urine (from the urea cycle). The glucose formed from gluconeogenic amino acids becomes the major source of blood glucose following depletion of liver glycogen stores. Complete oxidation of this glucose, as well as the ketone bodies formed from ketogenic amino acids, leads to a relative increase in the CO_2 and H_2O formed from amino acid carbon skeletons. Many amino acids are degraded and transaminated to yield citric acid cycle intermediates, including arginine, histidine, proline, glutamine to glutamate and then α-ketoglutarate, tyrosine and phenylalanine to fumarate, asparagine to aspartate, and then to oxaloacetate. Many, like cysteine, glycine, serine, and threonine can be converted to alanine and transaminated to pyruvate that directly contributes to gluconeogenesis (through pyruvate carboxylase and phosphoenolpyruvate carboxykinase).

366. The answer is a. *(Murray, pp 122–129. Scriver, pp 1327–1406.)* Although the same intermediates may appear in both anabolic and catabolic pathways, one path is not simply the reverse of the other, because irreversible enzymatic steps often occur in the beginning of the reaction sequence. However, many steps in both anabolic and catabolic pathways are reversible. The same enzymes often appear in many metabolic pathways, but regulatory steps are irreversible. A number of small precursors serve as the building blocks of anabolism, whereas large energy-storage molecules such as glycogen, lipids, and proteins give rise to smaller molecules during catabolic processes.

367. The answer is d. *(Murray, pp 231–236. Scriver, pp 1327–1406.)* Glucose is the major fuel for the brain in the well-fed state. The brain requires a continuous supply of glucose at all times. In fact, if glucose drops to a low level, convulsions may follow. However, during starvation or fasting, the brain is capable of obtaining approximately 75% of its energy from circulating ketone bodies. During the absorptive phase, ketone bodies such as acetoacetate and 3-hydroxybutyrate are low. Circulating amino acids are utilized for protein synthesis. Liver production of NADPH is at a high level because it is needed for fatty acid synthesis. Glucose is actively transported into all cells, including adipocytes, which require it to form glucose-3-phosphate for esterifying fatty acids into triacylglyceride.

368. The answer is b. *(Murray, pp 231–236. Scriver, pp 1471–1488.)* In the absorptive phase following a meal, the major source of glucose is glucose taken directly from the intestine into the blood system. Much of this glucose is absorbed into cells and, in particular, into the liver via the action of insulin, where it is stored as glycogen. Once the effects of daytime eating have subsided and all the glucose from absorption has been stored, the normal overnight fast begins. During this period, the major source of blood glucose is hepatic glycogen. Through the effects of glycogenolysis, which are mediated by glucagon, hepatic glycogen is slowly parceled out as glucose to the bloodstream, keeping blood glucose levels normal. In contrast, muscle glycogenolysis has no effect on blood glucose levels because no glucose-6-phosphatase exists in muscle and hence phosphorylated glucose cannot be released from muscle into the bloodstream. Following a more prolonged fast or in the early stages of starvation, gluconeogenesis is needed to produce glucose from glucogenic amino acids and the glycerol released by lipolysis of triacylglycerides in adipocytes. This is because the liver glycogen is depleted and the liver is forced to turn to gluconeogenesis to produce the amounts of glucose necessary to maintain blood levels.

369. The answer is d. *(Murray, pp 231–236. Scriver, pp 1471–1488.)* High blood levels of amino acids, in addition to glucose, promote the release of insulin through their action on receptors at the surface of the β-cells of the pancreas. Although insulin alone could lead to a hypoglycemic effect, hypoglycemia should not be observed because glucagon is also released in response to the elevated levels of circulating amino acids. The balance of glucagon and glucose tends to keep blood levels of glucose within normal ranges while amino acid transport into cells is promoted. Because of the normal insulin levels in the fed state, ketosis and depletion of liver glycogen are not observed. Both of these events occur during fasting and starvation due to the abundance of glucagon and epinephrine in the blood as opposed to the low levels of insulin.

370. The answer is e. *(Murray, pp 231–236. Scriver, pp 1471–1488.)* Following digestion, the products of digestion enter the bloodstream. These include glucose, amino acids, tri-acylglycerides packaged into chylomicrons from the intestine, and very-low-density lipoproteins from the liver. The hormone of anabolism, insulin, is also elevated because of the signaling of the glucose and amino acids in the blood, which allows release of insulin from the β-cells of the pancreas. Insulin aids the movement of glucose and amino acids into cells. In contrast, all the hormones and energy sources associated with catabolism are decreased in the blood during this time. Long-chain fatty acids and glycerol released by lipolysis from adipocytes are not elevated. Glucagon and epinephrine are not released. The only time glucose levels rise significantly above approximately 80 mM is following a well-balanced meal when glucose is obtained from the diet. The concentration of glucose reaches a peak 30 to 45 min after a meal and returns to normal within 2 hours after eating. This response of blood glucose after eating (mimicked by giving 50 g of oral glucose) is the basis for the glucose tolerance test. In the event of insulin deficiency (diabetes mellitus), the peak glucose concentration is abnormally high and its return to normal is delayed.

371. The answer is a. *(Murray, pp 153–162. Scriver, pp 1327–1406.)* Centrifugation of a cellular homogenate at a force of 100,000 X g will pellet all cellular organelles and membranes. Only soluble cellular molecules found in the cytosol will remain in the supernatant. Thus, the enzymes of glycolysis and most of those of gluconeogenesis, fatty acid synthesis, and the pentose phosphate pathway will be in the supernatant. Glucose-6-phosphate dehydrogenase, which results in the formation of 6-phosphoglucono-δ-lactone from glucose-6-phosphate, is the committed step in the pentose phosphate pathway. In the pellet will be the enzymes within mitochondria, including those of the citric acid cycle (aconitase), fatty acid β-oxidation (acyl CoA hydratase), and ketogenesis (hydroxybutyrate dehydrogenase). Enzymes of glycogen degradation and synthesis (glycogen synthetase) will also be in the pellet associated with glycogen particles.

372. The answer is b. *(Murray, pp 481–497. Scriver, pp 4029–4240.)* Calcium ions and calcium deposits are virtually universal in the structure and function of living things. In humans, calcium ions are required for the activity of many enzymes. Calcium is taken up from the gut in the presence of forms of vitamin D, such as cholecalciferol. Calcium is also primarily excreted through the intestine. When soluble, it is present as a divalent cation. When insoluble, it is found as hydroxyapatite (calcium phosphate) in bone. It is required by muscle cells for contraction and is sequestered into the sarcoplasmic reticulum during relaxation. It is actively transported by a calcium-ATPase across the sarcoplasmic reticulum.

373. The answer is e. *(Murray, pp 231–236. Scriver, pp 1471–1488.)* The enzyme phosphatidate phosphatase converts phosphatidic acid to diacylglycerol during synthesis of triacylglycerides. The function of adipose tissue is the storage of fatty acids as triacylglycerols in times of plenty and the release of fatty acids during times of fasting or starvation. Fatty acids taken in by adipocytes are stored by esterification to glycerol-3-phosphate. Glycerol-3-phosphate is derived almost entirely from the glycolytic intermediate dihydroxyacetone phosphate through the action of glycerol-3-phosphate dehydrogenase. Glycolytic enzymes are active in adipocytes during triglyceride synthesis, but those of glycogen degradation (low levels in adipocytes) and gluconeogenesis (i.e., glucose-6-phosphatase) are not. Glycerol kinase is not present to any great extent in adipocytes, so that glycerol freed during lipolysis is not used to reesterify the fatty acids being released. The enzyme triacylglyceride lipase is turned on by phosphorylation by a cyclic AMP–dependent protein kinase following epinephrine stimulation.

374. The answer is d. *(Murray, pp 153–162. Scriver, pp 1471–1488.)* Although the liver is the major site of the formation of free glucose to maintain blood glucose levels, the kidneys and intestinal epithelium (e.g., duodenum, jejunum, and ileum) may also release glucose. All of these tissues contain the enzyme glucose-6-phosphatase, an endoplasmic reticulum enzyme that dephosphorylates glucose and allows it to be transferred out of the cells. No other tissues in mammals contain this enzyme.

375. The answer is c. *(Murray, pp 231–236. Scriver, pp 1471–1488.)* There are certain properties of metabolism that are considered truisms. (1) Futile cycles involving useless synthesis and degradation of a fuel do not occur simultaneously. (2) Acetyl CoA or substances that produce it, such as fatty acids or ketogenic amino acids, cannot be precursors of glucose. (3) ATP is a major phosphate donor and energy source; it must be present in cells at all times in order for them to function. (4) Protein phosphorylation inactivates enzymes that store glycogen and fat and activates enzymes that increase blood glucose and fatty acids. (5) Low blood glucose stimulates gluconeogenesis and glycogenolysis. (6) Low energy levels stimulate glycolysis and lipolysis. (7) High energy levels inhibit glycolysis and β-oxidation of fatty acids. GTP can be a phosphate donor (e.g., in the phosphoenolpyruvate carboxykinase reaction of gluconeogenesis) but ATP is much more common. The acetylation of pyruvate to citric acid by pyruvate dehydrogenase rather than its reduction by lactate dehydrogenase is a key regulatory step between high energy yields of citric acid cycle/oxidative phosphorylation or lower energy yields of glycolysis.

376. The answer is a. *(Murray, pp 231–236. Scriver, pp 5467–5492.)* A diet high in carbohydrate and fats spares glucose use and inhibits gluconeogenesis, thereby preventing protein catabolism and nitrogen production. A major function of the kidneys is to excrete nitrogen catabolized from proteins in the form of urea. Indeed, the major clinical measures of renal function are products of protein catabolism [blood urea nitrogen (BUN) and blood creatinine]. A diet for a patient with renal failure should therefore minimize protein and nitrogen load. Although 3 L/d of fluid is a normal intake for adults with healthy kidneys, glomerular filtration and water excretion are decreased in renal failure. Water and salt intake (particularly potassium) must therefore be limited in renal failure. Excess water or salt intake in patients with renal disease is manifest clinically by edema (swollen eyelids, swollen lower limbs).

377. The answer is b. *(Murray, pp 474–497. Scriver, pp 1471–1488.)* Decreased insulin synthesis (juvenile onset, insulin-dependent type I diabetes) or increased resistance to insulin action (adult onset, type II diabetes) results in decreased glucose entry into extrahepatic tissues and increased serum glucose levels. Glucose can enter hepatic or pancreatic β-cells directly, regulating insulin release in the latter cells. Decreased glucose entry into extrahepatic tissues forces increased lipid catabolism with associated increases in serum cholesterol. The combination of increased cholesterol and perhaps hyperglycemia leads to the process of blood vessel damage called atherosclerosis. The blood vessel lining (intima) becomes damaged with buildup of plaques, deposit of cholesterol, and increased aggregation of platelets and other blood constitutents. The atheroma then blocks blood flow in the affected vessels, potentially causing coronary artery obstruction (coronary thrombosis) and myocardial infarction, carotid artery obstruction and strokes, or extremity artery obstructions with leg pains (claudication) and tissue hypoxia (nonhealing sores, gangrene).

378. The answer is d. *(Murray, pp 474–480. Scriver, pp 1623–1650.)* Milk intolerance may be due to milk protein allergies during infancy, but it is commonly caused by lactase deficiency in older individuals. Intestinal lactase hydrolyzes the milk sugar lactose into galactose and glucose, both reducing sugars that can be detected as reducing substances in the stool. The symptoms of lactose intolerance (lactase deficiency) and other conditions involving intestinal malabsorption include diarrhea, cramps, and flatulence due to water retention and bacterial action in the gut. In nontropical sprue, symptoms seem to result from the production of antibodies in the blood against fragments of wheat gluten. It seems likely that a defect in intestinal epithelial cells allows tryptic peptides from the digestion of gluten to be absorbed into the blood, as well as to exert a harmful effect on intestinal epithelia. Gallbladder inflammation (cholecystitis) usually presents with acute abdominal pain (colic) with radiation to the right shoulder. The normal composition of bile is about 5% cholesterol, 15% phosphatidylcholine, and 80% bile salt in a micellar liquid form. Increased cholesterol from high-fat diets or genetic conditions can upset the delicate micellar balance, leading to supersaturated cholesterol or cholesterol precipitates that cause gallstone formation. Removal of the gallbladder is a common treatment for this painful condition. Mobilization of fats with the production of ketone bodies occurs during fasting and starvation, but ketone production is well controlled. During uncontrolled diabetes mellitus, ketogenesis proceeds at a rate that exceeds the buffering capacity of the blood to produce ketoacidosis.

379. The answer is b. *(Murray, pp 180–189. Scriver, pp 2297–2326.)* A deficiency in carnitine, carnitine acyltransferase I, carnitine acyltransferase II, or acylcarnitine translocase can lead to an inability to oxidize long-chain fatty acids. This occurs because all of these components are needed to translocate activated long-chain (>10 carbons long) fatty acyl CoA across mitochondrial inner membrane into the matrix where β-oxidation takes place. Once long-chain fatty acids are coupled to the sulfur atom of CoA on the outer mitochondrial membrane, they can be transferred to carnitine by the enzyme carnitine acyltransferase I, which is located on the cytosolic side of the inner mitochondrial membrane. Acyl carnitine is transferred across the inner membrane to the matrix surface by translocase. At this point the acyl group is reattached to a CoA sulfhydryl by the carnitine acyltransferase II located on the matrix face of the inner mitochondrial membrane.

McArdle disease (deficiency of muscle glycogen phosphorylase) is one of several glycogen storage diseases. Muscle cramping and fatigue after exercise are characteristics of muscle glycogen storage diseases (types V and VII), whereas hypoglycemia, hyperuricemia, and liver disease are characteristics of liver glycogen storage diseases (types I, III, IV, VI, and VIII)—see Table 3.

Wood alcohol (methanol) is a cause of death or serious illness (including blindness) among patients who ignorantly substitute it for ethanol or mistakenly ingest it. Ingestion of automotive antifreeze (ethylene glycol) can also result in death if not treated. In both cases, death or serious injury can be averted by quickly administering an intoxicating dose of ethanol. The success of this treatment is based on the fact that methanol and ethylene glycol are not poisons as such. First, they must be converted by the action of the enzyme alcohol dehydrogenase to precursors of potentially toxic substances. Administration of large doses of ethanol inhibits oxidation of both methanol and ethylene glycol by effectively competing as a preferred substrate for the active sites of alcohol dehydrogenase. Over time, methanol and ethylene glycol are excreted.

One of the primary killers of children prior to immunization was upper respiratory tract infections by *Corynebacterium diphtheriae*. Toxin produced by a lysogenic phage that is carried by some strains of this bacteria causes the lethal effects. It is lethal in small amounts because it blocks protein synthesis. The viral toxin is composed of two parts. The B portion binds a cell's surface and injects the A portion into the cytosol of cells. The A portion ADP ribosylates a histidine-derived residue of the elongation factor 2 (EF-2) known as diphthamide. This action completely blocks the ability of EF-2 to translocate the growing polypeptide chain.

380. The answer is e. *(Murray, pp 231–236. Scriver, pp 1471–1488.)* In a normal postabsorptive patient, blood fuel values are 4.5 mM glucose, 0.5 mM free fatty acids, 0.02 mM ketone bodies, and 4.5 mM amino acids (choice a). Levels of ketone bodies are always low in a fed person. Following several days of starvation, a catabolic homeostasis has set in, such that free fatty acids (1.5 mM) have risen and production of ketone bodies (5 mM) by the liver is proceeding (choice c). At this point, glycogen stores have been depleted. Much of the blood glucose, which is maintained at about 4.5 mM throughout starvation, now comes from gluconeogenesis using increased concentrations of amino acids (4.7 mM) derived from protein breakdown.

Most of the brain's fuel supply still derives from glucose at this time. Because the brain accounts for at least 20% of the body's total consumption of fuel, this amount can be considerable. Following prolonged starvation, utilization of glucose and hence catabolism of protein are spared by the induction of increased amounts of brain enzymes to utilize ketone bodies. Thus, in prolonged starvation, the blood concentration of amino acids (3.1 mM) decreases, whereas that of free fatty acids (2 mM) and ketone bodies (8 mM) increases (choice e). Of course, blood glucose is maintained at about 4.5 mM. The lack of insulin in diabetics causes a stimulation of lipolysis, glycogenolysis, gluconeogenesis, and ketogenesis. Thus, the blood values of free fatty acids (2 mM), ketone bodies (10 mM), and amino acids (4.5 mM) should resemble those of a fasting or starving person with one major exception—the high level of blood glucose [12 mM (choice c)]. The lack of insulin does not allow the glucose to enter most cells.

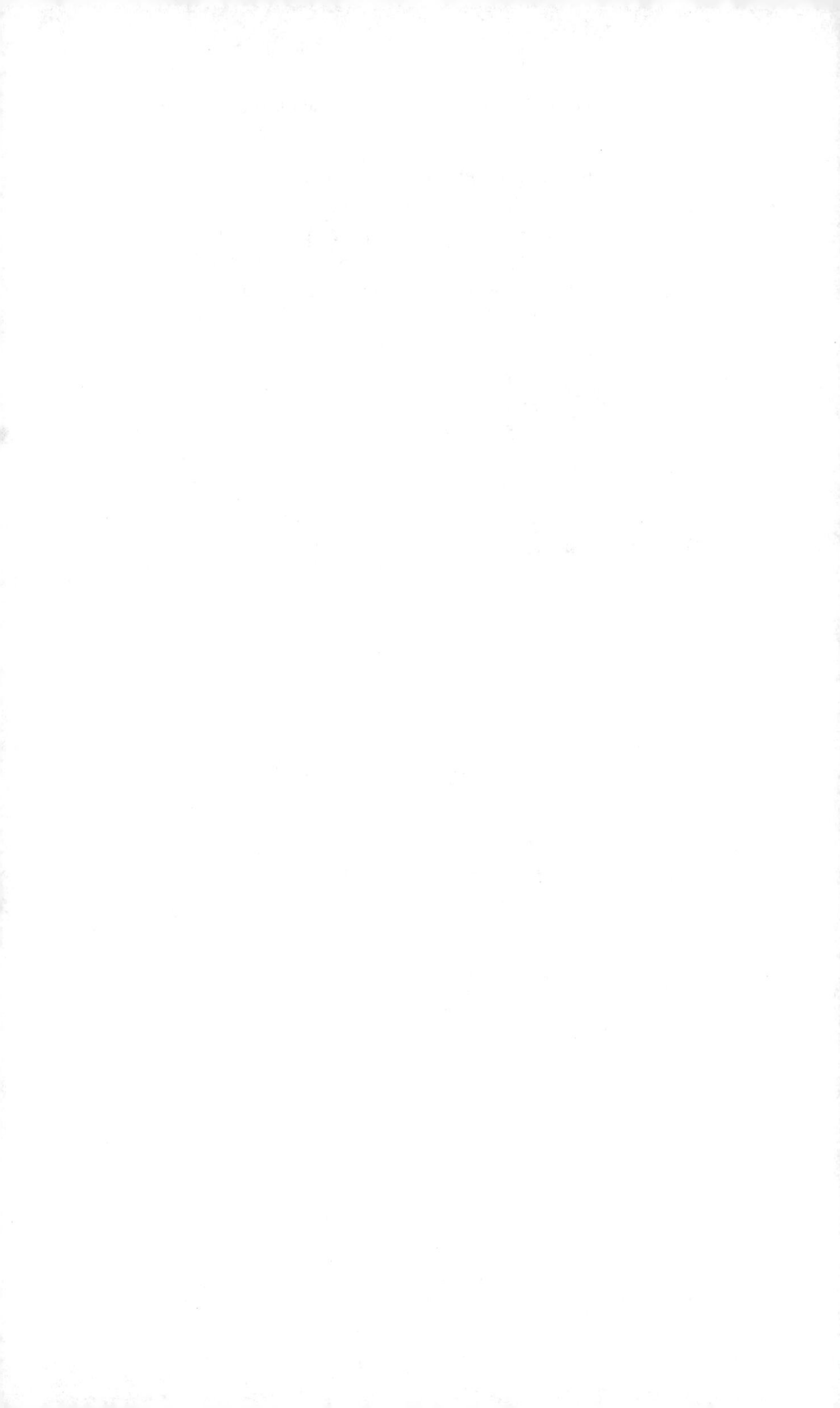

Inheritance Mechanisms and Biochemical Genetics

Inheritance Mechanisms/Risk Calculations

Questions

DIRECTIONS: Each item below contains a question or incomplete statement followed by suggested responses. Select the **one best** response to each question.

381. Amyotrophic lateral sclerosis (ALS, Lou Gehrig disease) usually has onset at older ages but is seen occasionally in young adults. Epidemiologic study indicates slight male predominance and slight excess of cases in the Western Pacific. Most cases are sporadic (i.e., are isolated) but occasional families have more than one individual affected with an autosomal dominant pattern. Which of the following is the best description of this disease?

a. Inherited
b. Genetic
c. Sporadic
d. Congenital
e. Familial

382. Diabetes mellitus is caused by insulin deficiency or resistance with decreased import of glucose into extrahepatic tissues. Juvenile-onset (type I) cases often follow a viral infection with inflammation of the pancreatic β cells. Adult-onset (type II) cases are strongly associated with obesity. Each type exhibits genetic predisposition with a 40–50% concordance rate in monozygous twins and clustering in families. Diabetes mellitus is best described as which of the following types of disorders?

a. Congenital disorder
b. Multifactorial disorder
c. Mendelian disorder
d. Sporadic disorder
e. Sex-limited disorder

383. Which of the following characteristics is most typical of multifactorial inheritance?

a. Sex predilection
b. Mitochondrial inheritance
c. Recurrence risks reflect the number of affected relatives
d. Major cause of miscarriages
e. Maternally derived

384. Assume that D and d alleles derive from a single locus and that the presence of one D allele causes deafness. Match the mating of a genotype Dd father with a genotype dd mother and their probabilities for genotypes in offspring.

a. 1 DD
b. ½ Dd, ½ dd
c. ¼ DD, ½ Dd, ¼ dd
d. ½ DD, ½ Dd
e. 1 dd

385. A couple has three girls, the last of whom is affected with cystic fibrosis. The first-born daughter marries her first cousin—that is, the son of her mother's sister—and they have a son with cystic fibrosis. The father has a female cousin with cystic fibrosis on his mother's side. Which of the following pedigrees represents this family history?

a. Diagram A
b. Diagram B
c. Diagram C
d. Diagram D
e. Diagram E
f. Diagram F
g. Diagram G
h. Diagram H

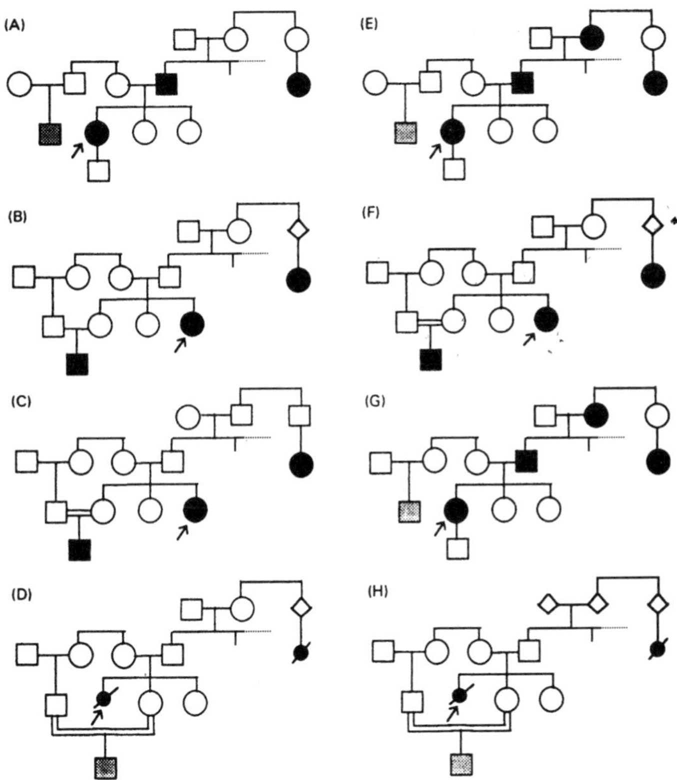

386. Huntington disease (143100) is an autosomal dominant, progressive neurodegenerative disease that causes uncontrolled physical movements and mental deterioration. A husband and wife have three children, two boys and one girl. The husband was diagnosed with Huntington disease in his mid-fifties, as was his father. The wife is normal, as were both her parents. What is the probability that all three of his children will eventually develop Huntington disease?

a. $\frac{1}{8}$
b. $\frac{1}{4}$
c. $\frac{1}{2}$
d. $\frac{3}{4}$
e. All three will develop Huntington disease

387. A couple is referred to the physician because their first three pregnancies have ended in spontaneous abortion. Chromosomal analysis reveals that the wife has two cell lines in her blood, one with a missing X chromosome (45,X) and the other normal (46,XX). Her chromosomal constitution is best described as which of the following?

a. Chimeric
b. Polyploid
c. Trisomic
d. Mosaic
e. Euploid

388. A child with cleft palate, heart defect, extra fifth fingers, scalp defect (absent skin exposing underlying flesh), and unusual face with narrow distance between the eyes is found to have 46 chromosomes with extra material on one homologue of the chromosome 5 pair. This chromosomal abnormality is best described by which of the following terms?

a. Polyploidy
b. Balanced rearrangement
c. Ring formation
d. Mosaicism
e. Unbalanced rearrangement

389. A 10-year-old boy is referred to the physician because of learning problems and some behavior changes. His family history is unremarkable. Physical examination reveals tall stature with few anomalies except for single palmar creases of the hands and curved fifth fingers (clinodactyly). The physician decides to order a karyotype. Which of the following indications for obtaining a karyotype best explains the physician's decision in this case?

a. A couple with multiple miscarriages or a person who is at risk for an inherited chromosome rearrangement
b. A child with ambiguous genitalia who needs genetic sex assignment
c. A child with an appearance suggestive of Down syndrome or other chromosomal disorder
d. A child with mental retardation and/or multiple congenital anomalies
e. A child who is at risk for cancer

390. A girl with early developmental and speech delay is able to progress to third grade but is failing fourth grade. Evaluation shows an elongated body habitus like her mother with somewhat lax joints. Genetic evaluation is suggested, and a chromosomal analysis reveals a 47,XXX karyotype with normal fragile X DNA studies. Which of the following descriptions best fits this abnormality?

a. A female with mosaicism
b. A female with polyploidy
c. Sex chromosome aneuploidy
d. A female with Turner syndrome
e. A female with X monosomy

391. The error in meiosis that produces a 47,XYY karyotype is best described by which of the following?

a. Meiosis division I of paternal spermatogenesis
b. Meiosis division I of maternal oogenesis
c. Meiosis division II of paternal spermatogenesis
d. Meiosis division II of maternal oogenesis
e. Meiosis division II in either parent

392. A physician evaluates a 16-year-old boy with a slightly unusual facial appearance and poor school performance. A peripheral blood chromosome study reveals a karyotype of 46,XY/47,XY,+8 mosaicism, with 10% of 100 examined cells showing the extra chromosome 8. Which of the following options is most appropriate for the physician during the counseling session that follows the chromosome result?

a. Recommend karyotyping of the parents
b. Explain that the recurrence risk for such chromosomal aberrations is about 1%
c. Urge that the school receive a copy of the karyotype since these boys often have behavior problems
d. Recommend special education
e. Inform the parents that their child will be sterile

393. A 4-year-old female presents with short stature, web neck, and other features suggestive of Turner syndrome, but also has mild mental disability. Her chromosome studies reveal 90,XX/92,XXXX with about 10% abnormal cells in blood and 20% in skin. These results can be described as which of the following?

a. Aneuploidy
b. Haploidy
c. Triploidy mosaicism
d. Tetraploidy without mosaicism
e. Trisomy with mosaicism

394. Which of the following is the proper cytogenetic notation for a female with Down syndrome mosaicism?

a. 46,XX,+21/46,XY
b. 47,XY,+21
c. 47,XXX/46,XX
d. 47,XX,+21/46,XX
e. 47,XX,+21(46,XX)

395. A female with Turner syndrome is denoted by which of the following cytogenetic notations?

a. 47,XX,+21
b. 45,X
c. 47,XXX
d. 46,XX,t(14;21)
e. 45,XX,–21

Questions 396–397. Refer to the figure below for the next two questions.

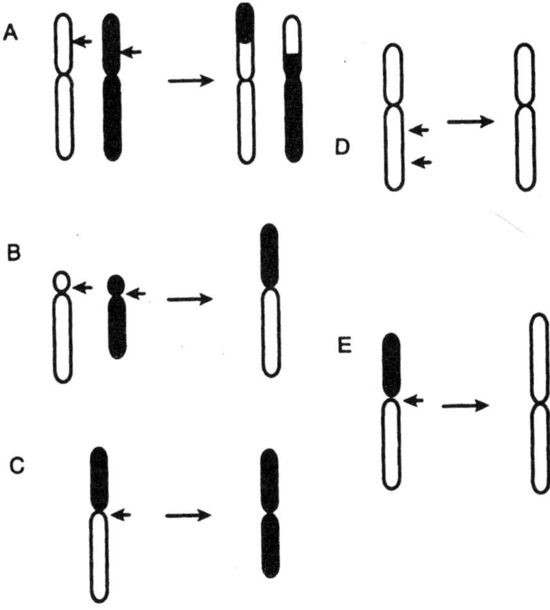

396. Which of the diagrams above depicts a reciprocal translocation?

a. Diagram A
b. Diagram B
c. Diagram C
d. Diagram D
e. Diagram E

397. A child with manifestations of Turner syndrome is found to have a karyotype described as 46,XX,i(Xq). This best fits with which of the lettered diagrams above?

a. Diagram A
b. Diagram B
c. Diagram C
d. Diagram D
e. Diagram E

Questions 398–400. Refer to the figure below to answer the next three questions.

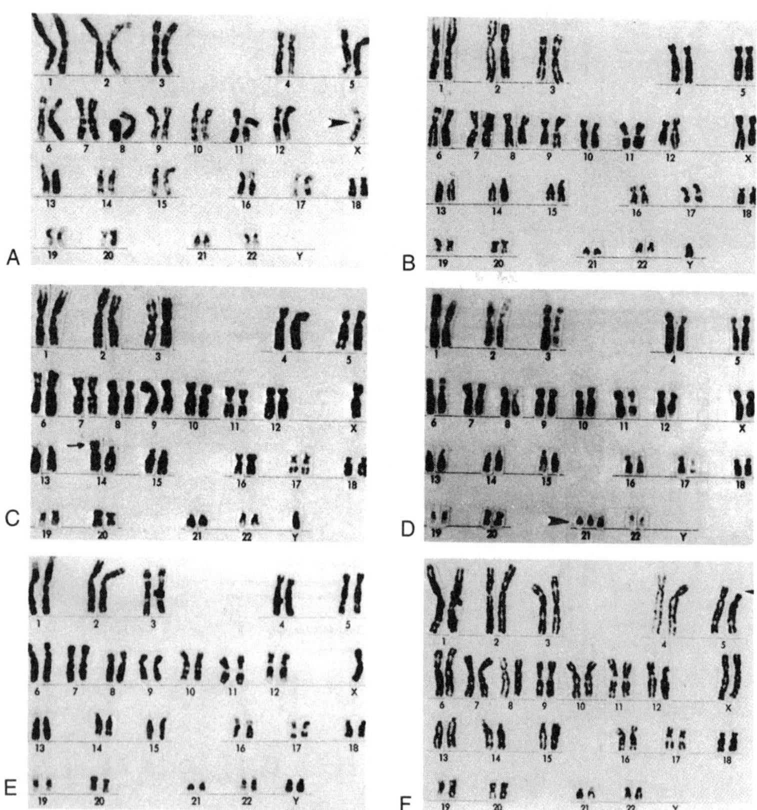

398. A newborn girl was noted to have swelling of the dorsal areas of her feet in the nursery, but this resolved and she did well during childhood. She later was noted to have delayed menstruation, broad neck and chest, mild short stature, and decreased peripheral pulses that suggested the possibility of coarctation of the aorta. Ovaries could not be seen on pelvic ultrasound, and the uterus was thin. Her physician suspected a chromosomal disorder and ordered a karyotype. Which of the results pictured above is most likely?

a. Result A
b. Result B
c. Result C
d. Result D
e. Result F

399. A newborn boy feeds poorly, turning blue and choking after breast-feeding. He is also very floppy (hypotonic), has a loud heart murmur, and has some unusual physical findings. These include a flat occiput (brachycephaly), folds over the inner corners of the eyes (epicanthal folds), single creases on the palms (single palmar creases), and a broad space between the first and second toes. Significant in the family history is that one of the parents' three prior children had Down syndrome. After obtaining a chromosome analysis, which of the results pictured above is most likely?

a. Result A
b. Result B
c. Result C
d. Result D
e. Result F

400. A 2-week-old baby is hospitalized for inadequate feeding and poor growth. The parents are concerned by the child's weak cry. An experienced grandmother accompanies them, saying she thought the cry sounded like a cat's meow. The grandmother also states that the baby doesn't look much like either parent. The physician orders a karyotype after noting a small head size (microcephaly) and subtle abnormalities of the face. Which of the results pictured above is most likely?

a. Result A
b. Result B
c. Result C
d. Result D
e. Result E

401. Children with type IV glycogen storage disease (232500) accumulate abnormal glycogen, causing them to have progressive liver damage in addition to the low blood glucose (hypoglycemia), increased triglycerides and cholesterol (hyperlipidemia), and high uric acid (hyperuricemic) due to deficient glycogenolysis (see High-Yield Facts Table 4). Type IV glycogen storage is autosomal recessive. Autosomal recessive conditions are correctly characterized by which of the following statements?

a. They are often associated with deficient enzyme activity
b. Both alleles contain the same mutation
c. They are more variable than autosomal dominant conditions
d. Most persons do not carry any abnormal recessive genes
e. Affected individuals are likely to have affected offspring

402. Gardner syndrome or adenomatous polyposis of the colon (175100) is an autosomal dominant condition characterized by retinal changes, extra teeth, skin cysts, and multiple colonic polyps with high rates of malignant transformation. A family is encountered in which a great-grandfather, grandmother, and father are affected with Gardner syndrome and develop intestinal cancer in their thirties. The father brags that none of his four children have inherited Gardner syndrome because they lack skin cysts and have not had cancer. The chance that at least one child has inherited the Gardner syndrome allele and the reason the children have not manifested cancer are which of the following?

a. $\frac{1}{4}$, ascertainment bias
b. $\frac{1}{2}$, variable cancer predisposition
c. $\frac{3}{4}$, early-onset disease manifestation
d. $\frac{13}{16}$, incomplete medical evaluation
e. $\frac{15}{16}$, later-onset disease manifestation

403. Ectrodactyly causes missing middle fingers (lobster claw malformation) and exhibits genetic heterogeneity with autosomal dominant and recessive forms. One type of ectrodactyly (split hand-foot malformation) is an autosomal dominant trait (183600). A grandfather and grandson have this form of ectrodactyly, but the intervening father has normal hands by x-ray. Which of the following terms applies to this family?

a. Incomplete penetrance
b. New mutation
c. Variable expressivity
d. Germinal mosaicism
e. Anticipation

404. A 4-year-old boy presents to the physician's office with coarse facies, short stature, stiffening of the joints, and mental retardation. His parents, a 10-year-old sister, and an 8-year-old brother all appear unaffected. The patient's mother is pregnant. She had a brother who died at 15 years of age with similar findings that seemed to worsen with age. She also has a nephew (her sister's son) who exhibits similar features. Based on the probable mode of inheritance, which of the following is the risk that her fetus is affected?

a. 100%
b. 67%
c. 50%
d. 25%
e. Virtually 0

405. A couple comes to the physician's office after having had two sons affected with a similar disease. The first-born son is tall and thin and has dislocated lenses and an IQ of 70. He has also experienced several episodes of deep vein thromboses. The chart mentions deficiency of the enzyme cystathionine-β-synthase, but a diagnosis is not given. The second son was treated from an early age with pyridoxine (vitamin B_6) and is less severely affected. No other family members are affected. While taking a family history, the physician discovers that the parents are first cousins. The 38-year-old mother is pregnant, and amniocentesis has demonstrated that the fetus has a 46,XY karyotype. What is the risk that the fetus will be affected with the same disease?

a. 100%
b. 67%
c. 50%
d. 25%
e. Virtually 0

406. Mr Smith is affected with Crouzon syndrome (123500) and has craniosynostosis (i.e., premature closure of the skull sutures) along with unusual facies that includes proptosis secondary to shallow orbits, hypoplasia of the maxilla, and a prominent nose. His son and brother are also affected, although two daughters and his wife are not. Mr and Mrs Smith are considering having another child. Their physician counsels them that the risk that the child will be affected with Crouzon syndrome is which of the following?

a. 100%
b. 67%
c. 50%
d. 25%
e. Virtually 0

407. A patient presents to the physician's office to ask questions about color blindness. The patient is color-blind, as is one of his brothers. His maternal grandfather was color-blind, but his mother, father, daughter, and another brother are not. His daughter is now pregnant. What is the risk that her child will be color-blind?

a. 100%
b. 50%
c. 25%
d. 12.5%
e. Virtually 0

408. Little People of America (LPA) is a support group for individuals with short stature that conducts many workshops and social activities. Two individuals with achondroplasia (100800), a common form of dwarfism, meet at an LPA convention and decide to marry and have children. What is their risk of having a child with dwarfism?

a. 100%
b. 75%
c. 50%
d. 25%
e. Virtually 0

409. A woman with cystic fibrosis (219700) marries her first cousin. What is the risk that their first child will have cystic fibrosis?

a. ½
b. ¼
c. ⅛
d. 1/16
e. 1/32

410. A woman with no family history of color blindness (304000) marries a color-blind man. What are the risks for this couple of having a son or daughter who is color-blind?

a. 100%
b. 75%
c. 50%
d. 25%
e. Virtually 0

411. A family presents with an unusual type of foot-drop and lower leg atrophy that is unfamiliar to their physician. The pedigree below is obtained. Based on the pedigree, what is the risk of individual III-3 having an affected child?

a. 100%
b. 75%
c. 50%
d. 25%
e. Virtually 0

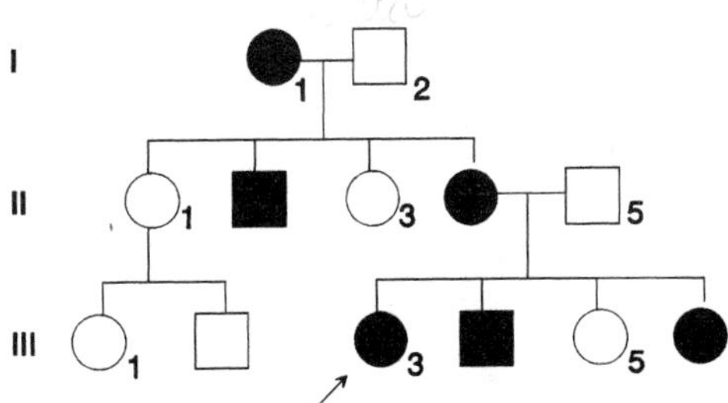

412. A child is evaluated by an ophthalmologist and is found to have retinitis pigmentosa, a disorder characterized by pigmentary granules in the retina and progressive vision loss. The pedigree below is obtained and the family comes in for counseling. What is the risk for individual II-2 of having an affected child if he mates with an unrelated woman?

a. 100%
b. 75%
c. 50%
d. 25%
e. Virtually 0

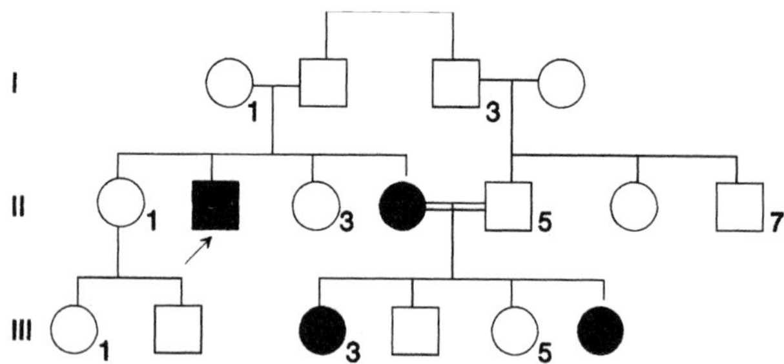

413. A different family with retinitis pigmentosa is encountered, and the pedigree shown below is documented. What is the risk that a son born to individual III-3 would be affected?

a. 100%
b. 75%
c. 50%
d. 25%
e. Virtually 0

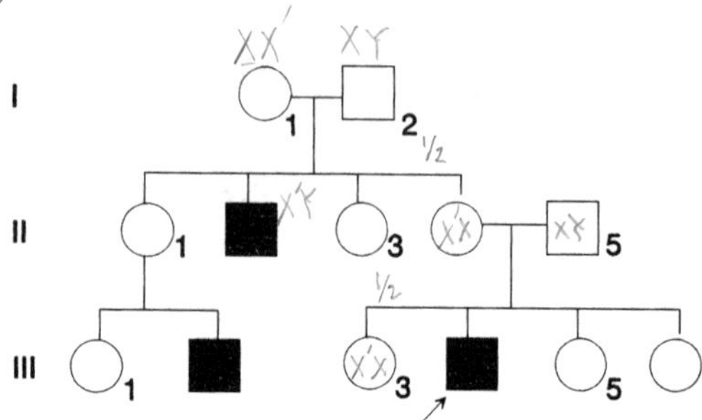

414. Osteogenesis imperfecta (166200) is an autosomal dominant disorder that causes thin, bluish sclerae (whites of the eyes), deafness, and multiple bone fractures. Parents have two children with osteogenesis imperfecta, but themselves exhibit no signs of the disease. Which of the following genetic mechanisms is the most likely explanation for two offspring of normal parents to have an autosomal dominant disease?

a. Variable expressivity
b. Uniparental disomy
c. New mutations
d. Germinal mosaicism in one parent
e. Incomplete penetrance

415. Females occasionally have symptoms of X-linked recessive diseases such as Duchenne muscular dystrophy, hemophilia, or color blindness. Which of the following is the most common explanation?

a. Nonrandom lyonization
b. X chromosome trisomy (47,XXX)
c. X autosome–balanced translocation that disrupts the particular X chromosome locus
d. Turner syndrome (45,X)
e. 46,XY karyotype in a female

416. Incontinentia pigmenti (308300) is an X-linked disorder that is lethal in utero for affected males. The findings vary in females and include pigmented skin lesions, dental abnormalities, patchy areas of alopecia, and mental retardation. Approximately 45% of cases are the result of new mutations. Which of the following descriptions of incontinentia pigmenti is most accurate?

a. X-linked recessive inheritance with spontaneous abortions and few isolated cases
b. X-linked dominant inheritance; 3:1 ratio of females to males in affected sibships
c. X-linked recessive inheritance with spontaneous abortions and many isolated cases
d. X-linked dominant inheritance, 1.5:1 ratio of females to males in affected sibships
e. X-linked dominant inheritance with spontaneous abortions and many isolated cases

417. A couple present for genetic counseling because three of their first four children have had pyloric stenosis, a narrowing of the valve between stomach and duodenum that presents with severe vomiting and loss of gastric hydrochloric acid (hypochloremic alkalosis). When parents with three affected children have a higher recurrence risk than parents with one affected child, the disease in question is likely to exhibit which of the following modes of inheritance?

a. Autosomal dominant inheritance
b. Autosomal recessive inheritance
c. X-linked recessive inheritance
d. X-linked dominant inheritance
e. Multifactorial determination

418. Two parents are both affected with albinism (203100, 203200), but have a normal child. Which of the following terms best applies to this situation?

a. Allelic heterogeneity
b. Locus heterogeneity
c. Variable expressivity
d. Incomplete penetrance
e. New mutation

419. Waardenburg syndrome (193500) is an autosomal dominant condition that accounts for 1.4% of cases of congenital deafness. In addition to deafness, patients with this condition have an atypical facial appearance, including lateral displacement of the inner canthi (eye corners), hypertelorism (widely spaced eyes), poliosis (white forelock), and white patches of skin on the ventral midline (partial albinism or piebaldism). A mother has Waardenburg syndrome, her husband is unaffected, and they plan to have a family with three children. What is the probability that one of the three children will be affected?

a. $\frac{1}{8}$
b. $\frac{1}{4}$
c. $\frac{3}{4}$
d. $\frac{1}{3}$
e. $\frac{1}{2}$

420. The major blood group locus in humans produces types A (genotypes AA or AO), B (genotypes BB or BO), AB (genotype AB), or O (genotype OO). For parents who are type AB and type O, what are the possible blood types of their offspring?

a. Type AB child
b. Type B child
c. Type O child
d. Type A or B child
e. Type B or AB child

421. Phenylketonuria (PKU—261600) is an autosomal recessive disease that causes severe mental retardation if it is undetected. Two normal parents are told by their state neonatal screening program that their third child has PKU. Assuming that the initial screening is accurate, what is the risk that their first child is a carrier for PKU?

a. 100%
b. 67%
c. 50%
d. 25%
e. Virtually 0

422. A couple presents for genetic counseling after their first child is born with achondroplasia (100800), a dwarfing syndrome. The physician obtains the following family history: the husband (George) is the first-born of four male children, and George's next oldest brother has cystic fibrosis (219700). The wife is an only child, but she had DNA screening because a second cousin had cystic fibrosis and she knows that she is a carrier. There are no other medical problems in the couple or their families. The physician should now draw the pedigree with the female member of any couple on the left. The generations are numbered with Roman numerals and individuals with Arabic numerals; individuals affected with achondroplasia or cystic fibrosis are indicated. Which of the following risk figures applies to the next child born to George and his wife?

a. Achondroplasia ½, cystic fibrosis ¼
b. Achondroplasia ½, cystic fibrosis ⅛
c. Achondroplasia virtually 0, cystic fibrosis ¼
d. Achondroplasia virtually 0, cystic fibrosis ⅙
e. Achondroplasia virtually 0, cystic fibrosis ⅛

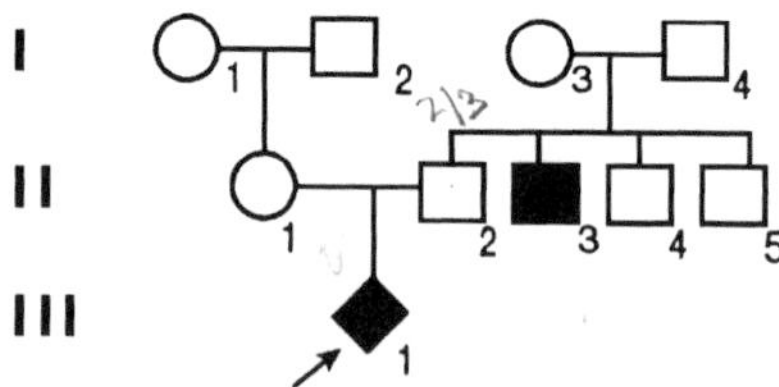

423. Tay-Sachs disease (272800) is a neurolipidosis that causes cherry red spots in the eye, "startle" responses in infancy, neurodegeneration, and death. The disorder is autosomal recessive, caused by deficiency of the lysosomal enzyme hexaminidase A with resultant accumulation of complex glycolipids in brain. What is the risk that the grandmother of an affected child is a carrier (heterozygote) for Tay-Sachs disease?

a. 100%
b. 67%
c. 50%
d. 25%
e. Virtually 0

424. Isolated cleft lip and palate is a multifactorial trait. The recurrence risk of isolated cleft lip and palate is which of the following?

a. The same in all families
b. Not dependent on the number of affected family members
c. The same in all ethnic groups
d. The same in males and females
e. Affected by the severity of the cleft

425. Individuals with achondroplastic dwarfism have about 80% fewer viable offspring than do normal persons, but the incidence of achondroplasia seems to have remained constant for generations. These observations imply which of the following?

a. Decreased fitness, negative selection, and relatively high mutation rates
b. Increased fitness, negative selection, and relatively high mutation rates
c. Decreased fitness, positive selection, and relatively low mutation rates
d. Increased fitness, positive selection, and relatively low mutation rates
e. Decreased fitness, positive selection, and relatively high mutation rates

426. A family is seen for routine prenatal counseling because the mother of two normal children is age 35, the arbitrary "advanced maternal age" when the approximate 1 in 100 risk for fetal chromosome disorders is deemed significant. Family history reveals that the mother's parents and her husband all have had onset of high blood pressure (hypertension) at early ages, and two of mother's grandparents died of strokes that may be hypertension-related. The mother also had some hypertension in the third trimester of her last pregnancy. Recognizing that hypertension is a multifactorial trait, which of the following is the most appropriate explanation and counseling for the couple?

a. Multifactorial determination indicates an interaction between the environment and a single gene, implying a 50% risk for eventual hypertension in mother and offspring
b. Multifactorial determination indicates an interaction between the environment and multiple genes, implying a 5–10% risk for eventual hypertension in mother and offspring
c. Multifactorial determination results from multiple postnatal environmental factors, implying a 75–100% risk for eventual hypertension in mother and a 5–10% risk to offspring
d. Multifactorial determination results from multiple pre- and postnatal environmental factors, implying a 75–100% risk for eventual hypertension in mother and a 5–10% risk to offspring
e. Multifactorial determination implies action of multiple genes independent of environmental factors, implying low risks for hypertension in mother's next pregnancy but a 5–10% risk for eventual hypertension in offspring

427. Availability of DNA testing for many single disease traits has allowed routine prenatal screening of couples for disorders prevalent in their ethnic group. Which of the following genetic disorders has a similar incidence in different ethnic groups and would not be subject to different criteria for screening?

a. Cystic fibrosis
b. Thalassemias
c. Tay-Sachs disease
d. Down syndrome
e. Sickle cell anemia

428. The incidence of a genetic form of diabetes insipidus (304800) in North Americans was hypothesized to be related to immigration of affected individuals on the ship Hopewell that arrived in Halifax Nova Scotia several hundred years ago. If the disease allele were known as A, and residents near Halifax had 10 times the frequency of this allele as did those on mainland Canada, which of the following terms best describes this phenomenon?

a. Selection for allele A
b. Linkage disequilibrium with allele A
c. Linkage to allele A
d. Founder effect for allele A
e. Assortative mating for allele A

429. Increased resistance to malaria is seen in persons with hemoglobin AS, where A is the normal allele and S is the allele for sickle hemoglobin. Which of the following terms applies to this situation?

a. Founder effect
b. Heterozygote advantage
c. Genetic lethal
d. Fitness
e. Natural selection

430. Assume that frequencies for the different blood group alleles are as follows: A = 0.3; B = 0.1; O = 0.6. What is the expected percentage of individuals with blood type B?

a. 7%
b. 13%
c. 27%
d. 36%
e. 45%

431. A male infant is being considered for adoption, and his older half-sister is known to have developed hydrocephalus, an accumulation of cerebrospinal fluid in the brain ventricles. Hydrocephalus is a multifactorial disorder, and the prospective parents wish to know the chance the boy will develop hydrocephalus. In order to estimate this risk, the physician must determine what proportion of genes the brother and half-sister will have in common?

a. One
b. One-half
c. One-fourth
d. One-eighth
e. One-sixteenth

432. A man whose brother has cystic fibrosis (219700) wants to know his risk of having an affected child. The prevalence of cystic fibrosis is 1 in 1600 individuals. Which of the following is the risk in this case?

a. $\frac{1}{8}$
b. $\frac{1}{16}$
c. $\frac{1}{60}$
d. $\frac{1}{120}$
e. $\frac{1}{256}$

433. An African American couple with a normal family history wants to know their chance of having a child with sickle cell anemia (603903). The incidence of sickle cell trait is 1 in 8 for African Americans. Which of the following is the risk in this case?

a. $\frac{1}{8}$
b. $\frac{1}{16}$
c. $\frac{1}{60}$
d. $\frac{1}{120}$
e. $\frac{1}{256}$

434. A woman who married her first cousin wants to know the risk of having a child with cystic fibrosis (219700) because her grandmother, who is also her husband's grandmother, died of cystic fibrosis. Which of the following is her risk?

a. $\frac{1}{8}$
b. $\frac{1}{16}$
c. $\frac{1}{60}$
d. $\frac{1}{120}$
e. $\frac{1}{256}$

Inheritance Mechanisms/Risk Calculations

Answers

381. The answer is e. *(Lewis, pp 1–20. Scriver, pp 193–202.)* The only accurate option given would be familial, since amyotrophic lateral sclerosis (ALS) is not always sporadic (isolated cases), not always inherited or genetic, and not present at birth (congenital). The question emphasizes the importance of terms when counseling families, for many assume that an isolated or new case in the family is not genetic—they need counseling about new mutations or new cases of autosomal/X-linked recessive disorders. Many disorders that are new to the family (not familial or inherited in a given pedigree) are in fact genetic, caused by chromosomal aberration or DNA sequence change. Multifactorial disorders often have exceptional familial cases with more severe manifestations and earlier onset: these derive from mutations in single genes of major effect. The superoxide dismutase gene may be mutated in rare cases of autosomal dominant amyotrophic lateral sclerosis (105400).

382. The answer is b. *(Lewis, pp 1–20, 135–134. Scriver, pp 1471–1488.)* Diabetes mellitus is associated with various risk factors, from autoimmune mechanisms with specific HLA haplotype associations to obesity. The multifactorial causation and hereditary tendency reflects multiple genes (polygenic inheritance) and environmental factors, termed multifactorial determination. Many common diseases are caused by a combination of environmental and genetic factors, and are described as multifactorial diseases. Examples include diabetes mellitus, schizophrenia, alcoholism, and many common birth defects such as cleft palate or congenital dislocation of the hip. The proportion of genetically identical monozygous twins who share (are concordant for) a trait such as diabetes mellitus provides a measure of the genetic contribution to etiology (heritability)—often 40–60% twin concordance in multifactorial disorders. Mendelian disorders are completely determined by the genotype of an individual and exhibit 100% concordance in identical twins.

383. The answer is c. *(Lewis, pp 1–20, 135–134. Scriver, pp 193–202.)* Disorders exhibiting multifactorial determination (polygenic inheritance plus environmental factors) frequently show sex predilection, an ill-defined pattern in pedigrees, higher but not 100% identical twin concordance, and empiric recurrence risks that increase as more affected family members are ascertained. Mitochondrial disorders can exhibit autosomal recessive or X-linked inheritance if they are affect nuclear gene products imported into mitochondria; they can exhibit maternal inheritance if they derive from alterations of the mitochondrial DNA (transmitted only from the mother). Over 60% of first trimester abortuses (miscarriages) are due to chromosome aberrations, although some will derive from multifactorial maternal conditions (lupus, toxemia) and some from single gene causes (mostly undefined).

Recurrence risks for multifactorial diseases are empiric, i.e., determined by population studies. An approximate risk of 3% applies to offspring of individuals affected with the majority of multifactorial diseases—a figure that is similar to the 2–3% risk for birth defects in the average pregnancy. This approximate risk can be tailored to the disease (i.e., 5% for a parent with juvenile diabetes) using appropriate tables, and increased if there are other relatives affected besides the parent (i.e., 10% risk to offspring of two parents with juvenile diabetes). It can also be tailored to the degree of relationship, falling off rapidly (as would befit the requirement for cotransmission of multiple causative alleles) with the affected being a twin (40–60% chance of concordance), parent or sibling (first degree relative, 3–5% risk), grandparent/aunt/uncle (second degree relative, 0.5–0.7% risk), or cousin (third-degree relative, close to background 0.1% incidence of many multifactorial diseases).

384. The answer is b. *(Lewis, pp 1–20, 75–94. Scriver, pp 3–45.)* The phenotype refers to individual traits or characteristics and the genotypes to gene combinations that determine them. Genetic loci are positions on chromosomes that contain genes; since all chromosomes are paired in humans except the XY of males, most genes are paired and have structures (now defined as DNA sequences) called alleles. During meiotic segregation, each parental gamete receives one paired gene (one allele) from every genetic locus (except males who receive paired alleles from the small homologous XY short arm regions and single alleles from the nonpaired X or Y. The probability of a parental allele being transmitted to offspring is thus one-half, and the probability of a given genotype appearing in offspring is the joint probability of maternal and paternal allele transmission.

For a paternal Dd versus maternal dd mating, the probability of maternal alleles D or d being transmitted is ½, and the probability of transmission of the paternal allele d is 1. The joint probability for an Dd genotype in offspring is thus one-half for D from mother multiplied by 1 for d from father = ½. A similar calculation would apply to the joint probability for the dd genotype, giving probabilities of one-half for Dd and one-half for dd, expected ratios of 1 Dd:1 dd in offspring, or a recurrence risk for father's deaf phenotype of one-half or 50%. More than 30 genes causing deafness have been characterized in humans, with over 75% exhibiting autosomal recessive inheritance rather than the dominant inheritance implied here.

385. The answer is f. *(Lewis, pp 1–20, 75–94. Scriver, pp 3–45.)* It is important that the pedigree be an accurate reflection of the family history and that information not be recorded unless specifically mentioned. Pedigree B in Fig. 41 omits the double line needed to indicate consanguinity, and pedigree C assumes that the father's affected cousin is the offspring of his uncle rather than being unspecified. Pedigree F correctly illustrates the birth order (third) of the affected female (indicated by arrow) and the consanguinity (double line) represented by the first-cousin marriage. Cystic fibrosis is an autosomal recessive disease that causes progressive lung disease and intestinal malabsorption due to deficiencies of multiple pancreatic enzymes (219700). Autosomal recessive diseases are much more common with consanguinity or inbreeding because the related couple has a greater chance to inherit the same rare allele.

386. The answer is a. *(Scriver, pp 5677–5702. Lewis, pp 216–225, pp 444–445.)* Since Huntington disease is autosomal dominant, both homozygotes and heterozygotes for the Huntington allele will develop the disease. The husband is a heterozygote, as his father had Huntington but his mother did not. The wife is most likely homozygous recessive, as she has not developed the disease. Thus the children each have a 50% chance (one-half) probability of having inherited the dominant Huntington allele from their father and a 100% chance of inheriting a recessive allele from their mother. Thus, the individual probability for each child developing Huntington disease is ½ and the probability that all three children will develop the disease is ½ × ½ × ½ = ⅛.

387. The answer is d. *(Lewis, pp 241–266. Scriver, pp 3–45.)* The case described represents one of the more common chromosomal causes of reproductive failure, Turner syndrome mosaicism. Turner syndrome involves short stature, anomalies including webbed neck (pterygium colli), heart defects such as coarctation of the aorta, short fourth and fifth knuckles (metacarpals),and streak ovary with infertility. Turner syndrome is produced by monosomy for all or a portion of the X chromosome, causing several genes to be present in a single rather than double dose (haploinsufficiency). Mosaicism (i.e., two or more cell lines with different karyotypes in the same individual) is common, including 46,XX/45,X or 46,XX/45,X/46,XY that poses risk for gonadal cancer due to the presence of a Y chromosome. Chimerism is extremely rare and occurs when two cell lines in an individual arise from different zygotes; some cases may reflect fraternal twins who do not separate.Trisomy refers to three copies of a chromosome rather than the normal two (e.g., 47,XXX), and monosomy to a missing chromosome as in the most common cause of Turner syndrome (45,X). Polyploidy refers to entire extra sets of haploid (23) chromosomes as in 69,XXX triploidy or 92,XXYY polyploidy; polyploidy occurs naturally in some tissues like liver. Euploidy refers to a normal chromosome number and composition.

388. The answer is e. *(Lewis, pp 241–266. Scriver, pp 3–45.)* Chromosomal abnormalities may involve changes in number (i.e., polyploidy and aneuploidy) or changes in structure (i.e., rearrangements such as translocations, rings, and inversions). Extra material (i.e., extra chromatin) seen on chromosome 5 implies recombination of chromosome 5 DNA with that of another chromosome to produce a rearranged chromosome. Since this rearranged chromosome 5 takes the place of a normal chromosome 5, there is no change in number of the autosomes (nonsex chromosomes) or sex chromosomes (X and Y chromosomes). The question implies that all cells examined from the patient (usually 11–25 cells) have the same chromosomal constitution, ruling out mosaicism. The patient's clinical findings are similar to those occurring in trisomy 13 or Patau syndrome, suggesting that the extra material on chromosome 5 is derived from the long arm of chromosome 13 (the acrocentric chromosomes 13–15 and 21–22 have small short arms that contain repetitive DNA). With this interpretation, or by comparing banding patterns of the extra and 13 material, the aberration would be more specifically described as duplication 13q—dup(13q)—or as partial trisomy for 13q.

389. The answer is d. *(Lewis, pp 241–266. Scriver, pp 3–45.)* The hallmarks of children with chromosomal anomalies are mental disability (developmental delay in children) with multiple congenital anomalies. The described individual has learning problems that are not yet described as mental disability, and many such children are mistakenly assumed to have poor motivation rather than cognitive problems that could be defined by IQ testing. Parents also may resist the classification as mental disability, particularly when the harsher term retardation is used. The hand changes can be classified as minor anomalies rather than major birth defects that cause cosmetic or surgical problems, but minor anomalies are significant in that several indicate abnormal development and an increased possibility of a birth defect pattern or syndrome. The physician was astute to suspect a chromosomal anomaly with subtle cognitive and physical changes, and this boy would be typical of 47,XYY individuals with tall stature, variable anomalies, and aggressive or antisocial behaviors. Other indications for peripheral blood chromosome studies include couples with three or more pregnancy losses, relatives of individuals with chromosome rearrangements, and children with ambiguous external genitalia. Fetal chromosomes will be considered with triple/quad screen and/or ultrasound abnormalities, while bone marrow/solid tumor chromosomes are now examined in most cancers as a guide to tumor type, chemotherapy, and prognosis.

390. The answer is c. *(Lewis, pp 241–266. Scriver, pp 3–45.)* The 47,XXX karyotype is an example of sex chromosome aneuploidy, which as a trisomy (47,XXX; 47,XXY; 47XYY) produces fewer anomalies and milder mental disability than autosomal trisomies like Down syndrome—e.g., 47,XX,+21 or trisomy 21; Patau syndrome—e.g., 47,XX,+13 or trisomy 13; and Edward syndrome—e.g., 47,XY,+18 or trisomy 18. Triploidy with a 69,XXX karyotype would be an example of a female with polyploidy, presenting as an spontaneous abortus or severely malformed, short-lived infant. Turner syndrome, most commonly 45,X, would be an example of a female with X monosomy and 45,X/46,XX an example of mosaicism—producing in this case a milder form of Turner syndrome that may have no abnormal signs or symptoms except for infertility.

391. The answer is c. *(Lewis, pp 241–266. Scriver, pp 3–45.)* The sex chromosomes with differently named homologues allow easy visualization of chromosome sorting during meiosis. Female meiosis only involves X chromosomes;

thus, Y chromosomal abnormalities must arise during paternal meiosis or occur spontaneously in offspring. During meiosis I, the newly replicated homologous chromosomes line up at the metaphase plate and then migrate to opposite poles of the cell. Nondisjunction at paternal meiosis I produces XY secondary spermatocytes and a 24,XY gamete. Fertilization with a 23,X ovum yields a 47,XXY individual (Klinefelter syndrome). In meiosis II, the replicated chromosomes line up at the equator of the cell and the sister chromatids separate. Thus, only nondisjunction at paternal meiosis II can produce a 24,YY gamete that yields a 47,XYY individual after fertilization.

392. The answer is b. *(Lewis, pp 241–266. Scriver, pp 3–45.)* The recurrence risk for simple extra or missing chromosomes (whole chromosome aneuploidies) is about 1% in addition to the maternal age-related risk. It is not known why the risk for aneuploidy increases slightly after an affected child is born, but parental karyotypes are almost always normal. Parental chromosome studies are thus not indicated in this case, especially with the low degree of mosaicism that might have arisen after conception. The empiric risk of 1% is comparable to that of women over 35 (ironically called advanced maternal age!) for fetal chromosome aberrations, so prenatal diagnosis should be discussed as an option for the parents. The school should not be given a copy of the karyotype unless the parents request it and sign a release of medical records. Some parents prefer to keep diagnoses of genetic disease or attention deficit-hyperactivity disorders confidential so their child will not be labeled as different by school personnel. Trisomy 8 mosaicism can have a very mild phenotype, so special education should not be recommended unless cognitive testing demonstrates a lower IQ (below 75 is often required for special education).

393. The answer is a. *(Lewis, pp 241–266. Scriver, pp 3–45.)* Aneuploidy involves extra or missing chromosomes that do not arise as increments of the haploid chromosome number n and thus would fit the 90,XX cell line since tetraploidy without aneuploidy would imply a 92,XXXX or 92,XXYY karyotype. Polyploidy involves multiples of n, such as triploidy ($3n = 69$,XXX) or tetraploidy ($4n = 92$,XXXX). Diploidy (46,XX) and haploidy (23,X) are normal karyotypes in gametes and somatic cells, respectively. A 92,XXXX/90,XX karyotype represents mosaicism with a tetraploid cell line and an aneuploid line with tetraploidy minus two X chromosomes, which was observed in a patient with features of Turner syndrome. The mental disability, unusual in Turner syndrome, may reflect the usual trend towards greater severity when sex chromosome aneuploidy involves more extra chromosomes (e.g., 47,XXY Klinefelter to 48,XXXY and 49,XXXXY Klinefelter variants).

394. The answer is d. *(Lewis, pp 241–266. Scriver, pp 3–45.)* Mosaicism occurs when a chromosomal anomaly affects one of several precursor cells of an embryo or tissue. The two or more karyotypes that characterize the mosaic cells are separated by a slash in cytogenetic notation. The notation 47,XX,+21 denotes a cell line typical of a female with trisomy 21 (Down syndrome), whereas 46,XX is the karyotype expected for a normal female.

395. The answer is b. *(Lewis, pp 241–266. Scriver, pp 3–45.)* Cytogenetic notation provides the chromosome number (e.g., 46), the sex chromosomes, and a shorthand description of anomalies. Examples include the following: 45,X indicates a female with monosomy X or Turner syndrome; 47,XX+21 indicates a female with trisomy 21 or Down syndrome; 46,XX,t(14;21) indicates a female with translocation Down syndrome; 45,XX–21 indicates a female with monosomy 21. Note the absence of spaces between symbols, and the use of 47,XXX for sex chromosomal aneuploidy ("triple X" syndrome) rather than the more awkward 47,XX+X. (Note also that 45,X is sufficient for X chromosome monosomy, since absence of an X is indicated by the convention of listing sex chromosomes). Translocations that join two chromosomes with minuscule short arms (acrocentric chromosomes—13, 14, 15, 21, and 22) are called Robertsonian translocations. The joined acrocentric chromosomes in a Robertsonian translocation have a single centromere between them and are counted as one chromosome. A normal person who "carries" a Robertsonian translocation therefore has a chromosome number of 45, as in 45,XX,t(14;21).

396. The answer is a. *(Lewis, pp 241–266. Scriver, pp 3–45.)* Reciprocal translocations (diagram A in Fig. 42) involve the exchange of segments between two chromosomes. Robertsonian translocations (diagram B) involve the joining of two acrocentric chromosomes by breakage and reunion of their short arms. Translocations that produce no duplication or deficiency are called balanced. Individuals who have balanced translocations are called "carriers"; they have normal phenotypes unless the translocation alters the expression of an important gene at the breakpoint region.

Isochromosomes involve duplication of short (diagram C) or long (diagram E) arms, which produces perfectly metacentric chromosomes deficient in long- or short-arm material, respectively. Paracentric inversions (diagram D) alter the banding pattern but not the shape of the chromosome because they do not involve the centromere.

397. The answer is e. *(Lewis, pp 241–266. Scriver, pp 3–45.)* The abbreviations i and t describe isochromosomes and translocation chromosomes, respectively. Isochromosomes create chromosomes with mirror-image duplications of the long arm (diagram E in Fig. 42) or short arm (diagram C). The child with 46,XX,i(Xq) would have an isochromosome composed of two X long arms fused together, thus having Xp material only on her normal chromosome and being haploinsufficient for those genetic loci. Individuals with isochromosome Xq and especially those with isochromosome Xp will have milder manifestations of Turner syndrome than those with full monosomy X. Reciprocal translocations (diagram A) involve exchange of segments between two chromosomes. A semicolon (;) indicates this exchange and is placed between the breakpoints, as in 46,XX,t (2;6)(q23;p14). Robertsonian translocations join together two acrocentric chromosomes to form a metacentric chromosome (diagram B). Carriers of balanced reciprocal translocations have a normal chromosome number, whereas carriers of balanced Robertsonian translocations have only 45 chromosomes.

398. The answer is a. *(Lewis, pp 241–266. Scriver, pp 3–45.)* A chromosome study or karyotype delineates the number and kinds of chromosomes in one cell karyon (nucleus). Blood is conveniently sampled, so most chromosomal studies or karyotypes are performed on peripheral leukocytes in blood. The buffy coat of leukocytes is removed after centrifugation, stimulated to grow in tissue culture media with lectins, arrested in metaphase with colchicine, swollen in hypotonic solution, dropped onto glass slides to rupture nuclei and spread metphase chromosomes, and stained with various dyes (usually Giemsa) to bring out bands (G-bands). Well-spread chromosomes are selected for karyotyping by eye (10–25, depending on the laboratory), representative photographs taken, and chromosome images arranged by computer) in order of size from the #1pair to the #22 pair; this ordered array is also called a karyotype. Except in cases of mosaicism (different karyotypes in different tissues), the peripheral blood karyotype is indicative of the germ-line karyotype that is characteristic for an individual. In most cases of Turner syndrome there is a lack of one X chromosome, as in panel A of Fig. 43, which shows one X (arrow) and no Y chromosome.

399. The answer is c. *(Lewis, pp 241–266. Scriver, pp 3–45.)* Panel C in Fig. 43 demonstrates normal X and Y sex chromosomes, but one pair of autosomes is not homologous (arrow). Given the family history of Down syndrome, the appearance of extra material on the short arm of chromosome 14 (arrow) can be interpreted as material from chromosome 21. Together with the two normal chromosomes 21, this extra 21 material would give three doses of chromosome 21 and result in Down syndrome. The abnormal chromosome 14 can thus be interpreted as a Robertsonian 14;21 translocation that was inherited by this child and by the previous child with Down syndrome [i.e., karyotypes of 46,XY,t(14;21) causing Down syndrome]. Karyotyping the parents would then be important to determine which was the carrier of the 14;21 translocation—45,XX,t(14;21) or 45,XY,t(14;21). Genetic counseling using the appropriate recurrence risk (5–10% for male carriers, 10–20% for female carriers) could include the option of prenatal diagnosis (fetal karyotyping) for future pregnancies.

400. The answer is e. *(Lewis, pp 241–266. Scriver, pp 3–45.)* Children with chromosome abnormalities often exhibit poor growth (failure to thrive) and developmental delay with an abnormal facial appearance. This baby is too young for developmental assessment, but the catlike cry should provoke suspicion of cri-du-chat syndrome. Cri-du-chat syndrome is caused by deletion of the terminal short arm of chromosome 5 [46,XX,del(5p), also abbreviated as 5p–] as depicted in panel E of Fig. 43. When a partial deletion or duplication like this one is found, the parents must be karyotyped to determine if one carries a balanced reciprocal translocation. The other karyotypes show (a) deletion of the short arm of chromosome 4 [46,XY,del(4p) or 4p–]; (b) XYY syndrome (47,XYY); (c) deletion of the long arm of chromosome 13 [46,XX,del(13q) or 13q–]; (d) Klinefelter syndrome (47,XXY). Most disorders involving excess or deficient chromosome material produce a characteristic and recognizable phenotype (e.g., Down, cri-du-chat, or Turner syndrome). The deletion of 4p– (panel A) produces a pattern of abnormalities (syndrome) known as

Wolf-Hirschhorn syndrome; deletion of 13q− produces a 13q− syndrome (no eponym). The mechanism(s) by which imbalanced chromosome material produces a distinctive phenotype is completely unknown.

401. The answer is a. *(Lewis, pp 75–94. Scriver, pp 1521–1552. Murray, pp 145–152.)* Autosomal recessive conditions tend to have a horizontal pattern in the pedigree. Men and women are affected with equal frequency and severity. Autosomal and X-linked recessive inheritance is seen in almost all metabolic diseases as illustrated by type IV glycogen storage disease (232500). Traits like deafness that can follow any of the three major Mendelian inheritance mechanisms (genetic heterogeneity) tend to be more severe in recessive rather than dominant forms, and recessive conditions are less variable than dominant phenotypes. Both alleles are defective but do not necessarily contain the exact same mutation. All individuals carry 6–12 mutant recessive alleles. Fortunately, most matings involve persons who have mutations at different loci. Since related persons are more likely to inherit the same mutant gene, consanguinity increases the possibility of homozygous affected offspring.

402. The answer is e. *(Lewis, pp 355–376. Scriver, pp 1063–1076.)* The father is affected with Gardner syndrome (175100), an autosomal dominant disease. Therefore, each of his four children has a half chance of receiving the allele that causes Gardner syndrome and a half chance of receiving the normal allele. The probability that none of his four children received the allele for Gardner syndrome is thus the joint probability of four independent events, computed by the product $\frac{1}{2} \times \frac{1}{2} \times \frac{1}{2} \times \frac{1}{2} = \frac{1}{16}$. The probability that at least one child has received the abnormal Gardner syndrome allele is thus $1 - \frac{1}{16} = \frac{15}{16}$. Gardner syndrome is one of many genetic disorders that may not be obvious in early childhood. Intestinal cancer in particular has a later onset, with 50% of patients being affected by age 30–35. More extensive evaluation of the children for internal signs of disease (e.g., the bony tumors) is required before the father can conclude that he has not transmitted the gene. The evaluations would be important, many patients choose colonectomy to avoid lethal colonic cancers. A recent option for the family would be DNA diagnosis for mutations in the adenomatous polyposis coli (APC) gene. Presymptomatic DNA diagnosis offers a new approach to genetic diseases of later onset, but is ethically controversial when minors are involved.

403. The answer is a. *(Lewis, pp 75–94. Scriver, pp 3–45.)* Incomplete penetrance applies to a normal individual who is known from the pedigree to have an allele responsible for an autosomal dominant trait. Variable expressivity refers to family members who exhibit signs of the autosomal dominant disorder that vary in severity. When this severity seems to worsen with progressive generations, it is called anticipation. A new mutation in the grandson would be extremely unlikely given the affected grandfather. The father could be an example of somatic mosaicism if a back-mutation occurred to allow normal limb development, but there is no reason to suspect mosaicism of his germ cells (germinal mosaicism). Split hand-foot malformation (183600) is one of many human birth defects that have been traced to mutations in developmental genes homologous to those in simpler organisms like the fruit fly—e.g., Sonic hedgehog (SHH—600725).

404. The answer is d. *(Lewis, pp 75–94. Scriver, pp 3421–3452. Murray, pp 197–204.)* The fact that the mother of the affected child has an affected brother and an affected nephew through her sister suggests X-linked recessive inheritance. This is made more likely because the symptoms suggest a mucopolysaccharidosis (storage of glycosaminoglycans) and because one type exhibits X-linked recessive inheritance [Hunter's syndrome or MPS type II (309900)]. When evaluating the possibility of an X-linked disorder, it is important to remember the pattern of inheritance of the X chromosome. Females have two X chromosomes, which are passed along in a random fashion. They pass any given X chromosome to 50% of their sons and 50% of their daughters. For an X-linked recessive condition, those daughters who inherit the affected allele are heterozygous carriers of the disorder but are not affected (in practice, some female carriers show mild expression). Since males have only one X chromosome, those who inherit the affected allele are affected with the disorder. Given X-linked recessive inheritance, the mother must have the abnormal allele on one of her X chromosomes (she is an obligate carrier) in order for her son and brother to be affected. The fetus thus has a $1/2$ chance of being a boy and a $1/2$ chance of being affected if male, resulting in a $1/4$ (25%) overall risk of being affected.

405. The answer is d. *(Lewis, pp 75–94. Scriver, pp 2007–2056. Murray, pp 249–269.)* The family history and the likelihood that the boys have a metabolic disease suggest autosomal recessive inheritance. Autosomal recessive conditions tend to have a horizontal pattern in the pedigree. Although there may be multiple affected individuals within a sibship, parents, offspring, and other relatives are generally not affected. Most autosomal recessive conditions are rare; however, consanguinity greatly increases the likelihood that two individuals will inherit the same mutant allele and pass it along to their offspring. The recurrence risk for the fetus will be that for an autosomal recessive condition with carrier parents—¼ or 25%. This risk is not affected by the sex of the fetus. The disease caused by cystathionine-β-synthase (CS) deficiency is homocystinuria (236300). S-Adenosylmethionine accepts methyl groups and is converted to S-adenosylhomocysteine, which yields homocysteine; homocysteine is converted to cystathionine by CS. Methionine and homocysteine (dimerized to homocystine) accumulate, and homocystine is excreted in urine. Pyridoxine is a cofactor for CS and is beneficial in some forms of homocystinuria. Other causes of homocystinuria include deficient methionine synthase, which can be ameliorated with its cofactors tetrahydrofolate and cobalamin (vitamin B_{12}).

406. The answer is c. *(Lewis, pp 75–94. Scriver, pp 6117–6146.)* In an autosomal dominant pedigree, there is a vertical pattern of inheritance. Assuming the disorder is not the result of a new mutation, every affected person has an affected parent. The same is true of X-linked dominant pedigrees. However, male-to-male transmission, as seen in this family, excludes the possibility of an X-linked disorder. A person with an autosomal dominant phenotype has one mutant allele and one normal allele. These people randomly pass one or the other of these alleles to their offspring, giving a child a 50% chance of inheriting the mutant allele and therefore being affected with the disorder. This risk is unaffected by the genotypes of the previous offspring.

407. The answer is c. *(Lewis, pp 75–94. Scriver, pp 3–45.)* Males always transmit their single X chromosome to their daughters. Therefore, a daughter of a male affected with an X-linked disorder is an obligate carrier for that disorder. When the condition is X-linked recessive, as with most forms of color-blindness, the daughter is unlikely to show any phenotypic evidence that she is carrying this abnormal gene. Offspring of female carriers are of four types: (1) female carrier with one normal and one mutant allele, (2) normal female with two normal alleles, (3) affected male with a single mutant allele, and (4) normal male with a single normal allele. The chance of having an affected child is thus one-fourth or 25%. If the obligate carrier female gives birth to a son, the chance of the son being color-blind is 50%.

408. The answer is b. *(Lewis, pp 75–94. Scriver, pp 5379–5398.)* The genotype of each dwarf can be represented as Aa, with the uppercase A representing the achondroplasia allele. The Punnett square below demonstrates that ¾ of the possible gamete combinations yield individuals with at least one A allele. Homozygous AA achondroplasia is a severe disease that is usually lethal in the newborn period. The increased likelihood of individuals with achondroplasia marrying each other because of their similar phenotypes is an example of assortative mating.

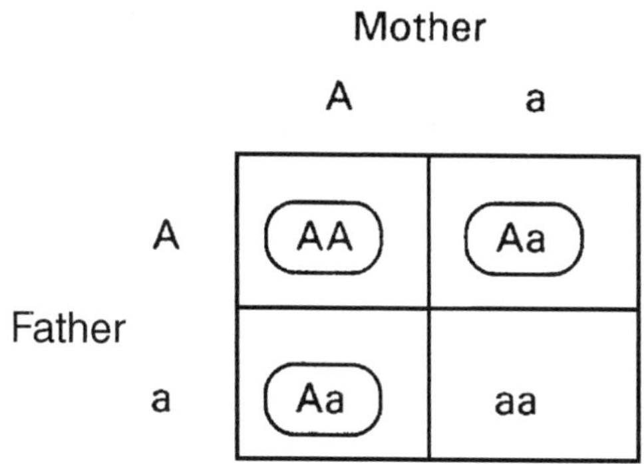

409. The answer is c. *(Lewis, pp 75–94. Scriver, pp 5121–5188. Murray, pp 415–433.)* The McKusick number for cystic fibrosis (219700) begins with 2, indicating an autosomal recessive disorder. The genotype of the affected woman with cystic fibrosis is therefore best represented as the two lowercase letters cc. Her parents are obligate carriers for the disorder (genotypes Cc), and one of her grandparents must also be a carrier (barring new mutations). Her first cousin then has a one-fourth chance of being a carrier, since one of their common grandparents is a carrier, one of his parents has a one-half chance of being a carrier, and he has a one-half chance of inheriting the c allele from his parent. The affected woman can only transmit c alleles to her fetus, while her cousin has one-half chance of transmitting his c allele if it is present. Thus, the probability that the first child will have cystic fibrosis is one-fourth (cousin is carrier) × one-half (cousin transmits c allele) = ⅛ (fetus has cc genotype).

410. The answer is e. *(Lewis, pp 75–94. Scriver, pp 5955–5976.)* The common forms of color blindness are X-linked recessive, as indicated by the initial 3 of the McKusick number (304000). The couple's daughters will be obligate carriers—that is, carriers implied by the pedigree. Using a lowercase c to represent the recessive color blindness allele, the woman is most likely X^CX^C, while her husband is X^cY. The Punnett square below indicates that all daughters will be carriers (X^cX^C), while sons will be normal (X^CY). Note again that loci on the X chromosome cannot be transmitted from father to son, since the son receives the father's Y chromosome.

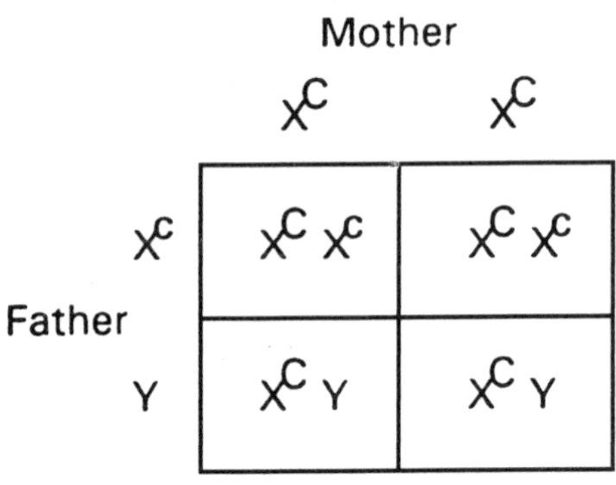

411. The answer is c. *(Lewis, pp 75–94. Scriver, pp 5759–5788.)* Autosomal dominant inheritance is suggested by the pedigree because of the vertical pattern of affected individuals and the affliction of both sexes. Autosomal recessive inheritance is ruled out by transmission through three generations, and X-linked recessive inheritance is made unlikely by the presence of affected females. Maternal inheritance should demonstrate transmission to all or most offspring of affected mothers. Polygenic or multifactorial inheritance is not associated with such a high frequency of transmission. Note that X-linked dominant inheritance would also be an explanation for the pedigree. Because the most likely mechanism responsible for the pedigree is autosomal or X-linked dominant inheritance, individual III-3 in the figure accompanying the question is affected with the disorder, and she has a 50% risk of transmitting the disease. Discrimination between autosomal and X-linked dominant inheritance could be made by noting the offspring of affected males, such as individual III-4. If X-linked dominant inheritance were operative, affected males would have normal sons and affected daughters. The likely diagnosis is an autosomal dominant form of Charcot-Marie-Tooth disease (118200). Charcot-Marie-Tooth disease exhibits genetic heterogeneity and can exhibit autosomal dominant, autosomal recessive (214380), and X-linked inheritance (302800). Note that the physician could provide counseling based on knowledge of genetics even though the disease is unfamiliar.

412. The answer is e. *(Lewis, pp 75–94. Scriver, pp 5903–5934.)* The presence of consanguinity (double line in the figure) is a red flag for autosomal recessive inheritance because, although disease-causing alleles are rare, the probability of a homozygous individual escalates dramatically when the same rare allele descends through two branches of a family. Using a lowercase r to denote the retinitis pigmentosa allele, the affected male (individual II-2 in the figure accompanying the question) has a genotype of rr. His prospective mate has a very low risk to be a carrier for this rare disease, making her genotype RR. Their children will all have genotypes Rr, making them carriers but not affected. Retinitis pigmentosa is another disease manifesting genetic heterogeneity, with autosomal dominant (180100), autosomal recessive (268000), and X-linked recessive (312650) forms. Carriers of autosomal recessive diseases are heterozygotes with one normal and one abnormal allele. Many autosomal recessive diseases involve enzyme deficiencies, indicating that 50% levels of enzymes found in heterozygotes are sufficient for normal function. The probability that an affected individual will encounter a mate who is a carrier is approximately twice the square root of the disease incidence. This figure derives from the Hardy-Weinberg law. Since most recessive diseases have incidences lower than 1 in 10,000, the risk for unrelated mates to be carriers is less than 1 in 50, and the chance of having an affected child is less than $\frac{1}{50} \times \frac{1}{4}$ = less than 1 in 200. Disorders that are fairly common in certain ethnic groups, such as cystic fibrosis, are exceptions to this very low risk.

413. The answer is d. *(Lewis, pp 75–94. Scriver, pp 5903–5934.)* X-linked recessive inheritance is characterized by a predominance of affected males and an oblique pattern. Transmission must be through females with no evidence of male-to-male transmission. The lack of affected females would make autosomal dominant inheritance less likely, and the sex ratio plus transmission through three generations would eliminate autosomal recessive inheritance. Polygenic inheritance usually exhibits less frequent transmission, although it is certainly not ruled out in this pedigree. The many normal offspring of affected females rule out maternal inheritance. Individual II-4 in the figure accompanying the question is an obligate carrier because she has an affected brother and affected son. This means that her daughter (III-3) has a one-half chance of inheriting the X chromosome with an abnormal allele and one-half chance of inheriting the X chromosome with the normal allele. If individual III-3 is a carrier, she has a one-half chance of transmitting her abnormal allele to her son. The risk that her son will be affected is thus one-half times one-half = one-fourth or 25%. Because the daughters of individual III-3 might be carriers (one-half chance) but will not be affected, individual III-3 has a one-half chance of having an affected child.

414. The answer is e. *(Lewis, pp 75–94. Scriver, pp 5241–5287.)* If two individuals in a sibship are affected with an autosomal dominant disease, then the usual implication is that one of the parents has the abnormal allele. Parents with one normal and one abnormal allele have a 50% chance of transmitting the abnormal allele with each pregnancy. Complicating the recognition of autosomal dominant inheritance are incomplete penetrance, where there are no signs of the disease phenotype after all relevant medical evaluations, and variable expressivity, where a parent may have more subtle disease than the offspring. Incomplete penetrance applies to this family because the parents have no signs or symptoms of disease. If a mutation occurs in the primordial germ cells, then these cells may have abnormal alleles despite the lack of these alleles in the rest of the body tissues (germinal mosaicism). Germinal mosaicism was thought to be very rare until testing for type I collagen gene mutations in osteogenesis imperfecta allowed verification of germinal mosaicism in this condition. Germinal mosaicism explained why autosomal recessive inheritance had been incorrectly postulated for families with normal parents and multiple affected children. Once a child has received the abnormal allele through the gamete of the mosaic parent, the child has the abnormal allele in all cells, with the usual 50% risk of transmission. The characterization of mutations in the $\alpha1$ or $\alpha2$ chains of type I collagen in the osteogenesis imperfectas allowed proof of germ-line mosaicism through paternal sperm studies and corrected the false impression that such families were examples of autosomal recessive inheritance.

415. The answer is a. *(Lewis, pp 75–94. Scriver, pp 3–45.)* Females have two alleles for each locus on the X chromosome because of their 46,XX karyotype. One normal allele is by definition sufficient for normal function in X-linked recessive disorders, so that females with one abnormal allele are carriers instead of affected individuals. Only when the companion normal allele is disrupted or missing does the abnormal allele cause disease. The Lyon hypothesis predicts that X inactivation is early, irreversible, and random, but some females inactivate only the X chromosome carrying the normal allele. X autosome translocations may disrupt an X chromosome locus and cause disease because the translocated autosome must remain active to avert embryonic death; nonrandom inactivation of the normal X chromosome thus ablates expression of its normal allele. Females with Turner syndrome, like males with 46,XY karyotypes, have only one X chromosome and can be affected with X-linked recessive diseases. Conversely, females with triple X or trisomy X syndrome have three alleles at each X chromosome locus and are not affected with X-linked recessive disorders. Since choices c, d, and e each require two genetic changes, they are less common than choice a.

416. The answer is e. *(Lewis, pp 75–94. Scriver, pp 3–45.)* Women who are heterozygous at an X-chromosome locus will have a one-half chance to transmit their abnormal allele to sons or daughters with each pregnancy. When heterozygous women show disease symptoms, they are considered affected and the disorder is considered to be X-linked dominant. When an abnormal X chromosome allele is sufficiently severe to affect heterozygous women, the hemizygous males often do not survive the embryonic period and present as unrecognized early losses or later miscarriages. If the disorder does not affect the in utero viability of females, twice as many females as males are born. The decreased survival of affected males and reduced reproductive fitness of affected females also implies a high rate of new mutations and means that many isolated cases will occur. In disorders such as incontinentia pigmenti (308300), where affected individuals have variable manifestations, careful examination of the mother is required before assuming that an affected daughter is a new mutation. A pregnancy history will also be helpful, in that a history of early pregnancy losses would suggest the mother was a mildly affected heterozygote. The distinction between X-linked dominant and X-linked recessive diseases is somewhat arbitrary, since heterozygous women may show mild symptoms in disorders such as Duchenne muscular dystrophy (310200) or hemophilia A (306700). Severe symptoms in some female heterozygotes, together with male lethality, are good criteria for classification as X-linked dominant (as for Goltz syndrome—305600, Aicardi syndrome—304050, and incontinentia pigmenti).

417. The answer is e. *(Lewis, pp 135–154. Scriver, pp 193–202.)* An increasing recurrence risk according to the number of relatives affected is characteristic of polygenic inheritance. The more affected relatives there are, the more evidence there is that an individual's genetic background is shifted toward the threshold for a particular trait; for example, the expectation for tall parents with tall grandparents is to have tall children. Inheritance risks for Mendelian disorders are unaffected by outcomes in prior offspring because they reflect segregation ratios for a known (or deduced) pair of alleles (chance has no memory). Pyloric stenosis was once a lethal disease but now is easily repaired by surgery (recently, by less invasive laparoscopic surgery). The diagnosis can be difficult, often requiring palpation of the abdomen for 20–30 minutes when the baby has vomited and is relaxed. The characteristic "olive" mass can be felt in the mid-abdomen and can now be confirmed by ultrasound study.

418. The answer is b. *(Lewis, pp 75–94. Scriver, pp 5587–5628.)* Albinism is one of many genetic diseases that exhibit locus heterogeneity, which means that mutations at several different loci can produce identical phenotypes. The two McKusick numbers provide a clue that there is more than one locus for albinism, both causing autosomal recessive disease. Each parent must be homozygous for a mutant allele from one albinism locus but heterozygous or homozygous normal at the other locus. Their child would then be an obligate carrier for each type of albinism. A new mutation in the child is also possible, converting one of the parental mutant alleles to normal, but this would be very rare. Autosomal dominant disorders often vary in severity within families (variable expressivity) but occasionally are clinically silent in a person known to carry the abnormal allele (incomplete penetrance).

419. The answer is c. *(Lewis, pp 75–94. Scriver, pp 6097–6116.)* For each pregnancy, the probability that the child will be affected is one-half. Therefore, the probability that all three children will be affected is the product of the three independent events—that is, $\frac{1}{2} \times \frac{1}{2} \times \frac{1}{2} = \frac{1}{8}$. The probability that all three children will be unaffected is the same. When evaluating the probability that one of the three children will be affected, it must be noted that there are three of eight possible birth orders that have one affected child (Www, wWw, wwW). For two of three children to be affected, there are also three of eight possible birth orders (WWw, WwW, wWW). The ventral midline hair and skin patches relate to the fact that neural crest cells provide melanin, and that migration of these cells from the dorsal midline (neural tube) of the embryo is slowed in disorders like Waardenburg syndrome (193500) and piebald trait (172800).

420. The answer is d. *(Lewis, pp 75–94. Scriver, pp 3–45.)* Diploid persons have two alleles per autosomal locus, with one being transmitted to each gamete (Mendel's law of segregation). The key to blood group problems is to recognize that a blood type is ambiguous regarding possible alleles—type A persons may have AA or AO genotypes. Once the possible genotypes are deduced from the blood types, potential offspring will represent all combinations of parental alleles. Parents with AB and OO genotypes can only have offspring with genotypes AO (type A) or BO (type B).

421. The answer is b. *(Lewis, pp 75–94. Scriver, pp 1667–1724.)* If the abnormal allele is represented as p and the normal as P, an infant affected with phenylketonuria (PKU) has the genotype pp. Parents must be heterozygotes or carriers (Pp) for the child to inherit the p allele from both the mother and father (assuming correct paternity and the absence of unusual chromosomal segregation). Subsequent children have a one-half chance of inheriting allele p from the mother and a one-half chance of inheriting allele p from the father; the chance that both events will occur to give genotype pp is thus $\frac{1}{2} \times \frac{1}{2} = \frac{1}{4}$ or 25%. A normal sibling may be genotype PP (one-fourth probability) or Pp (one-half probability since two different combinations of parental alleles give this genotype). The ratio of these probabilities results in a $\frac{2}{3}$ chance (67%) of genotype Pp. Note that genotype pp is excluded because a normal sibling (the first child) is specified. Neonatal screening is mandated for disorders like phenylketonuria (261600) because they are difficult to recognize clinically and early dietary treatment prevents severe mental disability.

422. The answer is d. *(Lewis, pp 75–94. Scriver, pp 5379–5398.)* The figure (Fig. 49) shows the correctly drawn pedigree with generations indicated by Roman numerals and individuals by Arabic numbers. As the McKusick numbers indicate, achondroplasia (100800) is autosomal dominant, cystic fibrosis (219700) autosomal recessive. Since neither parent is affected with achondroplasia, the risk for their next child to be affected is virtually zero (rare chances for germ-line mosaicism or incomplete penetrance are ignored). The person who prompted genetic concern is the proband (III-1). George has a brother with cystic fibrosis, making his parents (I–3, I–4) obligate carriers. He has a one-fourth chance of being normal, a two-fourths chance of being a carrier, and a one-fourth chance of being affected with cystic fibrosis. Since George's possibility of being affected is eliminated by circumstance (he is normal), his odds of being a carrier are two-thirds. George's wife is definitely a carrier, giving their next child a one-sixth chance to have cystic fibrosis (two-thirds chance George is a carrier X one-fourth chance the child is affected if both are carriers). Although the ΔF_{508} (three–base pair deletion of phenylalanine codon at position 508 in the cystic fibrosis transmembrane regulator gene) accounts for 70% of cystic fibrosis mutations in whites, George's family may have a different mutation than was detected by DNA analysis in his wife. Their child may therefore have a risk of being a compound heterozygote (two different abnormal cystic fibrosis alleles) but will still be affected. Current DNA analysis for cystic fibrosis would likely clarify this issue, since over 30 mutations can be screened in Caucasions.

423. The answer is c. *(Lewis, pp 75–94. Scriver, pp 3827–3876.)* Parents of children with autosomal recessive disorders are obligate carriers if nonpaternity and rare examples of uniparental disomy (inheritance of both chromosomal homologues from the same parent) are excluded. Normal siblings have a $^2/_3$ chance of being carriers because they cannot be homozygous for the abnormal allele. Grandparents have a one-half chance of being carriers because one or the other must have transmitted the abnormal allele to the obligate carrier parent. First cousins share a set of grandparents of whom one must be a carrier. There is a one-half chance for the aunt or uncle to be a carrier and a one-fourth chance for the first cousin. Half-siblings share an obligate carrier parent and have a one-half chance of being carriers. These calculations assume a lack of mutations (Tay-Sachs is rare) and a lack of coincidental alleles (no consanguinity).

424. The answer is e. *(Lewis, pp 135–154. Scriver, pp 193–202.)* Cleft lip with or without cleft palate [CL(P)] is one of the most common congenital malformations. Because of the genetic component of this trait, it tends to be more common in certain families. The more family members affected and the more severe the cleft, the higher the recurrence risk. In addition, CL(P) is more common in males and in certain ethnic groups (i.e., Asians > whites > African Americans).

425. The answer is a. *(Lewis, pp 267–282. Scriver, pp 3–45.)* If an abnormal allele is as likely to be transmitted to the next generation as its corresponding normal allele, it is said to have a fitness of 1. Loss of fitness (decrease in allele frequency after one generation) is also referred to as negative selection. The decreased fitness of achondroplast alleles that are eliminated by negative selection must be balanced by new mutations if the disorder has not disappeared or declined in incidence. Thus, the mutation rate of achondroplasia would be expected to be high relative to those of more benign dominant diseases.

426. The answer is b. *(Lewis, pp 135–154. Scriver, pp 193–202.)* Many common disorders tend to run in families but are not single-gene or chromosomal disorders. These disorders exhibit multifactorial determination, a theoretical mechanism envisioned as the interaction of multiple genes (polygenic inheritance) and environmental factors. For quantitative traits like height, it is easy to visualize how the alleles at multiple loci plus environmental factors (e.g., nutrition) might make additive contributions toward a given stature. For qualitative traits such as cleft lip/palate and other congenital anomalies, a threshold is envisioned that divides normal from abnormal phenotypes. Individuals with more clefting alleles, in combination with an unfavorable intrauterine environment, can cross the threshold and manifest the anomaly. Environmental factors in multfactorial determination are thus prenatal as well as postnatal. For adult diseases like coronary artery disease, strokes, or hypertension, the quantitative trait can be viewed as degree of artery occlusion or blood pressure and the threshold as events like myocardial or cerebral infarction. The likelihood of inheriting hypertension-promoting alleles is increased if there are several affected relatives as in the family under discussion, translating the usual 3–5% risk for a multifactorial disorder in a first-degree relative to the 5–10% risk estimated in answer b. Recurrence risks for multifactorial disorders are modified by family history because the multiple predisposing alleles cannot be determined by testing. Current research is attempting to find single nucleotide polymorphisms (SNPs) that travel with these multiple predisposing alleles, allowing more definitive susceptibility testing and risk prediction for the occurrence and transmission of multifactorial traits.

427. The answer is d. *(Lewis, pp 267–282. Scriver, pp 3–45.)* Down syndrome, a chromosomal disorder, has virtually the same frequency of 1 in 600 births in all ethnic groups. Screening for Down syndrome is carried out during pregnancy with triple test/quad screens offered to all individuals (with very poor sensitivity or specificity) and chorionic villus sampling/amniocentesis (with high accuracy but some miscarriage risk) to woman above age 35. Allele frequencies may differ among populations when there has been geographic isolation, founder effect, or selection for certain alleles based on different environments. Although African Americans have intermixed with whites in the United States for over 400 years, they retain a higher frequency of sickle cell alleles (603903), which are thought to protect individuals from malarial infection. Each ethnic group has frequencies of polymorphic alleles that reflect its origin; for example, Ashkenazi Jews have a higher frequency of Tay-Sachs alleles (272800); Greeks and other Mediterranean peoples of β-thalassemia alleles (603902); Asian peoples of α-thalassemia alleles (141800); and whites of cystic fibrosis alleles (219700). Specific genetic differences (polymorphisms) in the mitochondrial and Y chromosomes have allowed reconstruction of migrations that show correlations between genetic homogeneity and language.

428. The answer is d. *(Lewis, pp 267–282. Scriver, pp 3–45.)* Founder effects represent a special case of genetic drift in which rare alleles are introduced into a small population by the migration of ancestors. These founder mutant alleles can overcome selective disadvantage because they begin with high frequency in a small gene pool. Linkage disequilibrium describes an association between a particular polymorphic allele and a trait. Many autoimmune diseases exhibit association with particular human leukocyte antigen (HLA) alleles (i.e., HLA-B27 and ankylosing spondylitis). The association is not necessarily cause and effect (e.g., when viral infections that trigger a disease preferentially infect certain HLA genotypes). Genetic linkage implies physical proximity of the allele locus to the gene causing the disease. Linkage differs from allele association in that either allele A or a may be linked in a given family, depending on which allele is present together with the offending gene. Neither assortative mating (preferential mating by genotype) nor selection (advantageous alleles) applies to the situation under discussion. Later research using DNA polymorphisms has refuted the Hopewell hypothesis, showing that families with this form of diabetes insipidus (304800) are not related to ancestors from Halifax.

429. The answer is b. *(Lewis, pp 267–282. Scriver, pp 3–45.)* Sickle cell anemia (603903) is the classic example of a disorder with a high frequency in a specific population because of heterozygote advantage. Persons who are heterozygous for this mutant allele (hemoglobin AS) have increased resistance to malaria and are therefore at an advantage in areas where malaria is endemic. Founder effect is a special type of genetic drift. In these cases, the founder or original ancestor of a population has a certain mutant allele. Because of genetic isolation and inbreeding in populations such as the Pennsylvania Amish, certain disorders such as maple syrup urine disease (248600) are maintained at a relatively high frequency. Fitness is a measure of the ability to reproduce. A genetic lethal implies that affected individuals cannot reproduce and, therefore, cannot pass on their mutant alleles. Natural selection is a theory introduced by Charles Darwin, which postulates that the fittest individuals have a selective advantage for survival.

430. The answer is b. *(Lewis, pp 267–282. Scriver, pp 3–45.)* It is important to remember that individuals with blood type A can have either genotype AA or AO, and individuals with blood type B can have either genotype BB or BO. Therefore, the frequency of blood type A is the frequency of homozygotes—that is, 0.3×0.3—plus the frequency of heterozygotes—that is, $2\ (0.3) \times 0.6$—for a total of 0.45. The frequency of blood type B is $0.1 \times 0.1 + 2\ (0.1) \times 0.6$ for a total of 0.13. The frequency of individuals with blood type O is simply the frequency of homozygotes—that is, $0.6 \times 0.6 = 0.36$.

431. The answer is c. *(Lewis, pp 267–282. Scriver, pp 3–45.)* Although all individuals, other than identical twins, are genetically unique, each individual will have some genes in common with their relatives. The more closely related, the more genes individuals have in common. First-degree relatives, such as siblings, parents, and children, share one-half of their genes.

Second-degree relatives share one-fourth, and third-degree relatives share one-eighth. Full siblings will have half their genes in common, half-siblings (with only one common parent) one-fourth. Risks for multifactorial disorders like hydrocephalus fall off rapidly with decreasing degrees of relationship, with average figures of 3–5% for first degree relatives (sharing $\frac{1}{2}$ their genes), 0.5–0.7% for second-degree relatives (sharing one-fourth their genes as for this child and his sister), dropping to near baseline incidence (1–3 per thousand for congenital anomalies) for third-degree relatives like first cousins.

432. The answer is d. *(Lewis, pp 267–282. Scriver, pp 3–45.)* According to the Hardy-Weinberg equilibrium, the frequency of heterozygotes (2pq) is twice the square root of the rare homozygote frequency (q^2). The man in the question has a two-thirds chance of being a carrier. His wife has a one-twentieth chance of being a carrier. The rare homozygote frequency is $\frac{1}{600}$, so the square root is $\frac{1}{40}$ and the frequency of heterozygotes is thus $2 \times \frac{1}{40} = \frac{1}{20}$. His risk for an affected child is $\frac{2}{3} \times \frac{1}{20} \times \frac{1}{4} = \frac{1}{120}$.

433. The answer is e. *(Lewis, pp 267–282. Scriver, pp 4571–4636.)* The African American man and woman each have a one-eighth chance of having sickle trait. They have a $\frac{1}{64} \times \frac{1}{4} = \frac{1}{256}$ chance of having a child with sickle cell anemia. There is also a $\frac{1}{64} \times \frac{1}{2} = \frac{1}{128}$ chance that their child will have sickle trait.

434. The answer is b. *(Lewis, pp 75–94, 267–282. Scriver, pp 3–45.)* The grandmother has cystic fibrosis, so her children are obligate carriers. Each cousin therefore has a one-half chance of being a carrier. The woman's risk is $\frac{1}{2} \times \frac{1}{2} \times \frac{1}{4} = \frac{1}{16}$ chance of having an affected child. This illustrates the effects of consanguinity.

Genetic and Biochemical Diagnosis

Questions

DIRECTIONS: Each item below contains a question or incomplete statement followed by suggested responses. Select the **one best** response to each question.

435. A 48-year-old woman is diagnosed with Parkinson disease and there are no other cases in her family. She requests genetic counseling and/or testing to assess risks that her children will develop Parkinsonism. Her physician explains that 1% of people over 50 may contract the disease that monozygotic twins have a 1–2% concordance rate and that siblings of affected individuals have a 2–3% incidence of disease. Low levels of dopamine are found in the substantia nigra of the brains of people with Parkinson. Based on this information, the woman should be told which of the following regarding her children?

a. They have a 2–3% risk to develop the disease and that SNPs for loci controlling tyrosine metabolism might become available for future susceptibility testing
b. They have a 2–3% risk to develop the disease and that SNPs for loci controlling tyrosine metabolism might become available for future susceptibility testing
c. They have a 5–10% risk to develop the disease and that SNPs for loci controlling tyrosine metabolism might become available for future susceptibility testing
d. They have a 5–10% risk to develop the disease and that SNPs for loci controlling tryptophan metabolism might become available for future susceptibility testing
e. They have an indeterminate risk to develop the disease and that SNPs for loci controlling threonine metabolism might become available for future susceptibility testing

436. The strategy for therapy for dopamine deficiency in the substantia nigra of individuals with Parkinson disease is indicated by which of the following?

a. Feedback inhibition of dopamine oxidation
b. Competitive inhibition of biosynthesis from histidine
c. Provision of metabolites in the tyrosine pathway
d. Stimulation of monoamine oxidase
e. Provision of metabolites in the alanine pathway

437. A 3-year-old girl is scheduled for a tonsillectomy. As she is prepared for the operating room, her father becomes agitated and insists on accompanying her. He says that he lost a son several years ago when the child did not wake up after an operation. Which of the following options is the best response to the father's anxiety?

a. Postpone the operation until the psychiatric state of the father can be evaluated
b. Proceed after explaining that problems in the father's siblings are unlikely to be transmitted to his daughter
c. Proceed after reassuring the father that drug reactions are environmental and unlikely to have a genetic basis
d. Postpone the operation until a more detailed family history is obtained
e. Proceed after explaining that modern anesthetic procedures are much safer than in the past

438. In the operating room, a child receives succinylcholine as a muscle relaxant to facilitate intubation and anesthesia. The operation proceeds until it is time for recovery, when the child does not begin breathing. A hurried discussion with the father discloses no additional problems in the family, but he does say that he and his wife are first cousins. Which of the following is the most likely possibility?

a. An autosomal dominant disorder that interferes with succinylcholine metabolism
b. An autosomal recessive disorder that interferes with succinylcholine metabolism
c. An X-linked disorder that interferes with succinylcholine metabolism
d. A lethal gene transmitted through consanguinity that affects the respiratory system
e. Mismanagement of halothane anesthesia during the operation

439. Pharmacogenetics, or the study of drug-induced disease due to genetic variation, is receiving increased attention particularly with regard to population or at least preoperative screening. The frequency of heterozygotes for variant butyrylcholinesterase (BChE) alleles in Caucasians is about 4 per 100, implying an incidence of individuals with potential for severe apnea of which of the following?

a. 1 in 5000
b. 1 in 2500
c. 1 in 1250
d. 1 in 500
e. 1 in 50

440. A man with early-onset emphysema undergoes protein electrophoresis for analysis of α_1-antitrypsin (AAT) deficiency (107400). The result shows two electrophoretic bands that react with AAT, one at the normal position and one at an abnormal position. Which of the following best describes this result?

a. The man is homozygous and has normal AAT activity
b. The man is heterozygous and has normal AAT activity
c. The man is homozygous and has deficient AAT activity
d. The man is homozygous and has an altered AAT protein
e. The man is heterozygous and has an altered AAT protein

441. A girl seems normal at birth but begins flinching at loud noises (enhanced startle response) at age 6 months. Ophthalmologic examination reveals a central red area of the retina surrounded by white tissue (cherry red spot). The child initially can sit up, but then regresses so that she cannot roll over or recognize her parents. Her physician suspects a lipid storage disease (neurolipidosis). If the diagnosis is correct, what is the risk that the next child of these parents will be affected with the same disease?

a. $\frac{1}{2}$
b. $\frac{1}{4}$
c. $\frac{3}{4}$
d. $\frac{1}{12}$
e. $\frac{1}{24}$

442. The cause of Tay-Sachs disease (272800) is best described by which of the following?

a. Excess of a lysosomal enzyme in blood due to defective uptake
b. Deficiency of a lysosomal enzyme that digests proteoglycans
c. Deficiency of a membrane receptor that takes up proteoglycans
d. Deficiency of a mitochondrial enzyme that degrades glycogen
e. Deficiency of a mitochondrial triglyceride lipase

443. The frequency of Tay-Sachs carriers among Ashkenazi Jews is $\frac{1}{30}$. The frequency of Tay-Sachs carriers among whites of Western European descent is approximately $\frac{1}{300}$. If a mother is an Ashkenazi Jew and a father is a white from Western Europe, what is the chance that a child of this union will have Tay-Sachs disease?

a. $\frac{1}{120}$
b. $\frac{1}{240}$
c. $\frac{1}{3600}$
d. $\frac{1}{9000}$
e. $\frac{1}{36,000}$

444. The parents of a girl with Tay-Sachs disease decide to pursue bone marrow transplantation in an attempt to provide a source for the missing lysosomal enzyme. Preliminary testing of the girl's normal siblings is performed to assess their carrier status and their human leukocyte antigen (HLA) locus compatibility with their affected sister. What is the chance that one of the three siblings is homozygous normal (i.e., has a good supply of enzyme) and HLA-compatible?

a. $\frac{1}{2}$
b. $\frac{1}{3}$
c. $\frac{1}{4}$
d. $\frac{1}{6}$
e. $\frac{1}{12}$

445. A sibling donor is found for a patient with Tay-Sachs disease, and the physician writes to the patient's insurance company explaining the diagnosis of Tay-Sachs disease and the reasons for the bone marrow transplant. Not only does the insurance company refuse payment for transplantation, it also discontinues coverage for the family based on anticipated medical expenses. From the ethical perspective, these events fall under which of the following categories?

a. Patient confidentiality
b. Nondisclosure
c. Informed consent
d. Failure to provide ongoing care
e. Discrimination

446. A couple decide to have prenatal diagnosis because their previous child has Tay-Sachs disease. Which of the following prenatal diagnostic techniques is optimal for fetal diagnosis?

a. Chorionic villi sampling (CVS)
b. Percutaneous umbilical blood sampling
c. Amniotic fluid α-fetoprotein levels
d. Maternal serum α-fetoprotein (MSAFP)
e. Fetal x-rays

447. A patient with the Marfan syndrome (154700) is evaluated at a clinic. He is noted to have a tall, thin body habitus, loose joints, and arachnodactyly (spider fingers). Ophthalmologic examination reveals lens dislocation. Echocardiogram reveals dilation of the aortic root. A family history reveals that the patient's parents are medically normal, but that his paternal grandfather and great-grandfather died in their forties with lens dislocation and dissecting aortic aneurysms. A sister is found to have a similar body habitus, dilation of the aortic root, and normal lenses. The different findings in these different family members with the same disease are best described by which of the following terms?

a. Pleiotropy
b. Founder effect
c. Variable expressivity
d. Incomplete penetrance
e. Genetic heterogeneity

448. Marfan syndrome is caused by which of the following mechanisms?

a. Mutation that prevents addition of carbohydrate residues to the fibrillin glycoprotein
b. Mutation in a carbohydrate portion of fibrillin that interferes with targeting
c. Mutation that disrupts the secondary structure of fibrillin and blocks its assembly into microfibrils
d. Mutation in a lysosomal enzyme that degrades fibrillin
e. Mutation in a membrane receptor that targets fibrillin to lysosomes

449. The diagnosis of osteogenesis imperfecta (166200) is most accurately performed by which of the following?

a. PCR amplification and DNA sequencing of type I collagen gene segments to look for point mutations
b. Gel electrophoresis of labeled type I collagen chains synthesized in fibroblasts
c. PCR amplification and ASO hybridization to detect particular mutant alleles
d. Northern blotting to evaluate type I collagen mRNAs
e. Purification and trypsin digestion of type I collagen chains to visualize altered peptides after two-dimensional gel electrophoresis

450. Studies of the eye tumor retinoblastoma have revealed an Rb locus on the long arm of chromosome 13 that influences retinoblastoma occurrence. Patients with 13q–deletions often develop bilateral tumors (both sides), in contrast to more common forms of retinoblastoma that occur at one site. Which of the following phrases best explains this phenomenon?

a. Rb is an oncogene
b. Rb is a tumor suppressor gene
c. Rb mutations ablate a promoter sequence
d. Rb mutations ablate an enhancer sequence
e. Rb mutations must always involve chromosome abnormalities

451. In Burkitt lymphoma, there is increased expression of a hybrid protein with an amino-terminus similar to immunoglobulin (Ig) heavy chain and an unknown carboxyterminus. Which of the following best explains this phenomenon?

a. Chromosome translocation that brings together an Ig heavy chain with an oncogene
b. Chromosome duplication involving a segment with an oncogene
c. Chromosome translocation involving a segment with Ig heavy chains
d. Chromosome deletion removing an oncogene
e. Chromosome deletion removing a tumor suppressor gene

452. A couple request genetic counseling because the wife has contracted early-onset breast cancer at age 23. The husband has a benign family history, but the wife has several relatives who developed cancers at relatively early ages. Affected relatives include a sister (colon cancer, age 42), a brother (colon cancer, age 46), mother (breast cancer, age 56), maternal aunt (leukemia, age 45), maternal uncle (muscle sarcoma, age 49), and a nephew through the brother with colon cancer (leukemia, age 8). Which of the following is the correct conclusion from the family history?

a. No genetic predisposition to cancer since most individuals have different types of cancer
b. Possible autosomal dominant inheritance or multifactorial inheritance of cancer predisposition
c. Germ-line mutations in an oncogene, with somatic mutations that suppress the oncogene
d. Germ-line mutations in a tumor suppressor gene, with neoplasia from chemical exposure
e. Mitochondrial inheritance of tumor predisposition evidenced by the affected maternal relatives

453. A normal 6-year-old girl has a strong family history of cancer, including several relatives with Li-Fraumeni syndrome, an autosomal dominant condition that predisposes to breast and colon cancer. Her parents request that she have genetic testing for a possible cancer gene. Which of the following is the major ethical concern about such testing?

a. Nonmaleficence
b. Beneficence
c. Autonomy
d. Informed consent
e. Confidentiality

454. A 45-year-old male is hospitalized for treatment of myocardial infarction. His father and a paternal uncle also had heart attacks at an early age. His cholesterol is elevated, and lipoprotein electrophoresis demonstrates an abnormally high ratio of low- to high-density lipoproteins (LDL to HDL). Which of the following is the most likely explanation for this problem?

a. Mutant HDL is not responding to high cholesterol levels
b. Mutant LDL is not responding to high cholesterol levels
c. Mutant caveolae proteins are not responding to high cholesterol levels
d. Mutant LDL receptors are deficient in cholesterol uptake
e. Intracellular cholesterol is increasing the number of LDL receptors

455. A patient with myocardial infarction is treated with nitroglycerin to dilate his coronary arteries. Which of the following best describes the action of nitroglycerin?

a. Methylation occurs to produce S-adenosylmethionine
b. GTP hydrolysis accomplishes oxidation of LDL proteins
c. Arginine is converted to a neurotransmitter that activates guanyl cyclase
d. Acetyl CoA and choline are condensed to form a neurotransmitter
e. Tyrosine is converted to serotonin

456. A woman presents with fatigue, pallor, and pale conjunctival blood vessels. She gives a recent history of metrorrhagia (heavy menstrual periods). Which of the following laboratory findings is most likely?

a. High serum haptoglobin
b. High serum iron
c. High numbers of transferrin receptors
d. High saturation of transferrin
e. High serum ferritin

457. A man is evaluated for mild liver disease, arthritis, fatigue, and grayish skin pigmentation. A liver biopsy shows marked increase in iron. Which of the following laboratory values is most likely?

a. Low serum iron
b. High serum copper
c. Low saturation of transferrin
d. High serum ferritin
e. Low serum haptoglobin

458. The regulation of transferrin receptors is studied in tissue culture. There is increased synthesis of transferrin receptor protein with no changes in transferrin mRNA transcription. Which of the following is the most plausible explanation?

a. Change in amounts or types of transcription factors
b. Allosteric regulation of transferrin receptor function
c. Activation of transferrin receptor function by a protein kinase
d. Stabilization of transferrin mRNA
e. Increased GTP levels to accelerate protein elongation

459. A 2-year-old child is hospitalized for evaluation of poor growth and low muscle tone. The most striking physical finding is unruly, "kinky" hair, but the child also has increased joint laxity and thin skin. Which of the following laboratory findings is most likely?

a. High ceruloplasmin
b. High tissue copper
c. Low serum iron
d. Low saturation of transferrin
e. Low serum haptoglobin

460. Deletions of 11p13 may result in Wilm tumor, aniridia, genitourinary malformations, and mental retardation (WAGR syndrome). In some patients, however, not all features are seen. Additionally, individual features of this syndrome may be inherited separately in a Mendelian fashion. Limited features may also be seen in patients without visible chromosomal deletions. Which of the following is the most likely mechanism for this finding?

a. Mitochondrial inheritance
b. Imprinting
c. Germ-line mosaicism
d. Uniparental disomy
e. Contiguous gene syndrome

461. Polycystic kidney disease (173900) is a significant cause of renal failure that presents from early infancy to adulthood. Early-onset cases tend to affect one family member or siblings, whereas adult-onset cases often show a vertical pattern in the pedigree. Which of the following offers the best explanation of these facts?

a. Pleiotropy
b. Allelic heterogeneity
c. Locus heterogeneity
d. Multifactorial inheritance
e. Variable expressivity

462. A male child presents with delayed development and scarring of his lips and hands. His parents have restrained him because he obsessively chews on his lips and fingers. Which of the following is likely to occur in this child?

a. Increased levels of 5-phosphoribosyl-1-pyrophosphate (PRPP)
b. Decreased purine synthesis
c. Decreased levels of uric acid
d. Increased levels of hypoxanthine-guanosine phosphoribosyl transferase (HGPRT)
e. Glycogen storage

463. A couple request prenatal diagnosis because a maternal uncle and a male cousin on the wife's side were diagnosed with Lesch-Nyhan syndrome (308000). DNA analysis of the family is performed using Southern blotting with VNTR probes near the HGPRT gene, shown below. What is the chance that the fetus will have Lesch-Nyhan syndrome?

a. 100%
b. 50%
c. 33%
d. 25%
e. Virtually 0%

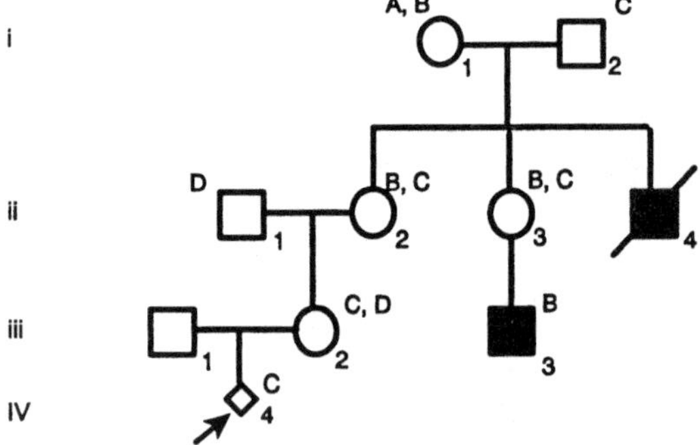

464. A 6-year-old girl is referred to a physician for evaluation. She is known to have mild mental retardation and a ventricular septal defect (VSD). On physical examination, the patient is noted to have some facial dysmorphism, including a long face, a prominent nose, and flattening in the malar region. In addition, the patient's speech has an unusual quality. Which of the following descriptions best explains the patient's condition?

a. Sequence
b. Syndrome
c. Disruption
d. Deformation
e. Single birth defect

465. A standard karyotypic analysis is ordered for a girl with heart defects, developmental delay, and an unusual appearance. The results are normal, but a colleague recommends performing fluorescent in situ hybridization (FISH) analysis on the patient's chromosomes, using probes for chromosome 22. Only one signal is seen for each chromosomal spread. Which of the following statements regarding these analyses is true?

a. The initial karyotype results are inconsistent with the FISH results
b. This is a normal result
c. A small deletion is present on one of the patient's number 22 chromosomes
d. FISH is only helpful when the initial karyotype results are abnormal
e. The chromosome with the positive signal is paternal in origin

466. As exemplified by HLA-DQβ haplotypes in type I diabetes mellitus, an individual's HLA status may be relevant to genetic counseling for certain multifactorial diseases. The relation of HLA haplotypes to disease and the use of this information in genetic counseling are referred to as which of the following?

a. Genetic linkage and the frequency of recombination
b. Allele association and risk modification
c. Positional cloning and gene isolation
d. Gene mapping and gene segregation
e. Genotyping and phenotypic correlation

467. Screening of an African American population in Minnesota yields allele frequencies of $^7/_8$ for the A globin allele and $^1/_8$ for the sickle globin allele. A companion survey of 6400 of these people's ancestors in central Africa reveals 4600 individuals with genotype AA, 1600 with genotype AS (sickle trait), and 200 with genotype SS (sickle cell disease—603903). Compared to their descendants in Minnesota, the African population has which of the following?

a. A lower frequency of AS genotypes consistent with inbreeding
b. A lower frequency of AS genotypes consistent with malarial exposure
c. A higher frequency of AS genotypes consistent with heterozygote advantage
d. A higher frequency of AS genotypes consistent with selection against the S allele
e. Identical A and S allele frequencies as predicted by the Hardy-Weinberg law

468. If all SS individuals in the Minnesota population were sterilized, the SS genotype frequency in the next generation would be which of the following?

a. Reduced by $^2/_3$
b. Reduced by $^1/_2$
c. Reduced by $^1/_3$
d. Reduced to 0
e. Approximately the same

469. A newborn infant presents with poor feeding, vomiting, jaundice, and an enlarged liver. The urine tests positive for reducing substances, indicating the presence of sugars with aldehyde groups. Which of the following processes is most likely to be abnormal?

a. Conversion of glucose to galactose
b. Conversion of lactose to galactose
c. Conversion of activated galactose to activated glucose
d. Excretion of glucose by the kidney
e. Excretion of galactose by the kidney

470. The frequency of galactosemia is approximately 1 in 40,000 live births. The frequency of the carrier state can be calculated as which of the following?

a. 1 in 50 live births
b. 1 in 100 live births
c. 1 in 200 live births
d. 1 in 500 live births
e. 1 in 1000 live births

471. A woman who has two brothers with hemophilia A (306700) and two normal sons is again pregnant. She requests counseling for the risk of her fetus to have hemophilia. What is the risk that her next child will have hemophilia?

a. 1
b. $\frac{1}{2}$
c. $\frac{1}{4}$
d. $\frac{1}{8}$
e. $\frac{1}{16}$

472. Which of the following statements about hemophilia A (306700) is true?

a. The extrinsic clotting pathway is impaired
b. The cleavage of fibrinogen is impaired
c. Tissue factor activation is impaired
d. Activation of factor XII is impaired
e. Activation of factor X is impaired

473. A woman who is at risk to be a carrier of hemophilia A desires prenatal diagnosis. She does not want her extended family to know about her pregnancy if the fetus is affected. Which of the following prenatal diagnostic techniques should be advised?

a. Amniocentesis with western blot analysis of factor VIII
b. Chorionic villus sampling with DNA analysis for factor VIII mutations
c. Percutaneous umbilical blood sampling with testing of factor VIII levels
d. Amniocentesis with DNA analysis for factor VIII mutations
e. Chorionic villus sampling with assay of factor VIII activity

474. The figure below shows a pedigree that includes individuals with Charcot-Marie-Tooth disease (CMT), a neurologic disorder that produces dysfunction of the distal extremities with characteristic footdrop. If individual III-4 becomes pregnant, what is her risk of having a child with CMT?

a. ½
b. ¼
c. ⅛
d. $\frac{1}{16}$
e. Virtually 0

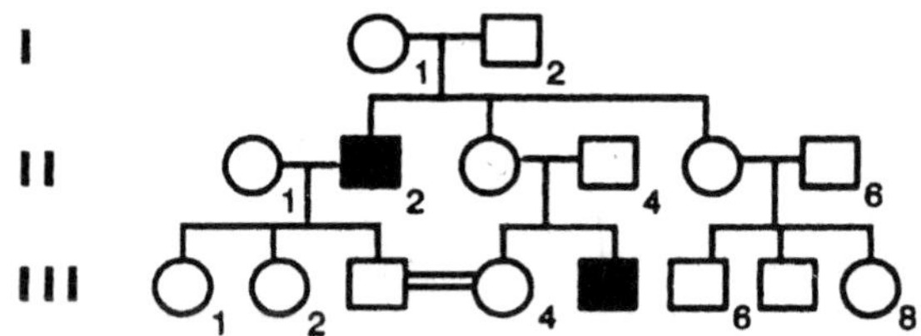

475. In another family with Charcot-Marie-Tooth disease (CMT), restriction analysis using sites flanking the CMT gene on 17 yields one large abnormal fragment and one smaller fragment that is seen in controls. What is the probable inheritance mechanism in this family?

a. X-linked recessive
b. Autosomal dominant
c. Autosomal recessive
d. Multifactorial
e. X-linked dominant

476. Prader-Willi syndrome involves a voracious appetite, obesity, short stature, hypogonadism, and mental disability. At least 50% of Prader-Willi patients have a small deletion on the proximal long arm of chromosome 15. In detecting the Prader-Willi deletion, which of the following techniques would be most accurate?

a. Standard karyotyping of peripheral blood leukocytes
b. Northern blotting of mRNAs transcribed from the deletion region
c. Restriction analysis to detect DNA fragments from the deletion region
d. Rapid karyotyping of bone marrow
e. Fluorescent in situ hybridization (FISH) analysis of peripheral blood lymphocytes using fluorescent DNA probes from the deleted region

477. A child is referred for evaluation because of low muscle tone and developmental delay. Shortly after delivery the child was a poor feeder and had to be fed by tube. In the second year, the child began to eat voraciously and became obese. He has a slightly unusual face with almond-shaped eyes and downturned corners of the mouth. The hands, feet, and penis are small, and the scrotum is poorly formed. The diagnostic category and laboratory test to be considered for this child are which of the following?

a. Sequence, serum testosterone
b. Single birth defect, serum testosterone
c. Deformation, karyotype
d. Syndrome, karyotype
e. Disruption, karyotype

478. A karyotype is performed on an obese child and is entirely normal. Because the physician suspects Prader-Willi syndrome, Southern blotting is performed to determine the origin of the patient's number 15 chromosomes. In the figure below, a hypothetical Southern blot with DNA probe D15S8 defines which of four restriction fragment length polymorphisms (RFLPs) are present in DNA from mother (M), child (C), and father (F). Based on the D15S8 locus, what is the origin of the child's two number 15 chromosomes?

a. One from the mother, one from the father
b. Both from the father
c. Both from the mother
d. From neither parent
e. Cannot tell because the locus is deleted in the child

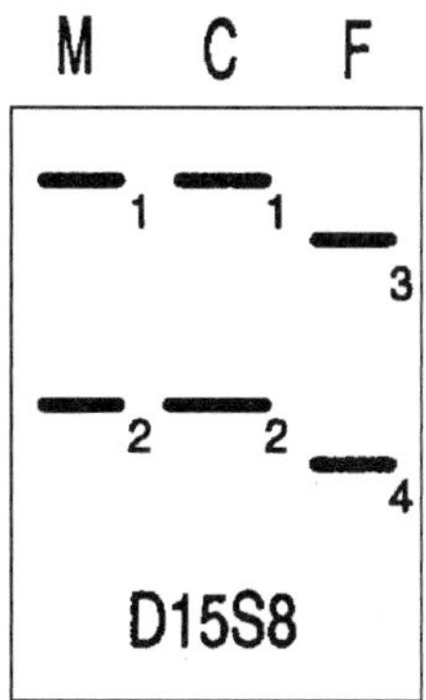

479. Because the figure in question 478 demonstrates that the child is missing both paternal chromosome 15 alleles, nonpaternity is a more plausible explanation than uniparental disomy. The hypothetical Southern blot shown below illustrates a DNA "fingerprinting" analysis to examine paternity, where maternal (M), child (C), and paternal (F) DNA samples have been restricted, blotted, and hybridized simultaneously to the probes D7Z5 and D20Z1. The distributions of restriction fragment alleles suggest which of the following?

a. The child is adopted
b. False maternity (i.e., baby switched in the nursery)
c. False paternity
d. Correct maternity and paternity
e. None of the above

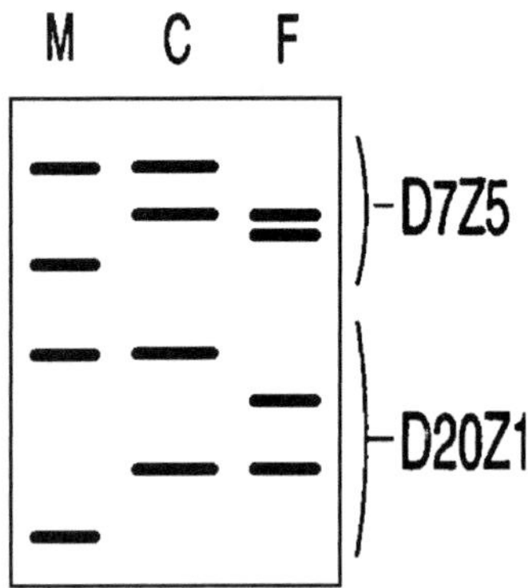

480. Many family studies employing DNA have the potential to demonstrate nonpaternity. If the physician ordering these analyses does not discuss this possibility with the couples involved, he or she is in violation of which of the following?

a. Patient confidentiality
b. Patient rights
c. Informed consent
d. Standards of care
e. Malpractice guidelines

481. The genesis of Prader-Willi syndrome by inheritance of two normal chromosomes from a single parent is an example of which of the following?

a. Germinal mosaicism
b. Genomic imprinting
c. Chromosome deletion
d. Chromosome rearrangement
e. Anticipation

482. A child with severe epilepsy, autistic behavior, and developmental delay has characteristics of a condition known as Angelman syndrome (105830). Because of the syndromic nature of the disorder and the developmental delay, a karyotype is performed that shows a missing band on one chromosome 15. Which of the following best describes this abnormality?

a. Interstitial deletion of 15
b. Terminal deletion of 15
c. Pericentric inversion of 15
d. Paracentric inversion of 15
e. $15q^-$

483. An infant with severe muscle weakness is born to a mother with mild muscle weakness and myotonia (sustained muscle contractions manifested clinically by the inability to release a handshake). The mother's father is even less affected, with some frontal baldness and cataracts. Worsening symptoms in affected individuals of successive generations suggest which of the following inheritance mechanisms?

a. Genomic imprinting
b. Heteroplasmy
c. Unstable trinucleotide repeats
d. Multifactorial inheritance
e. Mitochondrial inheritance

484. A child is born with spina bifida, a defect in the lower spinal cord and meninges that may cause bladder and lower limb dysfunction. The family history reveals that the father had a small spina bifida that was repaired by surgery. Which of the following is the most critical aspect of the medical evaluation as it pertains to genetic counseling?

a. A search for additional anomalies to determine if the child has a syndrome
b. A karyotype on the child
c. A serum folic acid level on the child
d. A spinal x-ray on the mother
e. A spinal x-ray on the father

485. Most isolated congenital anomalies exhibit which of the following?

a. Mendelian inheritance
b. Chromosomal inheritance
c. Multifactorial inheritance
d. Maternal inheritance
e. Atypical inheritance

486. Spina bifida exhibits female predilection and recurrence risks of 3% for first-degree relatives and 0.5% for second-degree relatives. A father and child have spina bifida, but the mother is normal. What is the risk that the couple's next child will have spina bifida?

a. >1%
b. <1%
c. >6%
d. <6%
e. 10%

487. Neural tube defects, such as spina bifida and anencephaly, are best diagnosed by which of the following laboratory tests?

a. Chorionic villus biopsy and karyotype at 10 weeks after the last menstrual period (LMP)
b. Maternal serum α-fetoprotein (MSAFP) levels and ultrasound at 16 weeks after conception
c. Amniotic fluid α-fetoprotein (AFP) levels and ultrasound at 16 weeks after the LMP
d. Amniotic fluid acetylcholinesterase levels at 16 weeks after conception
e. Amniotic fluid karyotype and ultrasound at 16 weeks after the LMP

488. Every prenatal evaluation should include which of the following diagnostic procedures?

a. Level I ultrasound
b. Chorionic villus sampling (CVS)
c. Doppler analysis
d. Amniocentesis
e. Genetic counseling

489. A couple has a child who has been diagnosed with medium-chain acyl coenzyme A (CoA) dehydrogenase deficiency (MCAD), a condition that affects the body's ability to metabolize medium-chain fatty acids. This couple is now expecting another child. What is the risk that this child will have MCAD?

a. $\frac{2}{3}$
b. $\frac{1}{2}$
c. $\frac{1}{3}$
d. $\frac{1}{4}$
e. $\frac{1}{5}$

490. A 1-year-old child develops fever and vomiting and is unable to keep food down for 2 days. The physical examination discloses no congenital anomalies, and the baby resembles his parents. Which of the following laboratory findings are most likely if the child has a disorder of fatty acid oxidation?

a. Hypoglycemia, acidosis, and elevated urine dicarboxylic acids
b. Alkalosis and elevated serum ammonia
c. Acidosis and elevated urine reducing substances
d. Hypoglycemia, acidosis, and elevated serum leucine, isoleucine, and valine
e. Hepatomegaly, elevated serum liver enzymes, and elevated tyrosine

491. Laboratory tests on a sick child reveal a low white blood cell count, metabolic acidosis, increased anion gap, and mild hyperammonemia. Measurement of plasma amino acids reveals elevated levels of glycine, and measurement of urinary organic acids reveals increased amounts of propionic acid and methyl citrate. Which of the following processes is most likely?

a. Diabetes mellitus
b. A fatty acid oxidation disorder
c. Vitamin B_{12} deficiency
d. Propionic acidemia
e. A disorder in glycine catabolism

492. In the treatment of propionic acidemia, which of the following is contraindicated?

a. Antibiotics
b. A diet high in fatty acids
c. Caloric supplementation
d. Aggressive fluid and electrolyte management
e. Hemodialysis

493. DNA analysis is performed on a family because the first child has propionic acidemia. The parents desire prenatal diagnosis, and the fetal DNA is also analyzed for polymorphic alleles A and B that are linked to the causative mutation (see the figure below). The results are shown below. Which of the following risk figures reflect the risk of the fetus being affected before and after testing?

a. $\frac{1}{2}$, virtually 0
b. $\frac{1}{4}$, $\frac{2}{3}$
c. $\frac{1}{4}$, $\frac{1}{2}$
d. $\frac{1}{4}$, $\frac{2}{3}$
e. $\frac{1}{4}$, virtually 0

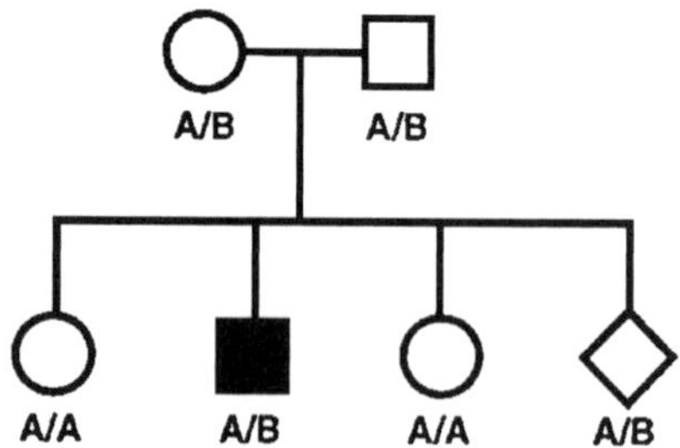

494. Neonatal screening is mandated in all states, but examines different numbers of diseases. Most commonly tested are phenylketonuria (PKU—261600), galactosemia (230400), congenital hypothyroidism, and sickle cell anemia (603903). Recently, a supplemental newborn screen using tandem mass spectrometry is being adopted by many states, allowing recognition of the more common organic acidemias and fatty acid oxidation disorders. Which of the following is the most important characteristic to qualify a disorder for newborn screening?

a. A highly accurate diagnostic test
b. A high frequency of disease
c. An advantage for treatment from early diagnosis
d. Use of microbial technology like the Guthrie method
e. A minimal incidence of false positive tests

495. The development of DNase therapy has dramatically improved survival and frequency/severity of lung infections in children with cystic fibrosis (219700). Over 30 common mutant alleles for Caucasions with cystic fibrosis have now been characterized at the DNA level, allowing screening of pregnant couples with high sensitivity. Which of the following techniques will be required for newborn screening of cystic fibrosis or other diseases using DNA-based technology?

a. Fluorescent *in situ* hybridization (FISH) for deletions surrounding the disease locus
b. Subtelomeric FISH analysis
c. DNA array or chip analysis
d. Southern analysis to display mutant alleles
e. Comparative genomic hybridization (CGH)

496. Which of the following is most likely in an untreated child with PKU?

a. Elevated tyrosine
b. Increased skin pigmentation
c. Decreased skin pigmentation
d. Normal phenylalanine hydroxylase levels
e. Elevated alanine

497. A newborn presents with ambiguous genitalia, having an enlarged clitoris or small phallus and labial fusion or hypoplastic scrotum. The newborn's sex can most reliably be established by which of the following?

a. Buccal smear to determine if there are one or two Barr bodies
b. Buccal smear to determine if there is one Barr body or none
c. Peripheral blood karyotype
d. Bone marrow karyotype
e. Polymerase chain reaction (PCR) using primers specific for the long arm of the Y chromosome

498. The dot-blot shown below examines DNA from a child with ambiguous genitalia after polymerase chain reaction (PCR) amplification and hybridization with DNA probes from the X and Y chromosome. In this case, the Y chromosome probe is from the SRY region of Yp that has recently been characterized as the male-determining region. DNA from control male and female patients is also applied to the dot-blot. Based on the dot-blot results, which is the most likely conclusion?

a. The proband is a genetic male
b. The proband is a genetic female
c. The proband is male
d. The proband is female
e. The proband is mosaic 46,XX/46,XY

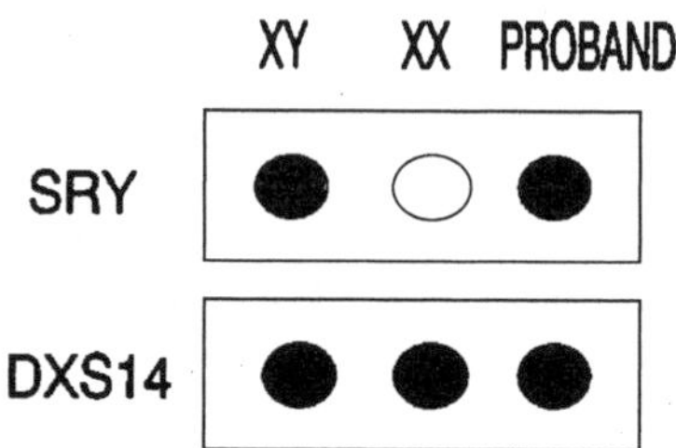

499. A child has ambiguous genitalia including an apparent small phallus and scrotum. The child's DNA hybridizes to probes from the sex-determining region of the Y (SRY). Based on the clinical findings and dot-blot analysis, which of the following terms applies?

a. Female pseudohermaphroditism
b. Male pseudohermaphroditism
c. True hermaphroditism
d. XY female
e. XX male

500. A newborn with ambiguous genitalia and a 46,XY karyotype develops vomiting, low serum sodium concentration, and high serum potassium. Which of the following proteins is most likely to be abnormal?

a. 21-hydroxylase
b. An ovarian enzyme
c. 5β-reductase
d. An androgen receptor
e. A testicular enzyme

Genetic and Biochemical Diagnosis

Answers

435. The answer is a. *(Lewis, pp 135–154. Scriver, pp 1366–1368.)* Parkinson disease shows some evidence of genetic predisposition that rules out pure environmental causation. It has higher incidence in identical twins and siblings than in the genetic population, but is puzzing because the identical twin concordance rate should be higher than that for siblings with multifactorial determination. The data suggest some type of selection against affected twins, or at least decreased ascertainment of affected twins (usually affected twins are notable and better ascertained in such studies). The most reasonable extrapolation from the data is that Parkinson disease is a multifactorial disorder in many instances, and that a 2–3% risk for primary or first-degree relatives (siblings) would imply the same risk for offspring of affected parents. Current research approaches to complex diseases include genome-wide searches for single nucleotide polymorphisms (SNPs occurring very 2–300 bp in human DNA) that associate with the phenotype. Given the connection of Parkinson disease with low dopamine, looking at SNPs near loci encoding enzymes of the phenylalanine/tyrosine/catecholamine/dopamine pathway would be a reasonable start. If a G for C nucleotide substitution was present in a certain allele, and a majority of those with Parkinson disease were G/G homozygotes or G/C heterozygotes, than the G SNP becomes a DNA marker for Parkinsonism susceptibility—more than 10 such loci have been found (168601). Another approach is to examine rare familial forms of Parkinsonism (e.g., 168601) for insights into disease causation, just as study of familial hypercholesterolemia (144010) highlighted elevated cholesterol as a risk factor for coronary artery disease.

436. The answer is c. *(Lewis, pp 397–416. Scriver, pp 1667–1724. Murray, pp 264–269.)* Dopamine is produced from L-dopa, which in turn is made from tyrosine. Therapy with the L-dopa precursor increases dopamine concentrations and improves the rigidity and immobility that occur in Parkinson disease. Dopamine is degraded in the synaptic cleft by monoamine oxidases A and B (MAO-A and MAO-B), producing 3,4-dihydroxyphenylacetaldehyde (DOPAC). DOPAC is in turn broken down to homovanillic acid, which can be measured in spinal fluid to assess dopamine metabolism. Inhibitors of MAO-A and MAO-B have some use in treating Parkinson disease. The metabolism of histidine or alanine is not related to that of dopamine, but phenylalanine is a precursor of tyrosine and L-dopa.

437. The answer is d. *(Lewis, pp 397–416. Scriver, pp 225–258. Murray, pp 396–414.)* A family history is an important precedent for anesthesia, and awareness of individual differences is important when administering any drug. Pharmacogenetics is the area of study that examines genetic influences on drug metabolism. The extensive human genetic variation revealed by DNA analysis has important implications for pharmacology, since drug effects often vary according to each patient's unique genome.

438. The answer is b. *(Lewis, pp 361–391. Murray, pp 396–414. Scriver, pp 233–238.)* Succinylcholine is metabolized by a plasma enzyme formerly called pseudocholinesterase [now called butyrylcholinesterase (BChE) to designate its favored substrate]. Approximately 1 in 100 individuals are homozygous for a variant of BChE that has 60% activity, whereas 1 in 150,000 individuals are homozygous for a variant with 33% activity. The latter group exhibits prolonged recovery from succinylcholine-induced anesthesia, a phenotype known as succinylcholine apnea (177400). As with most enzyme defects, succinylcholine apnea exhibits autosomal recessive inheritance. The parents will be heterozygous for a BChE variant but have not undergone anesthesia to display the phenotype.

439. The answer is b. *(Lewis, pp 267–282. Murray, pp 396–414. Scriver, pp 233–238.)* The Hardy-Weinberg law specifies that the distribution of genotypes, given frequencies of normal (p) and abnormal (q) alleles in an ideal population, will be p^2 for homozygous normal, 2pq for heterozygotes, and q^2 for homozygous abnormal. If the heterozygote frequence for butyrylcholinesterase variant alleles is 4 per 100 = 2pq, then pq = $^2/_{100}$. Since the frequency of abnormal alleles (q) is usually much less than that of normal (p), one can approximate p to 1 and assume q = 2 per 100 with q = $^4/_{10,000}$ or 1 in 2500. As a simplification, one can calculate carrier rates as the square root of disease incidence for autosomal recessive disorders. The proportion of individuals with susceptibility to severe consequences of anesthesia (1 in 2500) is similar to frequencies of common genetic diseases in Caucasions like cystic fibrosis (219700) and certainly deserves consideration for genetic screening.

440. The answer is e. *(Scriver, pp 5559–5586. Lewis, pp 377–396. Murray, pp 21–29.)* Serum protein electrophoresis separates proteins according to their structure and charge. Two bands for AAT in this man imply that two types of AAT protein with different structures or charges are present. The electrophoresis does not reveal whether the abnormal AAT protein has normal or abnormal activity. The McKusick number indicates that AAT deficiency is autosomal dominant, implying that two homologous loci encode AAT proteins. The man is thus heterozygous, one locus encoding a normal and one an abnormal protein. The AAT locus is located on chromosome 14 within a family of protease inhibitors called serpins. Altered AAT proteins termed M, S, or Z variants have normal inhibitory activity but are defective in their rates of secretion across the liver membrane into the blood. Lower levels of AAT protein apparently expose lung proteins to damage, causing emphysema. Heterozygotes are usually not affected, so the man may have emphysema because of cigarette smoking or other factors. Homozygous ZZ individuals may have liver disease in addition to lung disease because the abnormally secreted AAT accumulates in liver cells.

441. The answer is b. *(Lewis, pp 75–94. Scriver, pp 3827–3876.)* Metabolic diseases usually exhibit autosomal or X-linked recessive inheritance. Autosomal recessive inheritance is most likely because the affected patient is female. In this case, the parents are obligate carriers and there is a one-fourth chance (25% recurrence risk) that their next child will be affected. The symptoms suggest Tay-Sachs disease (272800), an autosomal recessive disorder involving severe neurodegeneration and early death.

442. The answer is b. *(Lewis, pp 75–94. Scriver, pp 3827–3876. Murray, pp 197–204.)* The lysosomal enzyme hexosaminidase A is deficient in Tay-Sachs disease. The enzyme cleaves aminohexose groups from gangliosides, complex lipids formed from ceramide (a derivative of sphingosine). Ceramide is synthesized in the endoplasmic reticulum from palmitoyl coenzyme A (16-carbon acyl CoA) and serine in a reaction catalyzed by pyridoxal phosphate. Uridine diphosphoglucose (UDP-glucose) or UDP-galactose moieties and sialic acid groups are then added in the Golgi apparatus and the gangliosides contribute to myelin in nerve cells. Neurolipidoses like Tay-Sachs disease lack certain lysosomal enzymes necessary to degrade the gangliosides, causing severe effects on nerve cells (neuro-degeneration). A parallel group of disorders called mucopolysaccharidoses result from the absence of lysosomal enzymes that degrade complex carbohydrate chains and their associated proteins (called proteoglycans). Proteoglycans are more widely distributed than gangliosides, occurring in the ground substance of many tissues.

Accumulation of the glycosaminoglycans from these proteoglycans thus causes a wide spectrum of symptoms including coarsening of the face and hair, cardiopulmonary problems, and bony deformities such as kyphosis (beaked spine). There is a specific lysosomal receptor that recognizes mannose-6-phosphate on certain lysosomal enzymes and targets them to lysosomes. Mutations in this receptor can cause increased blood levels and lysosomal deficiencies of several enzymes that are normally targeted to lysosomes. One such disease is I (inclusion) cell disease (252500). The slow accumulation of abnormal gangliosides in lipidoses and of abnormal proteoglycans in mucopolysaccharidoses causes a characteristic clinical course of normal early development that plateaus and then regresses. The age of regression and lifespan vary widely among the lysosomal storage diseases, with Tay-Sachs being one of the most severe.

443. The answer is e. *(Lewis, pp 75–94, 267–282. Scriver, pp 3827–3876.)* To determine the joint probability of two or more independent events, the product of their separate probabilities must be determined. If the parents were both Ashkenazi Jews, they would have a $^1/_{30}$ chance of carrying an abnormal gene for Tay-Sachs disease; for each pregnancy, they would have a $^1/_2$ chance of passing that gene along should they carry it. The probability that all of these four independent events would occur is $^1/_{30} \times ^1/_2 \times ^1/_{30} \times ^1/_2 = ^1/_{3600}$. The joint probability for a mother who is an Ashkenazi Jew and a father who is not is $^1/_{30} \times ^1/_2 \times ^1/_{300} \times ^1/_2 = ^1/_{36,000}$.

444. The answer is c. *(Lewis, pp 75–94, 267–282. Scriver, pp 3827–3876.)* The probability that any one sibling is homozygous normal is one-third.The human leukocyte antigen (HLA) cluster on chromosome 6 consists of several loci that are each highly polymorphic. Because the loci are clustered together, their polymorphic products form haplotypes (i.e., A1-B8-DR2 on one chromosome and A9-B5-DR3 on another chromosome).

Since recombination among HLA loci is unlikely, the chances of two siblings being HLA-identical are essentially those of inheriting the same parental chromosomes, that is, $\frac{1}{4}$. The chance for a sibling to be both homozygous normal for Tay-Sachs disease and HLA-compatible is $\frac{1}{3} \times \frac{1}{4} = \frac{1}{12}$. Since there are three siblings, the total chance is $\frac{1}{12} \times 3 = \frac{1}{4}$.

445. The answer is e. *(Lewis, pp 397–416. Scriver, pp 3827–3876.)* The physician is obligated to describe a patient's disease accurately in the medical record and to share such records with legally entitled entities, such as health insurance companies. Although care should be exercised that records containing confidential information are not shared inappropriately, there was no such breach of confidentiality in this case. If the physician had declined further care without appropriate notice, then this would be a breach of ongoing care. However, insurance companies and managed care plans have excluded patients because of prior conditions or excessive expenses (i.e., capitation limits). This does constitute discrimination, but application of the Americans with Disabilities Act to patients with genetic diseases is not yet routine. These dilemmas will grow dramatically with the increasing ability to test for genetic diseases and predispositions. Although the administration of exogenous normal enzyme (enzyme therapy) or transplantation to provide a cellular source of normal enzyme has been successful in correcting lysosomal deficiencies, the enzymes fail to cross the blood-brain barrier in sufficient amounts to remit neurological symptoms in patients with lipidoses. This form of enzyme therapy has the advantage of targeting the defective organelle via the mannose-6-phosphate residues on the enzyme. It is very expensive but effective in lipidoses that have few neurological symptoms, such as Gaucher disease (230800).

446. The answer is a. *(Lewis, pp 397–416. Scriver, pp 3827–3876.)* Most enzymes are expressed in chorionic villi or amniocytes and allow prenatal diagnosis of metabolic disorders through cell culture and enzyme assay. Percutaneous umbilical blood sampling (PUBS), or cordocentesis, offers another strategy if the enzyme is normally present in leukocytes. However, transabdominal aspiration of the umbilical cord is difficult and must be performed later in pregnancy (18+ weeks) than CVS (8–10 weeks). α-fetoprotein (AFP) is not known to be involved in any metabolic disorders, but it is used as an index of fetal tissue differentiation and integrity. Amniotic or maternal serum α-fetoprotein (MSAFP) is most often used to detect, respectively, neural tube defects or chromosomal disorders and would not be useful in a case of normal fetal development with hexosaminidase A deficiency.

447. The answer is c. *(Lewis, pp 377–396. Scriver, pp 5287–5312.)* Although a mutation at a single locus generally alters a single gene, the result being the abnormal synthesis or lack of production of a single RNA molecule or polypeptide chain, the results of this mutation may be far-reaching. When there are multiple phenotypic effects involving multiple systems, the result is referred to as pleiotropy. Penetrance is the all-or-none expression of an abnormal genotype, whereas expressivity is the degree of expression of that genotype. Incomplete or reduced penetrance implies that some individuals have a mutant allele with absolutely no phenotypic expression of that allele. Variable expressivity implies that all individuals with a mutant allele have some phenotypic effects, although the severity and range of effects differ in different people. Marfan syndrome (154700) exhibits pleiotropy of its single-gene mutation by causing lens dislocation, loose connective tissue (joint laxity, tall stature, sternal and vertebral deformities), and fragile aortic tissue that can lead to aortic valve insufficiency or aortic dissection. Individuals with the disease exhibit variable combinations and severity of these symptoms due to variable expressivity of this single gene.

448. The answer is c. *(Lewis, pp 377–396. Scriver, pp 5287–5312. Murray, pp 539–540.)* Mutations in structural proteins often exhibit autosomal dominant inheritance, while mutations in enzymes often exhibit autosomal recessive inheritance. Structural proteins such as collagen or fibrillin must interact to form scaffolds in the extracellular matrix of connective tissue. Mutation at one of the homologous autosomal loci can introduce an abnormal polypeptide throughout the scaffold much like a misshapen brick in a wall—the distorted polypeptide from the abnormal locus subverts that from the normal locus and weakens the connective tissue matrix, causing autosomal dominant disease. Sometimes the abnormal polypeptide complexes with normal polypeptides and causes them to be degraded, a mechanism called protein suicide. The suicidal effects of mutations at some loci are referred to generally as "dominant negative" mutations. Fibrillin is a glycoprotein used to form a scaffold in the connective tissue filaments called microfibrils. It is distributed in the suspensory ligament for the lens of the eye, the aorta, and the bones and joints, accounting for the symptoms of Marfan syndrome (154700). Similar pathogenetic mechanisms occur in the osteogenesis imperfectas (e.g., 166200) with multiple fractures and in the Ehlers-Danlos syndromes (e.g., 130060) with skin fragility (scarring) and vascular disease due to mutations in various collagens. The mutations disrupt the α-helix secondary structure of collagens, which is dependent on the glycine-X-Y triplet amino acid repeats; the distorted collagen polypeptides then disrupt the collagen fibrils with symptoms dependent on its tissue distribution (2 types of fibrillin and more than 15 types of collagen are known).

449. The answer is b. *(Lewis, pp 377–396. Scriver, pp 5241–5286. Murray, pp 396–414.)* The spectrum of mutations in collagen (and fibrillin) disorders is very broad, making it more efficient to evaluate electrophoretic mobility of their polypeptide chains as a clue to structural abnormality. Almost every patient with osteogenesis imperfecta (and other collagen disorders) has a different type of mutation. PCR amplification followed by allele-specific oligonucleotide (ASO) hybridation to detect specific alleles is thus impractical—hundreds of PCR/ASO reactions would be required to screen for all of the possible mutant alleles. Similarly, DNA sequencing would be extraordinarily time-consuming and give many false positives due to nucleotide polymorphisms or silent mutations that do not cause structural abnormalities in the polypeptide. Northern blotting would detect mutations that affect RNA processing and generate RNAs of altered size, but these are a small fraction of possible collagen mutations. As DNA chip technology becomes practical, screening for thousands of mutations at a locus may be possible. DNA chips contain thousands of different oligonucleotides embedded on a solid matrix. Hybridization of colored or labeled gene fragments with randomized sequences from that gene on a chip gives signals corresponding to the gene sequences that are present. The chip can then be washed and used again. Hybridization of the chip with suitably digested DNAs from patients and controls can thus detect any variant gene fragment (complementary oligonucleotide). Use of numerous control DNAs would separate true mutant alleles (sequence variants associated with disease) from polymorphisms or silent mutations.

450. The answer is b. *(Lewis, pp 355–376. Scriver, pp 521–524. Murray, pp 314–340.)* The two-hit hypothesis was developed by Knudsen to explain why patients with hereditary retinoblastoma [germ-line mutations (180200)] have multiple, bilateral tumors while those with sporadic tumors (no family history) have single tumors. A germ-line mutation (first hit) alters one Rb allele and confers enhanced susceptibility to retinoblastoma. A somatic mutation (second hit) inactivating the other homologous Rb allele can then occur in any tissue. If it occurs in the retina, a tumor is born. The multiple tumors thus represent the sites at which somatic mutations have occurred in the retina. In sporadic cases, two somatic mutational events must take place. Since these somatic mutations are relatively rare events, it is extremely uncommon for more than one tumor to develop. It is curious that, although retinoblastoma susceptibility is inherited in a dominant fashion, tumor development is a recessive event, requiring the inactivation of both alleles. Genes such as Rb are called tumor suppressor genes, in contrast to oncogenes, in which only one of the two homologous alleles must be altered to initiate malignant transformation. Alteration of an enhancer or promoter site on one Rb allele would thus not be sufficient to cause cancer, since the other Rb allele would not be affected. Obvious chromosome changes such as 13q–are rare compared to other mutations that alter Rb function.

451. The answer is a. *(Lewis, pp 355–376. Scriver, pp 521–552. Murray, pp 396–414.)* Chromosome translocations may often promote tumors in somatic cells by placing regulatory genes next to promoters that aberrantly increase their expression. Burkitt lymphoma, a B cell lymphoma that usually occurs in childhood, often involves reciprocal translocation of chromosomes 8 and 14. The result of this is to place the c-myc protooncogene from 8q24 into the immunoglobulin heavy chain locus at 14q32. Because immunoglobulin genes are actively transcribed, this move alters the normal regulatory control of c-myc. Another example is the Philadelphia chromosome, a shortened chromosome 22 caused by translocation t(9:22)(q34:q11). This translocation is seen in almost all patients with chronic myelogenous leukemia (CML) and in a percentage of patients with acute lymphoblastic leukemia (ALL). The Philadelphia chromosome is seen with increased frequency in individuals with Down syndrome.

452. The answer is b. *(Lewis, pp 355–376. Scriver, pp 521–552. Murray, pp 396–414.)* Genetic predisposition to cancer is best understood by the Knudsen hypothesis, where two independent mutations or "hits" are required to produce neoplasia of a somatic tissue. In many hereditary cancers, the "first hit" is a germ-line mutation that is transmitted in families. Individuals who inherit this mutation are much more likely to develop cancer through a "second hit" in their somatic cells. The second hit can be any mutation that removes the homologous allele (loss of heterozygosity); mechanisms include missense mutation, chromosome deletion, and chromosome nondisjunction. For tumor suppressor genes like those responsible for neurofibromatosis 1 (162200) or the Li-Fraumeni syndrome (114480), the first hit removes one suppressor allele and the second hit removes the homologous suppressor allele. The family in the question is an example of a "cancer family" that exhibits the bone, breast, colon, and blood cancers that are typical of Li-Fraumeni syndrome. The mechanism involves mutations in the src tumor suppressor gene.

453. The answer is d. *(Lewis, pp 355–376. Scriver, pp 521–552. Murray, pp 396–414.)* Presymptomatic DNA testing of individuals in cancer families is increasingly available. However, testing of minors is controversial because they may not be old or mature enough to understand the personal, medical, and financial implications. They therefore cannot give truly informed consent. Beneficence is the ethical imperative to do good for patients, while nonmaleficence is the imperative to do no harm. Autonomy refers to a patient's right to make decisions regarding his or her health care, and confidentiality to the privilege of doctor-patient communication.

454. The answer is d. *(Lewis, pp 135–154. Scriver, pp 2863–2914. Murray, pp 219–230.)* This man has familial hypercholesterolemia (143890), an autosomal dominant phenotype defined by studying men who experienced heart attacks at young ages. Mutations in the LDL receptor lead to decreased cellular cholesterol uptake and increased serum cholesterol. Since LDL has a high cholesterol content, the LDL fraction is elevated compared to the HDL fraction on lipoprotein electrophoresis. In normal individuals, the LDL is taken up by its specific receptor and imported via caveolae to the cell interior. Cholesterol then produces feedback inhibition on the rate-limiting enzyme of cholesterol synthesis (hydroxymethylglutaryl CoA reductase) and also leads to a decrease in the number of LDL receptors. In rare cases, two individuals with familial hypercholesterolemia marry and produce a child with homozygous familial hypercholesterolemia. These children develop severe atherosclerosis and xanthomas (fatty tumors) at an early age.

455. The answer is c. *(Lewis, pp 135–154. Scriver, pp 2863–2914. Murray, pp 219–230.)* Nitroglycerin causes release of nitric oxide (NO), which activates guanyl cyclase, produces cyclic GMP, and causes vasodilation. NO is formed from one of the guanidino nitrogens of the arginine side chain by the enzyme nitric oxide synthase. NO has a short half-life, reacting with oxygen to form nitrite and then nitrates that are excreted in urine. Coronary vasodilation caused by nitroglycerin is thus short-lived, making other measures necessary for long-term relief of coronary occlusion. The neurotransmitter formed by condensation of acetyl CoA and choline is acetylcholine, which does not play a role in dilation of coronary arteries.

456. The answer is c. *(Lewis, pp 135–154. Scriver, pp 2961–3062. Murray, pp 481–497.)* The symptoms are typical of iron-deficiency anemia, in this case caused by increased blood loss through menstruation. Transferrin is a glycoprotein that transports iron among tissues. Its amounts in serum can be measured as the total iron-binding capacity. Under conditions of iron deficiency, the percentage of transferrin saturated with iron (normally about 33%) is decreased. A specific transferrin receptor brings the iron-ferritin complex into cells, and it is regulated in response to iron stores. When iron is deficient, the number of transferrin receptors is increased. Ferritin is a protein that stores iron in tissues and is minimally present in serum unless there is iron excess. About 10% of the hemoglobin released by normal red cell destruction is bound by haptoglobin. The remainder is salvaged from damaged red cells that are degraded in the reticuloendothelial system. Haptoglobins are decreased in hemolytic anemias in which there is increased release of hemoglobin.

457. The answer is d. *(Lewis, pp 377–396. Scriver, pp 3127–3162. Murray, pp 580–597.)* The man has symptoms of hemochromatosis (235200), an autosomal recessive disorder with increased iron absorption from the small intestine. There is increased serum iron, higher saturation of transferrin, and increased amounts of ferritin-iron complex so that it appears in serum. The red cell lifetime is normal in hemochromatosis, resulting in normal release of hemoglobin and normal serum haptoglobin. Hemochromatosis is caused by mutations at a locus in the histocompatibility region of chromosome 6; the protein product is localized to the small intestine and influences iron absorption by an unknown mechanism.

458. The answer is d. *(Lewis, pp 377–396. Murray, pp 580–597. Scriver, pp 3127–3162.)* The regulation of mammalian gene expression is selective: specific genes are up- or downregulated by controls at the gene dosage, mRNA transcription, mRNA splicing, mRNA stability, or protein function levels. Under conditions of iron deficiency, transferrin receptor mRNA is stabilized so that more protein is synthesized. Regulation thus occurs at the protein translation level, without changes in transferrin mRNA transcription through transcription factors or transferrin receptor activity through interaction with small molecules (allostery) or through phosphorylation by protein kinases. Overall increases in rates of RNA transcription or protein elongation are not employed for gene regulation by mammalian cells.

459. The answer is b. *(Lewis, pp 377–396. Murray, pp 481–497. Scriver, pp 3105–3126.)* This child's kinky hair is a symptom of Menke disease, an alteration in a copper-binding ATPase. Dysfunction of the ATPase imprisons copper in cells and prevents its normal absorption from the intestine. Enzymes that use copper as cofactor have diverse roles in metabolism, including some that modify and degrade amino acids in collagen. This accounts for the connective tissue symptoms (lax joints, thin skin) in Menke disease. Wilson disease (277900) is also caused by mutations in a copper-binding ATPase that lead to copper storage in liver (causing hepatitis and cirrhosis) and the brain (sometimes causing psychosis). Ceruloplasmin, the major copper transporter in serum, is decreased in both diseases.

460. The answer is e. *(Lewis, pp 241–266. Scriver, pp 3–45.)* Contiguous gene syndromes, also known as microdeletion syndromes, occur when deletions result in the loss of several different closely linked loci. Depending on the size of the deletion, different phenotypes may result. Mutations in the individual genes may result in isolated features that may be inherited in a Mendelian fashion.

461. The answer is c. *(Lewis, pp 95–112. Scriver, pp 5467–5492.)* Polycystic kidney disease (173900) occurs in two distinctive genetic forms—adult-onset and infantile. Infantile disease is autosomal recessive, whereas adult-onset disease is autosomal dominant. Confusion between these types can occur due to variable expressivity in the adult, dominant form. Occasional onset in young children may occur in adult-type disease. Consistency of early onset, the presence of consanguinity, and the lack of vertical transmission distinguish the infantile, recessive form. Polycystic kidney disease is an example of genetic heterogeneity, in which different mutations may cause similar phenotypes. This may be further divided into allelic and nonallelic (locus) heterogeneity. Allelic heterogeneity implies that there are different mutations at the same locus that both result in similar disease [i.e., the many fibrillin mutations in Marfan syndrome (154700)]. In locus heterogeneity, mutations occur at different loci, yet the phenotype is similar. Locus heterogeneity also explains why certain disorders, such as polycystic kidney disease, Charcot-Marie-Tooth disease, sensorineural hearing loss, and retinitis pigmentosa may be inherited in several different fashions. A general rule predicts that the autosomal recessive forms of these diseases will be more severe, the autosomal dominant forms less so. It is especially important to recognize the possibility of genetic heterogeneity when counseling patients in regard to recurrence risks.

462. The answer is a. *(Lewis, pp 75–94. Scriver, pp 2537–2570. Murray, pp 293–302.)* The child has Lesch-Nyhan syndrome (308000), an X-linked recessive disorder that is caused by HGPRT enzyme deficiency. HGPRT is responsible for the salvage of purines from nucleotide degradation, and its deficiency elevates levels of PRPP, purine synthesis, and uric acid. PRPP is also elevated in glycogen storage diseases due to increased amounts of carbohydrate precursors.

463. The answer is e. *(Lewis, pp 377–396. Scriver, pp 2537–2570.)* Polymorphic DNA regions with variable numbers of tandem repeats (VNTRs) yield an assortment of DNA fragment sizes after restriction endonuclease digestion. The visualization of variable fragments (alleles) from a particular VNTR region can be performed by hybridization with a DNA probe after electrophoresis and transfer (Southern blotting). If the VNTR region is near (linked to) a disease locus, the VNTR alleles can be used to determine which accompanying allele at the disease locus is present. Transmission of VNTR allele B to the affected individual III-3 in the figure that accompanies the question (Fig. 50) establishes phase and indicates that the abnormal Lesch-Nyhan (L-N) allele is cosegregating with VNTR allele B in this family. Individual I-1 is an obligate carrier because both II-4 and III-3 received abnormal L-N alleles (the rare chance of two L-N mutations in one family is discounted). Individuals II-2 and II-3 are thus carriers by virtue of inheriting the B allele from their mother. Individual III-2 is not a carrier because she did not inherit the B allele, and her fetus is not at risk for L-N. These conclusions do not reflect the possibility of recombination between the VNTR allele and the abnormal L-N allele. If one of the affected individuals had a common mutant allele that could be detected by direct analysis of the HGPRT gene, then fetal DNA analysis could be performed without concern about recombination.

464. The answer is b. *(Lewis, pp 241–266. Scriver, pp 3–45.)* The child described in the question has multiple independent anomalies that are characteristic of a syndrome. Although they are likely to be causally related, they do not appear to be sequential. These problems do not appear to be caused by the breakdown of an originally normal developmental process as in a disruption, nor do they appear to be related to a nondisruptive mechanical force as in a deformation.

465. The answer is c. *(Lewis, pp 241–266. Scriver, pp 3–45.)* Fluorescent in situ hybridization (FISH) analysis is a technique in which molecular probes that are specific for individual chromosomes or chromosomal regions are used to identify these regions. FISH probes frequently identify chromosomal regions that are submicroscopic and therefore may be useful when standard karyotypic analysis is normal. In this case, the fact that only one signal is present, despite the fact that there are two number 22 chromosomes, indicates that a submicroscopic deletion has occurred. The parental chromosome of origin cannot be determined using this technique unless that parent also carries a similar deletion and his or her chromosomes are evaluated. Submicroscopic deletion at band 22q11 causes a spectrum of disorders ranging from DiGeorge anomaly to Shprintzen syndrome (192430).

466. The answer is b. *(Lewis, pp 135–154. Scriver, pp 193–202.)* Individuals affected with autoimmune disorders such as juvenile diabetes mellitus, ankylosing spondylitis, or rheumatoid arthritis often have increased frequencies of particular HLA alleles, termed allele associations. Genetic linkage differs from allele association in that the linking of allele and phenotype depends on the family context; one family may exhibit segregation of the nail-patella phenotype with allele A of the ABO blood group, whereas another family exhibits segregation with allele O. Allele association or linkage disequilibrium implies that the same allele is always seen at higher frequency in affected individuals from different families (e.g., HLA-B27 in ankylosing spondylitis). Allele association implies neither a genotype-phenotype relation between allele and disease nor a common chromosomal location for allele and disease. It may indicate a role for the allele in facilitating disease pathogenesis. In contrast, genetic linkage places a disease gene on the chromosome map, facilitating its isolation by positional cloning. Gene mutations in various individuals can then be characterized, allowing genotype-phenotype correlations. HLA testing for autoimmune disorders, like cholesterol testing for heart disease, exemplifies the use of risk factors to modify risks for multifactorial diseases.

467. The answer is c. *(Lewis, pp 267–282. Scriver, pp 4571–4636.)* Under certain conditions, the Hardy-Weinberg law allows one to interconvert genotype and allele frequencies in a population by using the formula $(p + q)^2 = p^2 + 2pq + q^2$. For a locus with two alleles, p represents the frequency of the more common allele, q of the less common allele, and $p + q = 1$. The Minnesota population therefore has $p^2 = 7/8 \times 7/8 = 49/64$ (4900 individuals) with the AA genotype, $2pq = 2 \times 7/8 \times 1/8 = 14/64$ (1400 individuals) with sickle trait (AS genotype), and $q^2 = 1/8 \times 1/8 = 1/64$ (100 individuals) with sickle cell disease (SS genotype). The African population has a higher frequency of AS and SS genotypes caused by heterozygote advantage for the AS genotype that confers resistance to malaria.

468. The answer is e. *(Lewis, pp 267–282. Scriver, pp 4571–4636.)* Even if SS individuals were prevented from contributing to the next generation by sterilization, breeding between AS individuals would replenish SS genotype frequencies. This stability of populations in accord with the Hardy-Weinberg law is often referred to as the Hardy-Weinberg equilibrium. During the decades of 1900 to 1920 in America, the eugenics movement succeeded in passing laws obligating sterilization of those with mental disabilities. These laws were based on two false premises—the idea that mental retardation is always due to Mendelian transmission (ignoring chromosomal and multifactorial disease) and the idea that elimination of affected people will always change gene frequencies.

469. The answer is c. *(Lewis, pp 377–396. Scriver, pp 1553–1588. Murray, pp 102–110.)* This infant may have galactosemia (230400), a deficiency of galactose-1-phosphate uridyl transferase (GALT). Galactose from lactose in breast milk or infant formula is phosphorylated by galactokinase, activated to uridine diphosphogalactose (UDP-galactose) by GALT, and converted to UDP-glucose by UDP-galactose epimerase. The elevation of galactose metabolites is thought to cause liver toxicity, and their urinary excretion produces reducing substances. Infants with the signs and symptoms listed are placed on lactose-free formulas until enzyme testing is complete. Deficiencies of epimerase or kinase can cause mild forms of galactosemia.

470. The answer is b. *(Lewis, pp 267–282. Scriver, pp 1553–1588. Murray, pp 102–110.)* The Hardy-Weinberg expansion, $p^2 + 2pq + q^2$, describes the frequency of genotypes for allele frequencies p and q. In the case of rare disorders ($q^2 < 1/10{,}000$), p approaches 1. The heterozygote frequency 2pq is thus approximately 2q. In this case, $q^2 < 1/40{,}000$, $q = 1/200$ and $2q = 1/100$. Since carriers are still quite rare compared with normal individuals, the matching of rare recessive alleles is greatly enhanced when there is common descent through consanguinity.

471. The answer is d. *(Lewis, pp 75–94. Scriver, pp 4367–4392. Murray, pp 598–608.)* The mother of the pregnant woman (consultand) is an obligate carrier since she has two affected sons with hemophilia. The consultand thus has a one-half chance of receiving the X that carries the abnormal gene and being a carrier. The risk for her fetus to have hemophilia A is thus $1/2 \times 1/4 = 1/8$.

472. The answer is e. *(Lewis, pp 75–94. Scriver, pp 4367–4392. Murray, pp 598–608.)* Hemophilia A is caused by deficiency of factor VIII and hemophilia B by deficiency of factor IX. Both factors are involved in the intrinsic blood coagulation pathway that results in activation of factor X. Alternatively, factor X can be activated by tissue factors through the extrinsic blood coagulation pathway. Activated factors X and V produce thromin from prothrombin, which in turn cleaves fibrinogen to produce fibrin monomers. The fibrin monomers are polymerized and cross-linked to produce a fibrin polymer, which interacts with platelets and other factors to produce a blood clot. The genes for factor VIII and factor IX are on the X chromosome, making hemophilia A and B X-linked recessive diseases.

473. The answer is b. *(Lewis, pp 75–94. Scriver, pp 4367–4392. Murray, pp 598–608.)* Chorionic villus sampling (CVS) is performed at 8–10 weeks' gestation, before a woman is obviously pregnant. This technique preserves the confidentiality of prenatal decisions because diagnostic results are available by 11–12 weeks' gestation rather than the 18–20 weeks for standard amniocentesis. DNA analysis must be employed because factor VIII is not expressed in chorion or amniotic cells. Percutaneous umbilical blood sampling (PUBS) must be performed later in gestation (18+ weeks). Because some factor VIII gene mutations may give normal amounts of structurally abnormal factor VIII, activity rather than amounts of factor VIII protein must be measured for diagnosis.

474. The answer is c. *(Lewis, pp 75–94. Scriver, pp 5759–5788.)* The predominance of affected males with transmission through females makes this pedigree (Fig. 51) diagnostic of X-linked recessive inheritance. Individual I-1 is an obligate carrier, as demonstrated by her affected son and grandson. Individual II-2 cannot transmit an X-linked disorder, although his daughters are obligate carriers. Individual II-3 must be a carrier because of her affected son, which results in a $\frac{1}{4}$ probability of recurrence of CMT in her offspring. Individual II-5 has a $\frac{1}{2}$ probability of being a carrier with a $\frac{1}{8}$ probability for affected offspring. Individual III-4 also has a $\frac{1}{2}$ probability of being a carrier; her risk for affected offspring is also $\frac{1}{8}$ despite the consanguineous marriage. Individual III-8 has a $\frac{1}{4}$ chance of being a carrier and a $\frac{1}{16}$ chance of having affected offspring. CMT is one of the disorders exhibiting genetic heterogeneity, with autosomal dominant (118200), autosomal recessive (214380), and X-linked recessive (302800) forms.

475. The answer is b. *(Lewis, pp 75–94. Scriver, pp 5759–5788.)* The large fragment could derive from a mutation ablating one flanking restriction site or from extra DNA inserted between the restriction sites. The fact that there are two DNA fragment sizes in the affected individual but one in controls suggests alteration of only one of the two homologous CMT regions on chromosome 17. The production of disease by alteration of one homologous locus (one abnormal allele) causes autosomal dominant inheritance. This form of CMT is caused by a duplication of the PMP22 gene, a gene encoding a peripheral myelin protein. The extra copy of PMP22 increases protein abundance and interferes with nerve conduction. DNA duplication is one form of atypical inheritance discovered through DNA analysis.

476. The answer is e. *(Lewis, pp 241–266. Scriver, pp 3–45.)* The Prader-Willi deletion is quite small and is not usually detected by standard metaphase karyotyping. Fluorescent *in situ* hybridization (FISH) is the most efficient and accurate method for detecting the deletion in Prader-Willi syndrome. Fluorescent DNA probes from the deletion region (chromosome band 15q11) give two signals in normal subjects and one signal in patients with a deletion. Detection of RNA or DNA fragments from this region would require quantitation to reveal one-half normal amounts, since genes on the homologous 15 chromosome would be normal. It is much easier to visualize one versus two fluorescent signals. Standard karyotypes typically display about 300 bands over the 23 chromosomes or about 10 bands on chromosome 10. This is adequate for detecting aneuploidy but inadequate for small deletions seen in conditions like Prader-Willi syndrome. Rapid karyotyping of bone marrow samples is possible because marrow contains actively dividing cells. Results are available in 2 to 3 h rather than the 2 to 3 days for standard karyotyping because peripheral blood T leukocytes must be stimulated to divide using lectins like phytohemagglutinin. Resolution of bone marrow karyotypes is usually even less than for standard karyotypes from blood, necessitating the use of FISH probes for accurate diagnosis. Newborns suspected of one of the common trisomies can have bone marrow karyotypes with FISH using probes from chromosomes 13, 18, and 21. Diagnosis is thus available in several hours, allowing guidance of management decisions.

477. The answer is d. *(Lewis, pp 241–266. Scriver, pp 3–45.)* This child has several minor anomalies, a major anomaly that affects the genitalia, and developmental delay. These multiply affected and embryologically unrelated body regions suggest a syndrome rather than a sequence. Because of the multiple anomalies and developmental delay, the first diagnostic test to be considered is a karyotype rather than a test for specific organ function, such as serum testosterone.

478. The answer is c. *(Lewis, pp 377–396. Scriver, pp 3–45. Murray, pp 396–414.)* The hypothetical probe D15S8 implies a unique DNA segment that recognizes a single locus on chromosome 15—the eighth such anonymous DNA probe to be isolated. Because normal individuals have two number 15 chromosomes, they should have two alleles visualized after DNA restriction and hybridization with probe D15S8. Because both parents are heterozygous for the D15S8 locus, as shown in the question, the child's result suggests that he has only received the maternal alleles (alleles 1 and 2) for locus D15S8. This implies that he has received both number 15 chromosomes from his mother. This is known as uniparental disomy and may occur due to correction of trisomy 15 conceptions through loss of the paternal number 15 chromosome.

479. The answer is d. *(Lewis, pp 377–396. Scriver, pp 3–45. Murray, pp 396–414.)* DNA fingerprinting is used in both paternity and forensic analyses and relies on highly variable DNA polymorphisms called variable numbers of tandem repeats (VNTRs). The multicopy repeats include $(CA)_n$ and minisatellite sequences that are present throughout the genome. The usual VNTR probe is directed against single-copy DNA that flanks these repeats and yields multiple restriction fragment sizes that reflect the number of intervening repeats. The hypothetical probes D7Z5 and D20Z1 shown in the question (Fig. 53) recognize VNTR loci on chromosomes 7 and 20 that yield at least three alleles. Because the child's two alleles for D7Z5 (and D20Z1) match those of the mother and father, correct maternity and paternity are established with a degree of error equal to the chance that these allele combinations would occur in an unrelated individual. In practice, at least five VNTR probes are employed so that the odds for paternity (or nonpaternity) are very high indeed.

480. The answer is c. *(Lewis, pp 377–396. Scriver, pp 3–45. Murray, pp 396–414.)* Informed consent requires that the patient be informed of all adverse effects that might result from a procedure. Evidence for nonpaternity may result from various types of DNA analysis and should be discussed with the concerned parties at the time of blood collection. Some physicians speak to the mother and father separately about this issue to maximize the opportunity for independent decision making.

481. The answer is b. *(Lewis, pp 241–266. Scriver, pp 3–45. Murray, pp 396–414.)* In humans and other mammals, the source of genetic material may be as important as its content. Mice manipulated to receive two male pronuclei develop as abortive placentas, whereas those receiving two female pronuclei develop as abortive fetuses. The different impact of the same genetic material according to whether it is transmitted from mother or father is due to genomic imprinting. The term imprinting is borrowed from animal behavior and refers to parental marking during gametogenesis—the physical basis may be DNA methylation or chromatin phasing. Both maternally derived and paternally derived haploid chromosome sets are thus necessary for normal fetal development. This is why parthenogenesis does not occur in mammals. The imprint is erased in the fetal gonads and reestablished based on fetal sex. Certain cases of Prader-Willi syndrome are disorders of imprinting with the absence of the paternally imprinted chromosome 15.

482. The answer is a. *(Lewis, pp 241–266. Scriver, pp 3–45. Murray, pp 396–414.)* A missing band suggests an interstitial (internal) deletion rather than removal of the distal short or long arm (known as a terminal deletion). The shorthand notation $15q^{-}$ implies a terminal deletion of the long arm of chromosome 15. Pericentric (surrounding the centromere) or paracentric (not including the centromere) inversions result from crossover of a chromosome with itself and then breakage and reunion to produce an internal inverted segment. Interstitial deletion 15q11q13 is seen in approximately 50% of patients with Prader-Willi and Angelman syndromes. Other patients with these syndromes inherit both chromosomes 15 from their mother (Prader-Willi) or both from their father (Angelman's), a situation known as uniparental disomy. Genomic imprinting of the 15q11q13 region is different on the chromosome inherited from the mother than on the chromosome inherited from the father. The normal balance of maternal and paternal imprints is thus disrupted by deletion or uniparental disomy, leading to reciprocal differences in gene expression that present as Angelman or Prader-Willi syndromes.

483. The answer is c. *(Lewis, pp 95–112. Scriver, pp 3–45.)* Anticipation refers to the worsening of the symptoms of disease in succeeding generations. The famous geneticist L.S. Penrose dismissed anticipation as an artifact, but the phenomenon has been validated by the discovery of expanding trinucleotide repeats. Steinert myotonic dystrophy is caused by unstable trinucleotide repeats near a muscle protein kinase gene on chromosome 19; the repeats are particularly unstable during female meiosis and may cause a severe syndrome of fetal muscle weakness and joint contractures. Variable expressivity could also be used to describe the family in the question, but the concept implies random variation in severity rather than progression with succeeding generations. Diseases that involve triplet repeat instability exhibit a bias for exaggerated repeat amplification during meiosis (e.g., women with the fragile X syndrome or myotonic dystrophy and men with Huntington chorea). The explanation for this bias is unknown.

484. The answer is a. *(Lewis, pp 397–416. Scriver, pp 3–45.)* Spina bifida is a defect of neural tube development that can be partially prevented by encouraging preconceptional folic acid supplementation in women desiring to become pregnant. Examination for subtle evidence of dysmorphology in children with major birth defects is necessary to rule out a syndrome. Syndromes often exhibit Mendelian or chromosomal inheritance.

485. The answer is c. *(Lewis, pp 135–154. Scriver, pp 193–202.)* When present as an isolated (rare) anomaly, spina bifida (meningomyelocele) exhibits multifactorial inheritance. Chromosomal inheritance usually causes a syndrome with predictable frequency rather than isolated anomalies. Atypical inheritance (genomic imprinting, trinucleotide repeat instability, mitochondrial inheritance) has not been implicated in neural tube defects.

486. The answer is c. *(Lewis, pp 135–154. Scriver, pp 193–202.)* The father and child are affected with spina bifida. The next child will be related to them as a primary (first-degree) relative. The existence of two affected primary relatives predicts a recurrence risk of >6%. Had the child had a Mendelian syndrome, the risk could have been as high as 25% from autosomal recessive inheritance.

487. The answer is c. (Lewis, pp 135–154, 397–416. Scriver, pp 193–202.) Any defect of the fetal skin may elevate the amniotic α-fetoprotein (AFP) level, causing a parallel rise of this substance in the maternal blood. Neural tube defects such as anencephaly or spina bifida elevate the AFP in amniotic fluid or maternal serum; other causes of increased AFP include fetal kidney disease with leakage of fetal proteins into amniotic fluid. Mild forms of spina bifida or meningomyelocele may be covered by the skin, so that the AFP is not elevated, and maternal serum AFP is less sensitive than amniotic fluid AFP for such cases. Ultrasound is required to detect covered neural tube defects that do not leak fetal AFP into the amniotic fluid and maternal blood. Acetylcholinesterase is an enzyme produced at high levels in neural tissue that is somewhat more specific than AFP for neural tube defects; it is used for confirmation rather than as a primary prenatal test. Chorionic villus biopsy is performed at about 10 weeks after the last menstrual period (LMP) and amniocentesis at 14–16 postmenstrual weeks. Because conception often occurs 2 weeks prior to the LMP, distinction between postconceptional and postmenstrual timing is important for early stages of pregnancy. Neural tube defects are usually localized, multifactorial anomalies rather than part of a malformation syndrome that can result from chromosomal aberrations. For this reason, documentation of the fetal karyotype by chorionic villus biopsy or amniocentesis does not influence the risk for neural tube defects.

488. The answer is e. *(Lewis, pp 397–416. Scriver, pp 3–45.)* Genetic counseling is an essential component of every prenatal diagnostic test. Couples must understand their risks and options before selecting a prenatal diagnostic procedure. There must also be adequate provisions for explaining the results. Because additional obstetric procedures, such as pregnancy termination, may follow prenatal diagnosis, obstetricians need to be comprehensive and thorough with the genetic counseling process.

489. The answer is d. *(Lewis, pp 377–396. Scriver, pp 2297–2326. Murray, pp 180–189.)* Assuming that nonpaternity or an unusual method of inheritance is not operative, the parents of a child with an autosomal recessive condition are obligate heterozygotes. Therefore, their risk of having a child with medium-chain acyl-coenzyme A (CoA) dehydrogenase deficiency (MCAD) is one-fourth or 25% for each future pregnancy.

490. The answer is a. *(Lewis, pp 377–396. Scriver, pp 2297–2326. Murray, pp 180–189.)* Catastrophic metabolic disease often begins after the first few feedings, when the baby is exposed to nutrients that cannot be metabolized and are toxic. Often there are misguided attempts to encourage feeding, which further poison the child. Inborn errors of carbohydrate, amino acid, or organic/fatty acid metabolism can present in the newborn period. They are characterized by a similar pattern of symptoms that include spitting up, vomiting, exaggeration of the usual physiologic jaundice, lethargy progressing to coma, hypoglycemia, acidosis, hyperammonemia, and, in the case of maple syrup urine disease or isovaleric acidemia, unusual odors. Disorders of fatty acid oxidation worsen during fasting to cause carnitine depletion, failure of fatty acid oxidation, and excretion of dicarboxylic acid intermediates. Deficiencies in medium-chain fatty acid oxidation are milder, and may present after a period of illness with calorie deprivation in children aged 2–6 years. Urea cycle disorders worsen during fasting (catabolic breakdown) or protein feeding, producing excess ammonia, rapid breathing, and respiratory alkalosis. Galactosemia worsens on exposure to lactose-containing formula, producing hypoglycemia, liver failure, and excretion of urinary sugars (reducing substances). Tyrosinemia and maple syrup urine disease are amino acid disorders that worsen after protein feeding and produce elevated levels of tyrosine or branch-chain amino acids (leucine, isoleucine, valine). Tyrosinemia is associated with severe liver failure and maple syrup urine disease with severe acidosis due to conversion of excess amino acids to ketoacids.

491. The answer is d. *(Lewis, pp 377–396. Scriver, pp 2297–2326. Murray, pp 249–263.)* Propionic acidemia (232000) results from a block in propionyl CoA carboxylase (PCC), which converts propionic to methylmalonic acid. Excess propionic acid in the blood produces metabolic acidosis with a decreased bicarbonate and increased anion gap (the serum cations sodium plus potassium minus the serum anions chloride plus bicarbonate). The usual values of sodium (~140 meq/L) plus potassium (~4 meq/L) minus those for chloride (~105 meq/L) plus bicarbonate (~20 meq/L) thus yield a normal anion gap of ~20 meq/L. A low bicarbonate of 6 to 8 meq/L yields an elevated gap of 32–34 meq/L, a "gap" of negative charge that is supplied by the hidden anion (propionate in propionic acidemia). Biotin is a cofactor for PCC and its deficiency causes some types of propionic acidemia. Vitamin B_{12} deficiency can cause methylmalonic aciduria because vitamin B_{12} is a cofactor for methylmalonyl coenzyme A mutase. Glycine is secondarily elevated in propionic acidemia, but no defect of glycine catabolism is present.

492. The answer is b. *(Lewis, pp 377–396. Scriver, pp 2297–2326. Murray, pp 249–263.)* In treating inborn errors of metabolism that present acutely in the newborn period, aggressive fluid and electrolyte therapy and caloric supplementation are important to correct the imbalances caused by the disorder. Calories spare tissue breakdown that can increase toxic metabolites. Because many of the metabolites that build up in inborn errors of metabolism are toxic to the central nervous system, hemodialysis is recommended for any patient in stage II coma (poor muscle tone, few spontaneous movements, responsive to painful stimuli) or worse. Dietary therapy should minimize substances that cannot be metabolized—in this case fatty acids, because the oxidation of branched-chain fatty acids results in propionate. Antibiotics are frequently useful because metabolically compromised children are more susceptible to infection.

493. The answer is c. *(Lewis, pp 377–396. Scriver, pp 2297–2326. Murray, pp 249–263.)* The proband in this case has inherited the A allele from one parent and the B allele from the other (Fig. 54). However, it is impossible to determine which allele came from which parent. The fetus has the same genotype as his affected brother. However, it cannot be determined if he inherited these alleles from the same parents as the affected boy and is thus affected, or from the opposite parents and is thus an unaffected noncarrier. It can be said that he is definitely not an unaffected carrier. Assuming no recombination has occurred, the risk for the fetus to be affected is one-half, or 50%.

494. The answer is c. *(Lewis, pp 397–416. Scriver, pp 175–192.)* Genetic screening requires not only a highly accurate diagnostic test but also one that can be adapted to testing of large numbers of individuals. Key for neonatal screening is that the disease can be ameliorated because of early diagnosis—some countries have tried screening for Duchenne muscular dystrophy (310200) but most do not because there is no treatment advantage from early diagnosis. Neonatal screening is set up so there will be more false positives than false negatives; this requires some work for pediatricians in obtaining and interpreting repeat screens, but is considered far preferable to missing a child with preventable disease consequences. The Guthrie test was the first to allow screening of large populations, as exemplified by the test for phenylketonuria (PKU—261600): infant blood from a heel or finger stick is placed on filter paper discs and mailed to the central screening laboratory. Discs are arrayed on agar plates containing a competitive inhibitor of bacterial growth (thienylalanine), which must be overcome by sufficient amounts of phenylalanine for bacterial colonies to be visible. Rapid scanning of agar plates with hundreds of filter discs is thus possible by eye, and discs surrounded by bacterial growth constitute a positive result. A recent problem for newborn screening is the trend towards early infant discharge (24 hours or less). If the infant blood sample is obtained too early before adequate dietary intake, blood levels of phenylalanine or other metabolites may not be elevated and a false negative result will be obtained. Many hospitals request that parents return with their infant for proper screening. The supplemental newborn screen by tandem mass spectrometry can be justified because the aggregate incidence of its 30 detected disorders is 1 in 5–6000, well above that for currently screened metabolic disorders such as PKU (1 in 10–12,000) and galactosemia (1 in 40,000).

495. The answer is b. *(Lewis, pp 397–416. Scriver, pp 5121–5188. Murray, pp 396–414.)* A method for rapid and inexpensive screening of multiple mutant alleles in large numbers of individuals will be required before genetic screening can be performed using DNA analysis. The likely method will involve DNA arrays or chips where thousands of DNA probes can be affixed to arrays on microbeads or glass slides, hybridized in replicate to individual DNAs, and passed through machines for reading of deficiencies.These techniques are undergoing explosive development, but cannot yet screen for thousands of potential mutant alleles in an individual (e.g., with neurofibromatosis—162200—or Marfan syndrome—154700), much less for multiple mutant alleles in each of the 3 million annual American newborns. Comparative genomic hybridization analyzes an individual DNA with probes across the genome, highlighting regions where there is extra or missing DNA. This technique is excellent for demonstrating extra or missing chromosome material but may not detect rearrangements. Fluorescent *in situ* hybrization may employ control and test labeled DNA probe to highlight their specific locus on a chromosome, showing two signals for individuals with paired autosomes. An absence of test signal on one chromosome when the control signal is present shows there is a submicroscopic deletion as in the DiGeorge or Williams syndromes. Subtelomere FISH analysis extends this to many DNA probes, highlighting all 44 autosome and the 2 X chromosome ends—subtle rearrangements will shift the position of the FISH signal, and deletions or duplications involving a target region will yield a missing or extra signal. Southern analysis is labor intensive and has limited use in this era of automated allele detection and DNA sequencing. The prime justification for newborn screening is that early diagnosis results in benefits through prevention or treatment. Although early identification of PKU carriers through diagnosis of their affected newborns is a benefit of newborn screening, its chief rationale is the prevention of mental retardation by early diagnosis and lowering of dietary protein intake. False-positive screens are the most frequent problem with screening, and repeat screens are sometimes needed for borderline results.

496. The answer is c. *(Lewis, pp 397–416. Scriver, pp 1667–1724. Murray, pp 249–263.)* Decreased melanin can occur in PKU because melanin is produced from phenylalanine and tyrosine. The defect in most children with PKU is deficiency of phenylalanine hydroxylase. Rare children have deficiency of biopterin cofactor due to a defect in its synthetic enzyme that is also autosomal recessive. Phenylalanine is converted to tyrosine by phenylalanine hydroxylase, so deficient tyrosine can occur in children on restrictive diets.

497. The answer is c. *(Lewis, pp 377–496. Scriver, pp 4077–5016. Murray pp 396–414.)* A peripheral blood karyotype provides the most reliable examination of the sex chromosomes. A bone marrow karyotype is more rapid (it uses rapidly dividing bone marrow cells) but usually has less resolution for defining subtle X and Y chromosome rearrangements. A buccal smear would theoretically show one Barr body in females (representing inactivation of one X chromosome) and none in males. In practice, this test is not very reliable and is rarely used. Detection of material of the Y long arm by polymerase chain reaction (PCR) would be useful but does not examine the Y short arm that contains the sex-determining region.

498. The answer is a. *(Lewis, pp 377–496. Scriver, pp 4077–5016. Murray pp 396–414.)* The dot-blot demonstrates hybridization of the proband's DNA with the DXS14 and SRY DNA probes and suggests the diagnosis of a genetic male. The presence of a Y rules out the possibility of the proband being a genetic female but not the rare occurrence of 46,XX/46,XY mosaicism. Gender assignment is not based solely on genetic testing but must include surgical and reproductive prognoses for male versus female adult function. For these reasons, the patient with ambiguous genitalia is a medical emergency that requires delicate management until gender assignment is agreed on. In the past, individuals judged not to have adequate phallic tissue for reconstruction of normal male genitalia underwent appropriate surgery for female gender assignment. However, recent follow-up studies suggest that at least some XY individuals who had feminizing surgery including orchiectomy have developed a male sexual identity. These findings make management more complex in that sexual identity may be at least partly determined during fetal life.

499. The answer is b. *(Lewis, pp 377–496. Scriver, pp 4077–5016. Murray pp 434–455.)* True hermaphroditism implies the presence of both male and female genitalia in the same patient and is extremely rare. Male pseudohermaphroditism implies a genetic male with incomplete development of his genitalia, as in the proband. Causes can range from abnormalities of the pituitary-adrenal-gonadal hormone axis to local defects in tissue responsiveness to testosterone. The XY female and XX male refer to phenotypically normal individuals whose genetic sex does not match their phenotypic sex. Examples include testicular feminization and pure gonadal dysgenesis (XY females) and offspring of fathers with Y translocations that inherit a cryptic SRY region without a visible Y chromosome (XX males).

500. The answer is a. *(Lewis, pp 377–496. Scriver, pp 4077–5016. Murray pp 434–455.)* Sex steroids are synthesized from cholesterol by side-chain cleavage (employing a P450 enzyme) to produce pregnenolone. Pregnenolone is then converted to testosterone in the testis, to estrogen in the ovary, and to corticosterone and aldosterone in the adrenal gland. The enzymes 3β-hydroxysteroid dehydrogenase, 21-hydroxylase, 11β-hydroxylase, and 18-hydroxylase modify pregnenolone to produce other sex and adrenal steroids. Deficiencies in adrenal 21-hydroxylase can thus lead to inadequate testosterone production in males and produce ambiguous external genitalia. Such children can also exhibit low sodium and high potassium due to deficiency of the more distal steroids corticol and aldosterone. 5β-reductase converts testosterone to dihydrotestosterone, and its deficiency produces milder degrees of hypogenitalism without salt wasting. Deficiency of the androgen receptor is called testicular feminization, producing normal looking females who may not seek medical attention until they present with infertility.

Bibliography

Lewis R. *Human Genetics: Concepts and Applications.* 5/e. New York, McGraw-Hill, 2003.

McKusick VA. *Mendelian Inheritance in Man.* 13/e. Baltimore, Johns Hopkins University Press, 1996. Internet address (updated monthly): *www3.ncbi.nlm.nih.gov/omim.*

Murray RK, Granner DK, Mayes PA, Rodwell VW. *Harper's Illustrated Biochemistry.* 26/e. New York, McGraw-Hill, 2003.

Scriver CR, Beaudet AL, Sly WS, Valle D. *The Metabolic and Molecular Bases of Inherited Disease.* 8/e. New York, McGraw-Hill, 2001.

The primary references cited in the key concepts and answers include the Murray and Scriver textbooks, which are more directed toward biochemistry, and the Lewis textbook that is more directed toward medical genetics.

Many genetic diseases cited in this book include a six-digit McKusick number that allows reference to the compendium of genetic diseases that is available in hard copy or online. This compendium is now maintained by the National Institutes of Health and lists more than 4000 genetic diseases and genetic loci (see *www.ncbi.nlm.nih.gov/omim/*). For all but the most recently entered disorders, the McKusick number provides the inheritance mechanism. Those numbers beginning with 1 designate autosomal dominant diseases, those beginning with 2 autosomal recessive diseases, those beginning with 3 X-linked recessive diseases, those beginning with 4 Y-linked diseases (so far only gene loci), and those beginning with 5 mitochondrial DNA–encoded diseases.

Appendix

OLIC-GENETIC DISORDERS INCLUDED AS EXAMPLES IN QUESTIONS

	Abnormality/ Deficiency	Clinical Information	Question Numbers
sorders			
mentosum	DNA repair defect with UV light sensitivity (278700)	Skin ulcers healing with brown pigment, photosensitivity, retinal disease	2, 18, 29
.0435)*	DNA mismatch repair defect (HNPCC—120435)	No colonic polyps, high incidence colon cancer	13, 20
e syndrome 400)	DNA repair/transcription factor defect	Growth failure, rapid aging, sunken eyes, sparse hair, old-age diseases as child	12
cers and cancer syndromes			
kitt lymphoma (113970)	Translocations involving MYC oncogene	Lymphoid proliferation (lymphoma) with secondary bone and immune disease	94, 451
Chronic myelogenous leukemia (608232)	Philadelphia chromosome (translocation 9/22)	Increased white blood cell count, bone marrow failure, chronic infections	5, 79
Gardner syndrome (175100)	Adenomatous polyposis coli (APC) gene	Unusual teeth, retinal lesions, multiple colon polyps, early-onset colon cancer	7, 20, 402
Li-Fraumeni syndrome (114480)	p53 oncogene	Predisposition to breast and colon cancers	452–3
Retinoblastoma (180200)	Rb tumor suppressor gene; origin of two-hit hypothesis	Retinal tumors	17, 450
Wilms tumor (194070)	WT-1 tumor suppressor gene	Renal tumors, sometimes with aniridia, genital anomalies, retardation (WAGR)	84, 86, 460

Triplet repeat amplification			
Fragile X syndrome (309550)	Fragile X mental retardation (FMR-1) gene	MR, long face, prominent ears and jaw, loose connective tissue, large testes	1, 11
Huntington chorea (143100)	Huntington gene	Tremors, staccato and slurred speech, degeneration	1, 386
Chromosomal and imprinting disorders			
Angelman syndrome (105830)	Deletion or abnormal parental origin at 15q11	Severe MR, seizures, jerking movements	482
Cri-du-chat syndrome	46,XX,5p- or 46,XY,5p-	MR, growth failure, microcephaly, cat-like cry, multiple congenital anomalies	400
Down syndrome	Trisomy 21 or translocation (2–3% e.g., 46,XX,(t14;21)	MR, short stature, eye, heart, thyroid, GI defects, atlantoaxial instability	394–5, 398–9
Klinefelter syndrome	47,XXY karyotype	Tall stature, gynecomastia, small testes, infertility, behavior differences	389
r-Willi syndrome 270)	Deletion or abnormal parental origin at 15q11	MR, early hypotonia, later hyperphagia and obesity	6, 477–9
drome (312750)	MECP protein	MR, gradual neurodegeneration, unusual hand wringing movements	26
DiGeorge	Submicroscopic deletion at band 22q11 (e.g., 192465)	MR, heart, palate, parathyroid, immune defects; schizophrenia in adults	464–5
Triple X ne	47,XXX karyotype	MR, variable short stature, occasional somatic defects	390

(Continued)

METAB GENETIC DISORDERS INCLUDED AS EXAMPLES IN QUESTIONS (Continued)

Di	Abnormality/ Deficiency	Clinical Information	Question Numbers
Turner	45,X, 46,XX/45,X mosaicism, ring X. etc.	Short stature, web neck, broad chest, ovarian dysgenesis, infertility	393, 395, 397–8
XYY	47,XYY karyotype	Tall stature, variable cognitive disability, and behavior differences	391
of membrane proteins			
osis (219700)	CFTR	Lung disease and pancreatic insufficiency due to viscous mucous	3, 37, 333, 385, 409, 432, 495
tes insipidus 25800)	Aquaporin	Water loss, hyperosmolar serum with hypernatremia, extreme thirst, polyuria	98
isorders of carbohydrate metabolism			
Diabetes mellitus (222100)	Multifactorial—insulin deficiency	Hyperglycemia, glucosuria, increased fat oxidation, ketoacidosis	4, 69, 97, 108, 177, 191, 280, 284, 345–6, 377, 382, 466
Essential pentosuria (260800)	Xylulose reductase	Pentose in urine without pathology	181
Galactosemia (230400)	Galactose-1-phosphate uridyl transferase	Neonatal illness with cataracts, jaundice, liver disease, reducing substances in urine	176, 469–70

Glucose-6-phosphate dehydrogenase deficiency (305900)	Enzyme of pentose phosphate shunt	Hemolytic anemia, particularly with exposure to antimalarial drugs or fava beans	77, 175, 188, 211
Hereditary fructose intolerance (229600)	Liver aldolase B	Hypoglycemia, acidosis, liver disease	166, 178, 196
Hypoglycemia	Multifactorial	Jittery babies; anxiety, tremors, fainting spells in adults	187
Liver GSD (see Table 3)	Defective glycogen breakdown or synthesis	Hypoglycemia, enlarged liver, elevated uric acid, cholesterol	123, 173, 179, 180, 200, 203–4, 339, 379, 401
scle GSD e Table 3)	Defective glycogen breakdown or synthesis	Muscle cramps, fatigue with exercise	168, 179, 200, 206
GSD able 3)	Lysosomal α-glucosidase (Pompe-232300)	Short PR interval on ECG, lethal cardiomyopathy with heart failure	183
Co... carbohydrate (mucopolysaccharide, glycosaminoglycan) storage diseases			
Hunte... syndrome (309...)	Iduronate sulfatase; type II mucopolysaccharidosis	Same as Hurler, males only, clear corneas.	81, 130, 272, 404
Hurler and ... syndrome...	Iduronidase; type I mucopolysaccharidosis	Neurodegeneration, cloudy corneas, coarse facies, hepatosplenomegaly	78, 130, 272
I-cell disease (2...2800) ...00)	Lysosomal transporter	Similar to Hurler, inclusion cells in fibroblasts	121

(Continued)

METABOLIC-GENETIC DISORDERS INCLUDED AS EXAMPLES IN QUESTIONS (Continued)

Disorder	Abnormality/ Deficiency	Clinical Information	Question Numbers
Fatty acid oxida...n disorders and organic acidemias			
Carnitine defici...s (e.g., 2121...)	Carnitine transporters	Muscle weakness, heart and liver failure due to defective fatty acid oxidation	228, 239
MCAD def...y (201450)	Medium chain CoA dehydrogenase	Lethargy, nonketotic hypoglycemia, heart and liver failure with fasting	228, 246, 249, 263, 339, 356, 489–90
Pr... acidemia ...0)	Propionyl CoA carboxylase	Acidosis with anion gap, hypoglycemia, moderate hyperammonemia, lethargy	491–2
...storage diseases			
...her disease (231000)	Glucosylceramide β-glucosidase	Organomegaly, fractures	78, 80
...-Sachs disease (272800)	Hexosaminidase A	Cherry red spot of the retina, exaggerated infantile startle reflex, neurodegeneration	272, 423, 441–5
Niemann-Pick disease (257220)	Sphingomyelinase	Organomegaly, neurodegeneration	268
Lipid transport diseases			
Abetalipoproteinemia (200100)	ApoB protein	Retinal changes, anemia with acanthocytes, low serum β-lipoprotein	54–55, 82–83
Familial hypercholesterolemia	LDL receptors	Xanthomas, hypercholesterolemia, early onset of atherosclerosis	266, 269–70, 282, 454–5
Familial hypertriglyceridemia	Abnormal VLDL metabolism	Hypertriglyceridemia, atherosclerosis	262

Hemoglobinopathies and anemias			
α-Thalassemia-MR syndrome	Altered transcription factor for the α-globin locus	Mental retardation, coarse facies, hypotonia, anemia	93
Hemoglobin lepore (141900)	Rearrangement of β-globin cluster	Anemia	34
Hexokinase deficiency (235700)	Hexokinase	Anemia	174, 241
Sickle cell anemia (603903)	β-globin point mutation	Anemia, vessel occlusion with pain and sequestration crises	15, 36, 41, 92, 112, 433, 467–8
Spherocytosis (182900)	Ankyrin erythrocyte protein	Anemia with small spherical red blood cells (spherocytes)	99
Thalassemias (e.g., 141900)	Imbalance of α-or β-globin chains	Severe anemia, growth failure, transfusion iron toxicity, bone changes	39, 43–46, 48, 51, 53, 58, 91, 113
Disorders of porphyrin, nucleic acid, or bile acid metabolism			
Bile acid synthesis disorders	Heme and bile degradative enzymes (e.g., 214950)	Liver disease, cholestatic jaundice with elevated bile acids	353
Gout (hyperuricemia)	Multifactorial disease	Hyperuricemia with joint nodules (tophi), kidney crystals, and joint pain	184, 296
Lesch-Nyhan syndrome (300322)	HGPRT	MR, self-mutilation to the degree of chewing off lips and fingers	291–2, 462–3
Neonatal jaundice	Multifactorial disease (unconjugated bilirubin)	Excess bilirubin produces yellow skin and yellow whites of eyes (sclerae)	257
Orotic aciduria (258900)	Uridine monophosphate synthase	Megablastic anemia unresponsive to vitamin B_{12}	290
Porphyrias (one form AD-176100)	Heme biosynthesis enzyme defects	Episodic abdominal pain, psychosis, skin rash	258, 295

(Continued)

METABOLIC-GENETIC DISORDERS INCLUDED AS EXAMPLES IN QUESTIONS (Continued)

Disorder	Abnormality/ Deficiency	Clinical Information	Question Numbers
Disorders of amino acid metabolism			
Albinism (203100)	Melanin synthesis	Pale skin and hair, nystagmus due to altered crossover of optic nerves	16, 418
Alkaptonuria (203500)	Homogentisic acid oxidase	Blackened urine on standing, black cartilage with arthritis (ochronosis)	116
Cystinosis (219800)	Lysosomal transporter	Childhood growth failure with eye and renal disease	105, 276
Gyrate atrophy (258870)	Ornithine aminotransferase	Retinal degeneration with vision and neurologic problems	76
Hartnup disease (234500)	Renal neutral amino acid transporter	Tryptophan and niacin deficiency with pellagra (rash, neurologic symptoms)	253, 318
Histidinemia (235800)	Histidine degrading enzyme	No symptoms or speech delay	128
Homocystinuria (236300)	Cystathionine synthase, others	Marfanoid habitus with tall stature, joint laxity, hernias, scoliosis, flat feet	251, 319, 405
Hyperprolinemia (239500)	Proline degrading enzyme	No symptoms or speech delay	128
Maple syrup urine disease (248600)	Branched-chain amino acid dehydrogenase	Seizures, acidosis, neurologic damage, death without low protein diet	126
Phenylketonuria (261600)	Phenylalanine hydroxylase	Mousy odor, pale skin, blond hair	106, 267, 421, 496
Urea cycle disorders	Citrullinemia (215700)	Neonatal lethargy, seizures, coma due to hyperammonemia	95, 120, 244–7, 294
Mitochondrial disorders			
Kearns-Sayre syndrome (530000)	Mitochondrial DNA point mutation	Ptosis, ataxia, muscle weakness	23

Respiratory chain disorders (e.g., Leigh syndrome, 256000)	Several encoded by mitochondrial or nuclear DNA	Low muscle tone, mental retardation, optic symptoms, lactic acidosis, ragged red fibers in muscle	197, 208–9, 231, 329
Disorders primarily affecting the nervous system			
Charcot-Marie-Tooth disease (e.g., 118200)	Peripheral myelin protein 22 in some forms	Peripheral neuropathy with characteristic "stepping" gait due to foot drop	411, 474–5
Deafness (e.g., 220290)	Many single gene forms, most commonly recessive	Sensorineural deafness	132
Hallervorden-Spatz disease (234200)	Pantothenic acid kinase	Insidious loss of cognitive and neural function, neurodegeneration	310
Menkes disease (309400)	Copper-transporting ATPase	Kinky hair, neurologic devastation, seizures, hypotonia, skeletal changes	81, 459
Retinitis pigmentosa (e.g., 180100)	Many genes, all Mendelian mechanisms	Variable onset of vision loss, beginning with night blindness	412–413
Succinyl choline apnea (177400)	Butyrylcholinesterase	Inability to recover from succinylcholine paralysis during anesthesia	438–9
Birth defects and birth defect syndromes			
Achondroplasia (100800)	Fibroblast growth factor receptor-3	Dwarfism, short proximal limbs (rhizomelia), hydrocephalus, scoliosis	408, 422
Cardiomyopathy (160760)	Cardiac myosin	Dilated heart with weakening cardiac muscles, sudden death from arrhythmia	124
Cleft lip/cleft palate	Multifactorial disease	Cleft of lip and/or palate, ear infections	424
Crouzon syndrome (123500)	Fibroblast growth factor-1	Premature fusion of the cranial sutures (craniosynostosis), no limb anomalies	406

(Continued)

METABOLIC-GENETIC DISORDERS INCLUDED AS EXAMPLES IN QUESTIONS (Continued)

Disorder	Abnormality/ Deficiency	Clinical Information	Question Numbers
Ectrodactyly (183600)	Several genes including *sonic hedgehog*	Split hand-split foot or lobster claw anomaly	403
Epidermolysis bullosa	Adhesive proteins of skin	Multiple blisters, similar to burns	115
Fetal warfarin syndrome	Multifactorial, defects in vitamin K synthesis	Short "fleur-de-lys" nose and skeletal changes	311
Hemophilia A (306700)	Factor VIII	Coagulopathy often presenting after circumcision, joint damage	471–3
Holoprosencephaly (e.g., 157170)	Many single gene and chrom-osome aberrations	Failure of forebrain development with facial cyclopia to midline cleft lip/palate	90, 341
Hydrocephalus	Multifactorial	Enlarged cerebral ventricles with macrocephaly	431
Incontinentia pigmenti (308300)	unknown	Skin lesions—vesicles, scaling, pigment patches—sparse hair, absent teeth	416
Marfan syndrome (154700)	Fibrillin	Tall stature, myopia, dislocated lens, high palate, heart defects, scoliosis, flat feet	114, 117, 447–8
Osteogenesis imperfecta (155210)	Type I collagen	Multiple fractures, deafness, blue-gray sclerae, large skull with Wormian bones	103, 118, 132, 242, 414, 449
Osteopetrosis (259730)	Carbonic anhydrase	Hardened, sclerotic bones and renal transport defect with acidosis	101
Pyloric stenosis (179010)	Multifactorial	Narrowing of pylorus with vomiting and hyperchloremic alkalosis	104, 417

Retinoic acid embryopathy	Prenatal exposure to retinoids (e.g., Accutane)	Brain, eye, limb, and craniofacial defects, usually with severe MR	89
Robert syndrome (268300)	Unknown	Cleft palate and congenital limb amputations	19
Spina bifida	Multifactorial	Failure of caudal neural tube closure with lower limb paralysis and incontinence	484–487
Stickler syndrome (108300)	Type II collagen	Retinal detachment, lax joints, arthritis, short stature	75, 119
Waardenburg syndrome (193500)	PAX genes	Deafness, hypertelorism, central white patches of hair (poliosis) and skin	419
Zellweger syndrome (214100)	Paroxysmal protein defects	Severe hypotonia, large fontanelle, liver disease, MR, short life span	283
Endocrine disorders			
Addison' disease (e.g., 103230)	Multifactorial due to adrenal insufficiency	Hypokalemia, hypoglycemia, muscle weakness, hypotension, fainting spells	342, 349
Ambiguous genitalia	Multifactorial, many single gene disorders	Incomplete development or sex reversal of external genitalia	497–500
Testicular feminization	Testosterone receptor (300068)	Female phenotype without uterus and ovarian tubes, infertile, XY karyotype	338
Cushing syndrome	Multifactorial due to ACTH or cortisol excess	Truncal obesity, "buffalo hump," striae of skin, hypertension, potassium loss	340
Diabetes insipidus	Multifactorial due to vasopressin (ADH) defect	Excessive thirst, dehydration, hypernatremia	98, 341, 428

(Continued)

METABOLIC-GENETIC DISORDERS INCLUDED AS EXAMPLES IN QUESTIONS (Continued)

Disorder	Abnormality/ Deficiency	Clinical Information	Question Numbers
Immune disorders			
AIDS (609423)	Viral infection with genetic susceptibility	Immune deficiency	25
Bruton agammaglobulinemia (300300)	Tyrosine kinase gene; deficiency of B-cells that fight bacterial infections	Severe and recurrent bacterial infections when maternal antibodies are cleared from system (age 3–6 months).	40, 111
Adenosine deaminase deficiency (102700)	Adenosine deaminase with stem cell immune defects	Viral, fungal, and bacterial infections due to B- and T-cell deficiencies	73
Organ system disorders			
Alcoholism	Multifactorial disease	Liver disease, cirrhosis, deficiencies of vitamins B_1 and B_{12}, psychosis	169, 172, 264, 316, 330
α1-Antitrypsin deficiency (107400)	Proteinase inhibitor PI, mutant S and Z alleles	Childhood liver and adult pulmonary disease	57, 72, 170, 440
Cholera	Bacterial infection with *Vibrio cholerae*	Diarrhea, dehydration, shock	237
Crohn disease	Multifactorial	Inflammatory bowel disease with bloody diarrhea, cramping, malabsorption	304
Ethylene glycol intoxication	Environmental poisoning	Acidosis, liver failure	259
Polycystic kidney disease (e.g., 173900)	Polycystin—dominant and recessive forms	Cysts in kidneys and liver with propensity to strokes	461

Multiple sclerosis	Multifactorial with abnormal CNS lipids	Waxing and waning neurologic symptoms with incoordination, ataxia, depression	261
Prematurity	Multifactorial	Lung and liver immaturity, deficient fatty acid and iron stores	260
Disorders of vitamin and mineral metabolism			
Multiple carboxylase deficiency (253260)	Biotinidase	Intermittent acidosis, hair loss, skin rashes, neutropenia	312
Hemochromatosis (e.g., 235200)	Proteins encoded by HFE, HFE2A, HFE 2B genes	Abnormal iron transport and storage with accumulation in heart and liver	303, 457–8
Mineral deficiencies (see Table 7)			324
Vitamin deficiencies (see Table 6)			230, 286, 301, 305–8, 314, 316, 318, 320–2, 325–8, 332–7

*Online Mendelian Inheritance in Man (OMIM) number provided for single gene disorders—some multifactorial or chromosomal diseases will have an OMIM number to list genes implicated in pathogenesis/susceptibility; HNPCC, hereditary nonpolyposis colorectal cancer; AD, autosomal dominant; AR, autosomal recessive; MR, mental retardation; GI, gastrointestinal; CFTR, cystic fibrosis transmembrane conductance regulator; GSD, glycogen storage diseases; ACTH, adrenocortical hormone; ADH, antidiuretic hormone; HGPRT, hypoxanthine-guanine phosphoribosyltransferase; AIDS, acquired immunodeficiency syndrome.

Index

A

AA genotypes, 430
Abetalipoproteinemia, 112, 270
Acetaminophen, 344
Acetosalicylic acid, 344
Acetyl-CoA carboxylase, 247
Acetyl coenzyme A (acetyl CoA), 22, 313
Achondroplasia
  cause of, 193
  inheritance of, 391
  risk calculations, 384, 390
Acid-base equilibria, 10–13
Acidemias, 250, 265
Acid hydrolysis, 159
ACP (Acyl carrier protein), 312
Activated sugars, 283
Acylcarnitines, 250
Acyl carrier protein (ACP), 312
ADA (Adenosine deaminase) deficiency, 107
Addison disease, 338, 340
Adenine, 2
Adenomatous polyposis coli (APC), 62, 382
Adenosine, 2
Adenosine deaminase (ADA) deficiency, 107
Adenosine diphosphate (ADP), 244
Adenosine monophosphate (AMP), 2
Adenosine triphosphate (ATP)
  generation of, 245, 248, 268
  in glycolysis, 23
  synthesis of, 244
  yield of, 250
Adipocytes, 245, 348
ADP (Adenosine diphosphate), 244
Adrenal cortex, 338, 340
Adrenal medulla, 340
Adrenal tumor, 340
African Americans, 430
AIDS, 71
Alanine, 14, 38, 94
Albinism, 67, 388
Albumin, 161
Alcohol, metabolism of, 211
Alcohol abuse, 210
Aldehydes, 430
Aldolase B, 213
Alimentation solutions, 274
Alleles, 157, 374
Allopurinol, 280
Alpha1-antitrypsin deficiency, 102, 107, 421
Alpha-globin, 100, 117
Alpha-helices, 149
Alpha-ketoglutarate, 263
Amanitin, 94
Ambiguous genitalia, 440–441
Amenorrhea, 318
Amino acids
  activation of, 103
  aromatic, 162
  blood levels, 350
  in collagen, 156–157, 161
  and collagens, 157
  definition of, 13
  elevated, 154
  identification of, 152–153, 160, 275
  labeling of, 263
  metabolism of, 38–40
  pathways, 156
  phosphorylation of, 188
  and scurvy, 156
  side chains of, 152, 157, 160
  (*See also* Proteins)

Aminoacyl-tRNA, 105
Ammonia, 38, 157
Amniocentesis, 383
AMP (Adenosine monophosphate), 2
Amphibolic pathways, 346
Amphipathic lipids, 31
Amylopectinosis, 27
Amyotrophic lateral sclerosis, 373
Anabolism, 18
Andersen disease, 27
Androgen insensitivity syndrome, 337
Anemia
  cause of, 212
  and deficiency in alpha-globin chains, 117
  diagnosis of, 74, 155, 212
  hemolytic, 216
  sickle cell, 66, 93, 117, 439
Anencephaly, 318, 436
Anesthesia, 420
Angelman syndrome, 435
Aniridia, 427
Ankyrin, 149
Antibodies, 16
Anticoagulants, 311
Antiinflammatory steroids, 342
Antimalarial drug, 216
Antioxidants, 268
Anxiety attacks, 340
APC (Adenomatous polyposis coli), 62, 382
Apnea, 421
Apobetalipoproteinemia, 112
Apolipoprotein, 101–102
Aquaporin-2 gene, 149
Arachidonic acid, 31, 344
Arachnoactyly, 423
Arginase, 264
Arginine, 14, 279
Argininosuccinate, 264
Arterial blood gas, 183
Ascorbic acid, 46
AS genotypes, 430
Ashkenazi Jews, 422
Asparagine, 14
Aspartate, 264
Aspartate transcarbamoylase, 280
Aspartic acid, 14
Ataxia, 112
ATP. *See* Adenosine triphosphate (ATP)
Autism, 310
Autosomal dominant diseases, 53
Autosomal recessive diseases, 53
Azidothymidine (AZT), 71

B

Bacteremia, 154
Basal metabolic rate (BMR), 43
Base excision-repair, 7
Bases, 2
B-cell lymphoma, 67
B-cells, 95, 107
Beriberi, 312
Beta-cell lymphoma, 67
Beta-globin
  locus, 74
  mutation in, 66, 93, 97–99, 117
  in sickle cell anemia, 66, 93, 97–98
  (*See also* Hemoglobin)
Beta-thalassemia, 103
Bicarbonate, 148
Bilateral tumors, 424
Bile acids, 35, 342
Bilirubin, 35, 212
Biochemical diagnosis, 55
Bioenergetics, 25–29
Biological oxidation, 29
Biotin, 46, 311
Biotinidase, 311
Blistering skin, 156

Blood glucose
in infants, 209, 216
sources of, 347
storage as glycogen, 220, 337
tissues contributing to, 348
(*See also* Glucose)
Blood levels, 350
Blood types, 389, 393
Blood urea nitrogen, 152
BMR (Basal metabolic rate), 43
Bohr effect, 16
Brachycephaly, 381
Branch-chain amino acids, 160
Breast cancer, 425
Breast feeding, 209
Brittle bone disease, 151
Bromo-deoxyuridine triphosphate, 66
Bronchitis, 211
Bruton agammaglobulinema, 95, 154
Bruton kinase assay, 154
Burkitt lymphoma, 424
Butyrylcholinesterase, 421

C

CAC. *See* Citric acid cycle (CAC)
Calciferol, 45
Calcium, 47, 348
Calcium channel regulators, 184
Cancers, 113, 425
Carbohydrate metabolism, 22–23
Carbohydrates, 20–21, 210
Carbon dicarboxylic acids, 266
Carbon dioxide, 148
Carbonic acid, 148
Carbonic anhydrase, 150
Carbon monoxide, 249
Cardiac arrythmia, 215, 338
Caretaker genes, 113
Carnitine, 250, 266
Cathepsins, 38
CDKs (Cyclin-dependent protein kinases), 4
Cellulose, 216
Ceramide, 31
Charcot-Marie-Tooth (CMT) disease, 432
Chloride, 47
Cholera toxin, 249
Cholesterol, 35, 279
Cholic acid, 342
Chromium, 48
Chromosomes
abnormalities in, 376–381
chemical basis of, 1–6
of mammalian cells, 63
non-coding region of, 61
satellite regions on, 99
sequence, 73
terminal deletion of, 61, 110
Chronic hypoxia, 211
Chronic myeloid leukemia, 61, 110
Chronic steroid therapy, 342
Chylomicrons, 36, 269
Cirrhosis, 38, 309
Citric acid cycle (CAC), 22–24
catalysts, 219
and cyanide ingestion, 218
enzyme reactions of, 219
high-energy phosphates from, 217
intermediates, 240, 276, 279, 345
link with urea cycle, 345
in mitochondria, 220–221
Cleft lip, 391
Cleft palate, 68, 391
Clinitest, 218
Clinodactyly, 377
Cloning, 72
CMP (Cytidine monophosphate), 2
CMT (Charcot-Marie-Tooth) disease, 432
CoA (Coenzyme A), 312

Cobalamin, 46
Cobalt, 48
Cockayne syndrome, 65
Coenzyme A (CoA), 312
Coenzyme Q, 248
Coenzymes, 315
Collagen
  amino acids in, 156–157, 161
  labeling of, 263
  mutations in, 151
  synthesis of, 162
  type II, 108
Colon cancer, 65, 69, 425
Colonoscopy, 69
Color blindness, 384, 385
Complex lipids, 31
Congenital anomalies, 436
Congenital deafness, 388
Congenital hypothyroidism, 439
Congestive heart failure, 343
Copper, 48
Copper oxidases, 30
Cori disease, 27
Coronary artery disease, 277
Cotinine, 243
Craniosynostosis, 339, 384
Creatinine, 152
Crohn disease, 309
Crouzon syndrome, 384
CTP (Cytidine triphosphate), 282
Cushing syndrome, 338
Cyanide, 218, 249
Cyanosis, 148
Cyclic AMP, 25
Cyclin-dependent protein kinases (CDKs), 4
Cyclins, 4
Cystathione-beta-synthase, 383
Cysteamine, 194
Cysteine, 14
Cystic fibrosis
  cause of, 60, 94
  inheritance of, 375, 385, 390
  risk calculations, 394
Cystinosis, 194
Cytidine, 2, 61
Cytidine monophosphate (CMP), 2
Cytidine triphosphate (CTP), 282
Cytochrome P450, 243
Cytogenetic notation, 55
Cytosine, 2

D

Debrancher enzyme deficiency, 214
Dehydrogenases, 243
Delayed menstruation, 381
Delta wave, 184
Deoxyribonucleotides, 1–2
Derived lipids, 31
Diabetes, 187
  in children, 214
Diabetes insipidus, 393
Diabetes mellitus, 278
  carbohydrate substitute in, 213
  and fetal growth, 106
  hypoglycemia in, 339
  long-term effects of, 349
  types of, 373
Diabetic ketoacidosis, 153, 278
Diarrhea, 209
Dicumarol, 311
Digestive enzymes, 194
2,4–Dinitrophenol, 249
Diphosphoglycerate mutase, 186
Diphtheria, 105
Disaccharides, 20
Dissociation constant, 11–13
DNA diagnosis, 55
DNA fingerprinting, 70, 434
DNA polymerases, 3, 63
DNA repair, 3–7, 54, 72

DNA replication, 3–6
double-stranded, 69
leading and lagging strands in, 69
DNAse therapy, 439
DNA structure, 1–3
Dolichol, 35
Dopamine, 420
Dot blot, 440
Double-strand break repair, 7
Double-stranded DNA replication, 69
Down syndrome, 192, 378, 381
Dwarfism, 384

E

Ectrodactyly, 382
Edema, 150
Ehlers-Danlos disease, 161
Eicosanoids, 31
Electron transport, 219
Elevated liver enzymes, 266
Elongase, 31
Emphysema, 211
Emulsification, 277
Endergonic reactions, 26
Endonucleases, 95
Energy metabolism, 25–29, 348
Enzymes
allosteric interaction, 193
classes of, 30–31
digestive, 194
function of, 16
in metabolism, 19
noncompetitive inhibitor of, 191
in oxidation reactions, 30
preproteins of, 194
reaction velocity, 190, 194
substrate concentration, 190, 194
vitamins as reactive agents, 314
(*See also* Amino acids; Metabolism; Proteins)
Epidermis bullosa, 156
Epigenesis, 3
Epinephrine, 52, 340
Erythrocytes, 149
Erythromycin, 104
Essential fatty acids, 345
Essential minerals, 44, 47–48
Ethanol, 210
Eukaryotic cells, 1
Eukaryotic protein synthesis, 106
Exergonic reactions, 26
Extracellular matrix, 162

F

FAD (Flavin adenine dinucleotide), 248
FAD dehydrogenases, 30
Fasting, 51, 220, 343, 347
Fatty acid oxidation disorders, 246, 270, 437
Fatty acids, 31–33
biosynthesis of, 266, 275–276
blood levels, 350
essential, 345
oxidation of, 275, 279, 343
as supplements, 269
Ferric chloride test, 153
Fetal chromosome disorders, 392
Fetal warfarin syndrome, 311
FGFR3 (Fibroblast growth factor-3), 193
Fibrillin, 155, 424
Fibroblast growth factor, 339
Fibroblast growth factor-3 (FGFR3), 193
Fibroblasts, 54, 162
FISH (Fluorescent *in situ* hybridization) analysis, 74, 429
Flavin adenine dinucleotide (FAD), 248
Flavoprotein oxidases, 30
Fluorescent *in situ* hybridization (FISH) analysis, 74, 429
Fluoride, 48

Fluorouracil, 189
FMN dehydrogenases, 30
Folate, 279
Folic acid, 46, 279
Foot-drop atrophy, 385
Forbes disease, 27
Fragile X syndrome, 59, 64
Frame-shift mutation, 94
Free radical oxidation, 30
Frequent feeding, 343
Frontal bossing, 117
Fructose
  as carbohydrate substitute, 213
  intolerance, 213
  sensitivity to, 209
Fumarate, 240

G
Galactose, 21, 283
Galactosemia, 430, 439
Gametes, 53
Gangliosides, 278
Gardner syndrome, 62, 382
Gastroenteritis, 151
Gaucher disease, 110
Gene expression, 6–10
Gene methylation, 115
Gene regulation, 10
Gene repair, 72
Genes, 53
Gene therapy, 107
Genetic code, 9, 93, 114
Genetic diagnosis, 55
Genetic testing, 425
Genotypes, 374, 389
Globin, 74, 96–99
Glucagon, 52, 220
Glucocorticoids, 338
Gluconeogenesis, 24–25
  phosphoenol pyruvate in, 217
  primary substrate for, 218
  in starvation, 346
  triacylglycerols in, 245
Glucose, 20–21
  absorption of, 341
  blood levels, 350
  conversion of, 244
  glycolysis of, 216
  ketose isomer of, 215
  metabolism, 217
Glucose-6–phosphate, 244
Glucose-6–phosphate dehydrogenase deficiency, 212, 241
Glucosuria, 184–187
Glutamate, 38, 187
Glutamic acid, 14, 117
Glutamine, 14, 38
Glutathione, 268
Glycerol-ether lipids, 31
Glycerophospholipids, 31, 33–38
Glycine, 14, 161, 438
Glycogen, 24–25
  activated sugars in, 283
  donors of glucose molecules in, 220
  structure of, 220–221
Glycogenesis, 25, 26
Glycogenolysis, 25, 26, 337
Glycogen phosphorylase, 159, 192
Glycogen storage diseases
  in children, 212, 214
  diagnosis of, 210, 214, 218
  types of, 27–28, 215, 382
Glycogen synthase, 25
Glycolysis
  definition of, 22
  energy-requiring step of, 218
  generation of ATP in, 216, 243
  pathway of, 23
  phosphorylation of substrates, 245
  (*See also* Metabolism)
Glycoprotein, 283
Glycosaminoglycans, 161, 274

Glycosides, 209
Glycosphingolipids, 31, 33
GMP (Guanine monophosphate), 2
Gout, 215, 282
Group II signal transduction hormones, 277
Growth factors, 277
GTP (Guanine triphosphate), 104
Guanine, 2
Guanine monophosphate (GMP), 2
Guanine triphosphate (GTP), 104
Guanosine, 2
Gyrate atrophy, 108

H

Hallavorden-Spatz disease, 311
Hardy-Weinberg law, 55
Hartnup disease, 267
HDLs (High density lipoproteins), 35–36, 112, 425
Heart diseases, 184–187
HELLP syndrome, 266
Hematemesis, 271
Hematochezia, 270
Hemiballismus, 267
Hemihypertrophy, 113
Hemoglobin
  affinity for oxygen, 188
  mutation in, 93
  oxygen-binding curve of, 16
  primary structure of, 155
  properties of, 183
  and resistance to malaria, 393
  structure of, 154–155
Hemoglobinopathies, 97, 155, 158
Hemolysis, 109, 242, 266
Hemolytic anemia, 216
Hemophilia, 431
Henderson-Hasselbach equation, 12–13
Hepatitis, 309
Hepatocytes, 219
Hepatosplenomegaly, 110
Hereditary nonpolyposis colon cancer (HNPCC), 65, 69
Hers disease, 28
Heteregenous RNA (HnRNA), 6–8
Heterochromatin, 1
Heterozygotes, 390, 421
Hexaminidase A, 390
High density lipoproteins (HDLs), 35–36, 112, 425
Histidine, 14
HLA (Human leukocyte antigen), 422
HLA haplotypes, 429
HNPCC (Hereditary nonpolyposis colon cancer), 65, 69
HnRNA (Heteregenous RNA), 6–8
Homocystinuria, 267
Hormones, 31, 44, 50
Human genome, 1
Human leukocyte antigen (HLA), 422
Human plasma lipoproteins, 36
Hunger strike, 350
Hunter syndrome, 111
Huntington chorea, 59
Huntington diseases, 376
Hurler syndrome, 109
Hydrocephalus, 394
Hydroperoxidases, 30
Hydroxylysine, 38
Hydroxyproline, 38
Hyperalimentation, 274
Hyperammonemia, 38, 265, 438
Hypercholesterolemia, 187, 271, 273
Hyperglycemia, 106
Hyperinsulinemia, 106
Hyperlipidemia, 215
Hypernatremia, 149, 338
Hyperoxaluria, 103
Hypertelorism, 388
Hypertension, 340, 392

Hyperuricemia, 280, 282
Hypochloremic alkalosis, 388
Hypoglycemia, 214, 339
Hypothalamic-pituitary axis, 116
Hypotonia, 147, 278, 316, 381
Hypoxanthine, analogue of, 282
Hypoxia, 97, 211

I

Ibuprofen, 344
I-cell disease, 158
IDDM (Insulin-dependent diabetes mellitus), 61
IDLs (Intermediate-density lipoproteins), 269
Iduronidase, 109
Immunoglobin, 424
Inclusion cell disease, 158
Incontinentia pigmenti, 387
Inheritance, 53–54
Inosine monophosphate, 42
Insomnia, 314
Insulin
  actions of, 339
  description of, 339
  and fetal growth, 106
  in glycogenolysis, 25
  and weight-loss diets, 343
Insulin-dependent diabetes mellitus (IDDM), 61
Integrated metabolism, 50–52
Intermediary metabolism, 18–19
Intermediate-density lipoproteins (IDLs), 269
Intestinal bowel resections, 309
Intestinal cancer, 382
Intrahepatic cholestasis, 342
Introns, 96
Iodine, 48
Iron, 48, 309, 426
Isoleucine, 14

J

Jinga beans, 347

K

Karyotype, 55, 377–378, 381
Kearns-Sayre syndrome, 70
Keratins, 156
Ketoacidosis, 153
Ketoglutarate, 263
Ketone bodies, 278, 350
Ketones, 153
Ketonuria, 278
Ketose sugar, 222
K_m (Michaelis constant), 17
Kussmaul respirations, 148, 278
Kyphosis, 161

L

Lactate dehydrogenase (LDH), 184
Lactic acid, 239
Lactic acidemia, 316
Lactic acidosis, 214, 313
Lactose, 213
Lactose operon, 116
LDH (Lactate dehydrogenase), 184
LDLs. *See* Low density lipoproteins (LDLs)
Learning problems, 377
Lesch-Nyhan syndrome, 42, 280, 282, 428
Leucine, 14
Leukemia, 61, 73, 425
Leukocytes, 275
L-iduronidase, 109
Li-Fraumeni syndrome, 425
Limit dextrinosis, 27
Lineweaver-Burk plot, 17–18, 189–190
Linoleic acid, 31
Linolenic acid, 31
Lipids, 29–31
  catabolism, 33–38

emulsification of, 277
synthesis of, 32–33
transport, 33–38
(*See also* Fatty acids)
Lipogenesis, 267
Lipolysis, 33–38
and glycogenolysis, 337
inhibition of, 343
regulation of, 245
(*See also* Metabolism)
Lipoproteins, 36, 112, 269
Live cells, homogenate of, 347
Liver enzymes, 309
Lou Gehrig disease, 373
Low density lipoproteins (LDLs), 36
in apobetalipoproteinemia, 112
in heart diseases, 425
in hypercholesterolemia, 273
ranking in density, 269
Low-fat diets, 271
Lymphoblasts, 73
Lysine, 14

M

Magnesium, 47
Malaria, 393
Malonyl coenzyme A, 313
Mammalian chromosomes, 63, 73
Mannose, 21
Mannose-6–phosphate groups, 158
Marasmus, 150
Marfan syndrome, 155, 423
cause of, 424
MCAD (Medium-chain acyl coenzyme A), 437
McArdle syndrome, 27, 222
Meconium ileus, 274
Meconium peritonitis, 274
MECP gene, 71
Medium-chain acyl coenzyme A (MCAD), 437
Megavitamin supplements, 310
Meiosis, 377
Melanin
Mendelian diseases, 53
Messenger RNA (mRNA)
codon assignments in, 6–9
stimulin, 94
synthesis of, 100
Metabolic inhibitors, 241
Metabolic pathways, 346
Metabolism, 18–19
amino acids, 38–40
hormones, 44, 50
integrated, 50–52
intermediary, 18–19
lipids, 33–38
nucleotides, 40–43
porphyrins, 40–43
Methionine, 14
Methotrexate, 314
Methyl citrate, 438
Methylene-tetrahydrofolate, 189
Methylmalonic acid, 195
Methylmalonyl CoA mutase, 195
Metrorrhagia, 426
Mevalonate, 37
Mevastatin, 277
Michaelis constant (K_m), 17
Michaelis-Menton equation, 17
Microcephaly, 381
Micronutrients, 44
Mineralocorticoids, 338
Minerals, 44, 47–48
Mismatch repair, 7
Mitochondrial syndrome, 70
Monosaccharides, 20
Monozygotic twins, 419
mRNA. *See* Messenger RNA (mRNA)
Multifactorial inheritance, 374, 391–392
Multiple sclerosis, 270

Muscle contraction, 195
Muscle sarcoma, 425
Muscular dystrophy, 243
Mutation, 65
Myasthenia gravis, 338
Myelin, 311
Myeloid leukemia, 61
Myocardial infarction, 184, 426
Myoglobin, 16, 160
Myopathy, 112
Myophosphorylase deficiency, 27
Myotonia, 435
Mystagmus, 313

N

N-acetylgalactosamine, 275
NAD (Nicotinamide adenine nucleotide), 248, 250, 283
NAD^+ dehydrogenases, 440–441
NADH (Nicotinamide dinucleotide), 23, 250
NADP (Nicotinamide adenine nucleotide diphosphate), 283
Neonatal screening, 439
Nephrogenic diabetes insipidus, 149
Neural tube defects, 318, 436
Neuritis, 314
Neurodegenerative diseases, 311
Neurolipidosis, 421
Neurotransmitters, 162
Neutrotransmitters, 162
Niacin, 45, 267, 283
Nicotinamide, 283
Nicotinamide adenine nucleotide (NAD), 248, 250, 283
Nicotinamide adenine nucleotide diphosphate (NADP), 283
Nicotinamide dinucleotide (NADH), 23, 250
Nicotine addiction, 243
Niemann-Pick disease, 272
Nitroglycerin, 426
Nonessential amino acids, 38
Non-Mendelian inheritance, 55
Nonpaternity, 434
NOR (Nucleolar organizing regions), 99
Nucleolar organizing regions (NOR), 99
Nucleosides, 2
Nucleotide excision-repair, 7
Nucleotides, 2, 100, 283
Nutrition, 43–44

O

Oligomycin, 245
Oncogenes, 113
Ophthalmoplegia, 313
Ornithine, 264
Ornithine transcarbamoylase, 264
Orotate phosphoribosyltransferase, 280
Orotic aciduria, 280
Osteogenesis imperfecta
  cause of, 161
  diagnosis of, 157, 263, 424
  inheritance of, 387
  types of, 151
  (*See also* Collagen)
Osteomyelitis, 154
Osteopetrosis, 150
Oxaloacetate, 276
Oxalosis, 103
Oxidation, 29
Oxidative phosphorylation, 248
Oxygen, 147–148
Oxygenases, 30

P

P450 cytochromes, 243
P57 gene, 115
Pancreatic juice, secretion of, 341

Pantothenic acid, 46, 311, 318
Parkinson disease, 419–420
Partial pressure of oxygen, 147–148
PCR (Polymerase chain reaction), 440
PDH (Pyruvate dehydrogenase), 22
Pedigree patterns, 54
Pedigree symbols, 54
Pellagra, 267, 313
Pentose phosphate pathway, 217, 241
Peptidases, 38
Peptide bond, 10
Peritonitis, 274
Peroxisome, 278
Pharmacogenetics, 421
Phenols, 156
Phenotypes, 63
Phenylalanine, 60, 94, 272
Phenylketonuria, 389, 439
Pheochromocytoma, 340
Philadelphia chromosome, 61, 110
Phophoribosylpyrophosphate (PRPP), 41–42
Phophorylase kinase deficiencies, 28
Phophorylases, 25
Phosphoenolpyruvate, 217
Phosphoenolpyruvate carboxylase, 24
Phospholipids, 31
Phosphorus, 47
Phosphorylation, 188
Phylloquinone, 45
Piebaldism, 388
Plasma cholesterol, 273
Plasmalogens, 278
Platelets, 266
PMC (Proopiomelanocortin) gene, 116
Point mutation, 93
Poliosis, 388
Polycystic kidney disease, 427
Polydipsia, 149, 187
Polymerase chain reaction (PCR), 440
Polysaccharides, 20
Polyuria, 149, 187
Pompe disease, 27, 215
Porphyrias, 40, 281
Porphyrins, 40–43, 268
Potassium, 47
Prader-Willi syndrome, 61
  diagnosis of, 432
  genetic aspects of, 433
  inheritance of, 435
Pregnancy, 392
Prenatal diagnosis, 55, 392, 423, 437
Primaquine, 216
Projectile vomiting, 152
Proline, 14, 94
Proopiomelanocortin (PMC) gene, 116
Propionic acid, 438
Propionic acidemia, 438
Prostaglandins, 340
Proteases, 38
Proteasome, 38
Protein electrophoresis, 421
Proteins, 13–18
  amino acids in, 14
  metabolism, 346, 347
  regulatory, 162
  structures, 13–15, 160, 162
  synthesis of, 102, 106
Proteolytic enzymes, 159
PRPP (Phophoribosylpyrophosphate), 41–42
Purines, 41–42, 281, 282
Purpura, 315
Pyloric stenosis, 388
Pyridoxine, 46, 383
Pyrimidines, 41–43, 281, 282
Pyruvate, 217
Pyruvate carboxylase, 24, 311
Pyruvate dehydrogenase (PDH), 22

R
Radiation therapy, 73
Reciprocal translocation, 379
Recombinant cloning, 72
Red blood cells, hemolysis of, 109
Redox pairs, 242
Redox potential, 29
Regulators, 116
Regulatory proteins, 162
Renal failure, 348
Replication, 3–6, 69
Respiration, rate of, 248
Respiratory chain
  carriers, 242
  disorders, 219, 248
  inhibitors, 249
  uncouplers, 249
Restriction endonuclease, 95
Restriction fragment length polymorphism (RFLP), 63, 433
Retinitis pigmentosa, 386
Retinoblastoma, 67, 424
Retinoic acid embryopathy, 116
Retinols, 45
Retinopathy, 112
Rett syndrome, 71
RFLP (Restriction fragment length polymorphism), 63, 433
Riboflavin, 45, 248
Ribosomal RNA (rRNA), 6–8
Ribosomes, 103–105
Rigor mortis, 194
Risk calculations, 53–54
RNA molecules, 72, 99
RNA polymerases, 6–8
Roberts syndrome, 68
rRNA (Ribosomal RNA), 6–8

S
Sanger method, 62
SCID (Severe combined immune deficiency), 107
Scleral icritus, 149
Scurvy, 38, 156
Selenium, 48
Sensorineural deafness, 161
Sepsis, 160
Serine, 14
Serum cholesterol, 273
Serum glucose, 244
Serum glutamine-oxalate aminotransferase (SGOT), 188
Serum immunoglobin deficiency, 118
Severe combined immune deficiency (SCID), 107
Sex hormones, 337
SGOT (Serum glutamine-oxalate aminotransferase), 188
Sickle cell anemia
  cause of, 66, 93
  mutation in, 117
  neonatal screening for, 439
  risk calculations, 394
  (*See also* Anemia)
Sickle cell hemoglobin, 187
Sickle globin allele, 430
Sickle hemoglobin, 393
Signal transduction hormones, 277
Simple lipids, 31
Skeletal dysplasia, 339
Skeletal muscle, 195, 247
Slow-reacting substance of anaphylaxis (SRS-A), 344
snRNAs (Small nuclear RNAs), 6–8
SOD (Superoxide dismutase), 192
Southern blotting, 96, 428, 433
Spherocytosis, 149
Sphingolipids, 274
Sphingophospholipids, 31
Spina bifida, 318, 436
Spontaneous abortion, 376
SRS-A (Slow-reacting substance of anaphylaxis), 344
SS genotypes, 430

Starvation, 150, 346
Statin therapy, 271
Stem cells, 95
Steroid digitalis, 343
Stickler syndrome, 108
Stimulin gene, 94
Stridor, 105
Substantia nigra, 419–420
Succinate, 240
Succinylcholine, 420
Sugars, 20–21
Sulfonamide, 109
Superoxide dismutase (SOD), 192

T
Tachypnea, 147–148, 344
Tarui disease, 28
Tay-Sachs disease
  cause of, 422
  diagnosis of, 275
  genetic aspects of, 422
  insurance coverage for, 423
  prenatal diagnosis, 423
  risk calculations, 390, 422
T-cells, 107
Telomere FISH analysis, 74
Telomeres, 73
Tendons, 162
Testicular feminization, 337
Testosterone, 337
Thalassemias, 94, 98, 101
Thanatophoric dwarfism, 193
Theonine, 14
Thiamin, 45
Thymidine, 2
Thymidine monophosphate (TMP), 2
Thymidylate synthase, 189
Thymine, 2
TMP (Thymidine monophosphate), 2
Tocopherols, 45
Topoisomerases, 313
Transaminases, 24, 263, 342
Transcription, 100, 106
Transferrin receptors, 426
Transfer RNA (tRNA), 6–9
Transient hypoglycemia, 216
Transketolase, 313
Translation, 9
Triacylglycerides, 246–247
Triacylglycerols, 35, 245
Trihydroxycoprostanic bile acid, 342
tRNA (Transfer RNA), 6–9
Tryptophan, 14, 313
Turner syndrome, 378–379
Tyrosine, 14

U
Ubiquinone, 248
Ubiquitin, 38
UMP (Uridine monophosphate), 2
Uracil, 2
Urea, 38
Urea cycle, 39
  intermediates, 345
  link with citric acid cycle (CAC), 345
Urea cycle disorders, 157, 264–265, 281
Urea synthesis, 276
Uridine, 2
Uridine monophosphate (UMP), 2
Urinary ketones, 187

V
Valine, 14, 187
Ventricular septal defect, 429
Very low density lipoproteins (VLDLs), 35–36, 112, 269
Vitamin A, 310, 316
Vitamin B12, 195, 310
Vitamin B6, 383
Vitamin C, 185
Vitamin D, 310
Vitamin K, 316

Vitamins, 44–46
  deficiency in, 315–319
  as electron acceptors, 317
  as reactive agents, 314
VLDLs (Very low density lipoproteins), 35–36, 112, 269
Von Gierke disease, 27

W

Waardenburg syndrome, 388
WAGR syndrome, 427
Warfarin, 311
Water, 10, 153
Weight loss, 249
Weight-loss diets, 343
Wernicke-Korsakoff syndrome, 313
Western blotting, 187
White blood cells, 438
Wilms tumor, 113, 115
Wolff-Parkinson-White syndrome, 184

X

X chromosome, 64, 71, 111, 117
Xeroderma pigmentosum, 60, 68
X-linked inheritance, 53
X-linked mental retardation, 111
X-linked recessive diseases, 387

Z

Zellweger syndrome, 278
Zinc, 48
Zwitterions, 13